P9-DVU-663

WITHDRAWN

Metabolical

Also by Robert H. Lustig, MD, MSL

Fat Chance

The Fat Chance Cookbook

The Hacking of the American Mind

Sugar Has 56 Names

Metabolical

The Lure and the Lies of Processed Food,
Nutrition, and Modern Medicine

ROBERT H. LUSTIG, MD, MSL

HARPER WAVE
An Imprint of HarperCollins*Publishers*

HarperCollins books may be purchased for educational, business, or sales promotional use. For information, please email the Special Markets Department at SPsales@harpercollins.com.

Endnotes and Bibliography can be found online at **Metabolical.com**

FIRST EDITION

Library of Congress Cataloging-in-Publication Data

Lustig, Robert H., author.
Metabolical : the lure and the lies of processed food, nutrition, and modern medicine / Robert H. Lustig, MD, MSL.
Description: New York, NY : HarperWave, [2021] | Includes index. | Summary:
"The NYT bestselling author of Fat Chance, Dr. Robert Lustig explains the eight pathologies that underlie all chronic disease, and how they are not 'druggable,' but how they are 'foodable'—meaning, medication can't cure what nutrition can—by following two basic principles: protect the liver and feed the gut"— Provided by publisher.
Identifiers: LCCN 2021002178 (print) | LCCN 2021002179 (ebook) | ISBN 9780063027718 (hardcover) | ISBN 9780063027732 (ebook)
Subjects: LCSH: Chronic diseases—Nutritional aspects. | Chronic Diseases—Treatment.
Classification: LCC RC108 .L87 2021 (print) | LCC RC108 (ebook) | DDC 616/.044—dc23
LC record available at https://lccn.loc.gov/2021002178
LC ebook record available at https://lccn.loc.gov/2021002179

21 22 23 24 25   LSC   10 9 8 7 6 5 4 3 2

I retired clinically from UCSF in 2017 after forty years practicing medicine, with the notion that I could spend more time doing what I wanted to do. But as usual, Man plans and God laughs. It's been a rough five years for many reasons, including personal, professional, and health concerns—I've had my share. But my family is with me, and for pulling me through, this book is dedicated to them. Daughters Miriam and Meredith, wife Julie, sister Carole Berez, thank you—indeed, this book is the product of your love and patience, especially this past year. And to my extended family, neighbors Marcia and Mark Elias, my cookbook coauthor Cindy Gershen, my UCSF friends Elissa Epel and Jack Glaser, Walt Miller and Sindy Mellon, Ivy and Fred Aslan, and my editor Amy Dietz, for buoying me up when I needed it most. This book is your handiwork as much as mine.

Contents

Introduction

It's been a rough day, you're finally home after a long commute, and you're starving. You sit down at the kitchen table, turn on the TV, and inadvertently consume a plate of poison. It looks like food, it tastes like food, maybe it tastes *even better* than food. But what if something had been done to poison it?

No—this isn't an episode of *Game of Thrones*; it's what's happening to most of us every day, every meal, every snack. In bygone times, kings employed food tasters and cupbearers to sample their food and drink first to determine if it had been poisoned. Those poor peons knew that each bite might be their last. But our food today is safe, right? Your cart at the grocery store is full of vacuum-wrapped, refrigerated or frozen, hermetically sealed, spoilage-resistant, irradiated, pathogen-tested, screened-at-the-border products that meet all USDA and FDA standards. But what if that food has been altered or adulterated in some fashion by some ne'er-do-wells before it's even been harvested, while it's being cooked, or even after it's been packaged, in order to kill you? And by design? Not because they want your life—just your wallet?

We occasionally hear about *E. coli* in hamburger meat, *Salmonella* in eggs, *Listeria* in spinach, or even melamine in infant formula; a recall is announced, and the matter is forgotten. So our food's safe, right? But what if it acts more like a slow poison, like cigarettes—one won't kill you, but ten thousand consumed over ten years might? Unlike *Salmonella*, you won't be feeling the effects immediately. But eventually, you'll feel it . . . everywhere. In your heart, muscles, bladder, brain, and especially your wallet. What if this consumable poison is laced with additives that toy with your brain's reward center, leading to addiction and needing ever more of it? Kind of like the pusher in the schoolyard who offers you your first toke for free—and then he's got you. And the bigger and the more chronic the dose—the quicker you die.

Let's take it a step further: what if this poison doesn't just kill you chronically, but sets you up to be susceptible to acute illness—say, a viral pandemic—that could kill you even quicker? What if the USDA and FDA are aware that this slow consumable poison is sold in grocery stores nationwide, and they allow it to be promoted heavily? What if the entire world is exposed to the same toxic and addictive consumable poison, and has now started to get sick, too?

And finally—what if this slow consumable poison looks like everything else in the store? How do you protect yourself?

This is not a Stephen King novel. It's real life and it's happening now. This consumable poison is called *processed food*.

Food writer Mark Bittman has said that since food is defined as "a substance that provides nutrition and promotes growth" and poison is "a substance that promotes illness," then "much of what is produced by industrial agriculture is, quite literally, not food but poison." He was talking primarily about pesticide use versus sustainable farming, arguing that we have *laced* our food with poison. Yes, pesticides are one aspect of food toxicity—but only the tip of the iceberg, maybe about 10 percent of what ails us. The other 90 percent is due to the procedures of the processing, which has morphed what was food into this new slow-acting poison. Your box of cereal may tout that it's "organic" and "all natural"—but it still may be poison. What's important is the alchemy of how the food *itself* has become poison. Until you understand that, you can't understand what has happened to our food—and to us. This book will explain it's not what's *in the food*—it's what's *been done to the food* that counts. And you can't learn that from your doctor, dietitian, advertisement, internet blog, or even a Nutrition Facts label. Nope, you're going to have to learn that yourself.

Nutrition is not the same as food science. Nutrition is what happens to food between the mouth and the cell. Food science is what happens to food between the ground and the mouth. Each is dependent on the other, yet both are "opaque" to the public. That's on purpose—because the food industry and the government don't want you to know that it's the food processing that's rendered the current concepts of nutrition moot.

Food processing isn't listed on the Nutrition Facts food label. The label tells you *what's in the food*. This is mostly irrelevant—what you really need to know is *what's been done to the food*, and no label tells you that. In this book, I will make both nutrition and food science transparent. Essentially, all you need to know are two precepts, six words total: *1) protect the liver, 2) feed the gut.* Those foods that satisfy both precepts are healthy; those that do neither are poison, and those that do one or the other are bad (but less bad)—no matter what the USDA and FDA allow to be stated on the package. Only items that meet both of these criteria qualify as Real Food, i.e., that hasn't been stripped of its beneficial properties and sprinkled with toxins that will hasten our demise.

So buckle up—I'm going to take you on a ride. Now that you're strapped in, we are going on a journey from the ultra-micro to the ultra-macro—from molecule to planet, and everything in between. We're going to get both the subcellular and the thirty-thousand-foot view. And we're going to travel through time, over the last fifty years. The reason for this bottom-to-top and backward-to-forward excursion is to answer these questions: why has our health status declined, our healthcare system devolved, and our climate immolated?

Some might argue that these alterations are unrelated to each other. But it all starts with the changes in our food supply chain that shifted five decades ago in order to support the production and consumption of processed food. To make and bolster this case, I've connected several dots for you: the food to the biochemistry; the biochemistry to the disease; the disease to the medicine; the medicine to the demographics; the demographics to the economy; the economy to the agriculture; the agriculture to the climate; the climate to the planet; and the planet back to the food yet again.

I know this sounds like a nightmare ride on an academic Tilt-A-Whirl, but I'm asking you to hold on to your seat. When you see how these factors are all interlinked with one another, two incontrovertible truths emerge. First, the change in food processing, starting about fifty years ago, has fueled a slow but unrelenting medical, economic, and climate vortex downward. It's picked up speed with time and overwhelmed our medical resources, now evidenced and accentuated by the social disparities of the coronavirus pandemic. It threatens to overwhelm our planetary resources to boot. Second, in today's society, food is the only possible lever that we can apply immediately to effect change. If *you* do not fix *your* food, you continue to court chronic disease and death. If *we* do not fix *our* food, we continue to court societal and planetary oblivion. This book explains what's needed to fix *both*.

Most nutrition authors have a diet to sell to you, a single axe to grind, don't take care of patients, can't provide a diagnosis or medical advice, and think that there's one diet that fits all. They can't or won't address nutritional issues based on age, sex, or race, because they only know one aspect of nutrition, and can't meld it into context for individual readers. Frankly, we have a right to view them as co-opted.

Conversely, clinical health professionals are supposed to keep you healthy, but they can't do that if they haven't been taught how. For decades, the combined healthcare professions have subscribed to the inevitability of chronic disease and aging, and have been consistently dissuaded from keeping you healthy with the "lure of cure," and more recently the "temptation of treatment"—because they don't know otherwise. Doctors and dietitians and dentists have been part of the problem, but we can be part of the solution—but only by changing the paradigm. By elaborating the science and pathways of chronic disease in this book, I will demonstrate that our current processed food model is *prima facie* defective, and must be discarded in favor of a Real Food model.

Many people think Real Food is effete and snobbish, and that I must've had a privileged upbringing to eschew the Standard American Diet. Nothing could be further from the truth. My mother worked two jobs, by day a New York City school secretary, and by night the agent for my grandparents' rental properties. I heated up and ate a whole lot of Swanson TV dinners (I hated the Salisbury steak). I also was a stress eater, and in medical school I was the master of the three-second lunch, as I would have to inhale a sandwich while transitioning from one clinic to another. Hardly a diet to be envied.

I didn't just stumble into this problem, but like you, originally I yielded to the siren song of mainstream nutrition dogma. I majored in nutritional biochemistry at MIT, graduating in 1976. I was fascinated by how micronutrients such as vitamins could fix certain diseases, but not others. I was also intrigued by the tabloid headlines proclaiming that some people who consumed high-protein formula shakes for weight loss were dying from kidney failure. It was clear to me then that the science and the physiology of nutrition actually mattered. Then I went to Cornell University Medical College in New York City, where despite having one of the most distinguished nutritionists in the world on faculty (Professor Maurice Shils, 1914–2015), there was no nutrition curriculum, and they beat my scientific interest in it out of me. I was told that my undergraduate training was irrelevant in dealing with how to take care of patients. I succumbed to the "common wisdom" of calories, obesity, and the inevitability of aging—they taught that it was all about *calories in and calories out*, and I believed what I was told, even though it was the opposite of what I'd learned just one year prior. Hey, these were the doctors, the experts, and my parents were paying a big tuition bill for learning and incorporating the expertise of those doctors.

So, mea culpa—I practiced medicine for my first twenty years as a pediatric endocrinologist (glandular and hormone problems in children) without a real clue of what was truly right or wrong when it came to disease. Match the diagnosis to the disease, and then the treatment to the diagnosis. A big game of Clue: Colonel Mustard in the Conservatory with the Candlestick. And then throw some medicines at it. My colleagues eschewed seeing the obese children who were my patients, because they were steeped in that same common wisdom—it's about energy balance; the kids eat too much and exercise too little; it's all their fault. When I was at the University of Tennessee in the late 1990s, one divisional colleague sent a form letter to outside providers admonishing them for referring such patients, to dispel their belief that an endocrinologist could somehow cure obesity—such sacrilege!—that a doctor could somehow upend the first law of thermodynamics, which espouses a simple mantra: *a calorie is a calorie*. That mantra, recited with almost religious fervor, has set medicine back at least fifty years, and maybe more.

My own research showed me the inconsistencies of this mainstream nutritional dogma, and the true path forward. At UCSF we have a motto, "In God we trust, everyone else has to produce the data." I guess everyone else trusted. But I produced the data. And it didn't match the party line. The science said that not all calories are created equal; and it's the food quality, not the quantity, that matters. I didn't know it at the time, but that was my only salvation in terms of my reputation, personal integrity, and sanity. It also set up the second half of my career to be an iconoclast, relegated to the outside of both the medical establishment and the government.

You can therefore consider this book as both my act of contrition to you, the public, and my act of medical disobedience to the medical establishment. Perhaps I had to wait until I was retired from clinical practice to write this book, for no ivory tower academic bastion would want to take credit for the "medical heresy" that you'll find sandwiched within these pages.

Doing the research myself was like taking the red pill from *The Matrix* (1999)—and now I know just how far down the rabbit hole goes. Iconic chef Anthony Bourdain, even in the face of his own personal demons, relished telling the full truth about his profession. My favorite Bourdain quote: "An ounce of sauce covers a multitude of sins." That might as well be the motto of the entire food industry. And the health-care industry. And the medical industry. And the pharma industry.

And the chemical industry. And the insurance industry. And government, which is its own industry. But the truth will set you free. This book is my contribution to the truth—my *Clinician Confidential*. By educating you, the reader, this book is my attempt to eventually bring the medical profession to *heel*, and to *heal*.

There are two keys to understanding the breakdown of our health and healthcare model. The first key is the one the *medical establishment doesn't want you to know*—that their drugs can't and don't treat chronic disease; they only treat the *symptoms*. Oh yes, they can treat the high blood pressure, high blood glucose, high blood lipids—but not the actual *cause* of any of these conditions. Modern Medicine has gotten the treatment of certain diseases right, such as infectious diseases (like polio), genetic diseases (like childhood leukemia), and some surgeries (like gallbladder or appendix removal). But for chronic noncommunicable diseases (NCDs)—such as diabetes, heart disease and stroke, fatty liver disease, cancer, and dementia, which kill more people, at earlier ages, and in the most debilitating of ways (think amputation, dialysis, blindness) and eat up 75 percent of all healthcare dollars— Modern Medicine has gotten it all wrong.

This book will explain in layman's terms the science behind chronic disease. There are eight subcellular pathologies that underlie all chronic conditions—and all of them are *nutrient-sensing* (Chapters 7 and 8), meaning that they respond positively or negatively to specific components in food; yet none of these are considered diseases themselves. When you look carefully at the science of these eight pathologies, you realize that none are *druggable*, which is why they don't respond to our current medications, and why people keep getting sicker despite the doctors' best efforts. But they are all *foodable* (Chapter 10). Despite the billions of dollars poured into pharmaceutical research, no drug can fix or treat any of these eight pathologies, because drugs are not nutrients. Only Real Food works. In fact, Big Pharma is adept at covering up this subterfuge by advertising directly to the consumer, pretending the symptoms are the disease. They're not. And of course, the public wants to know—are these eight pathologies *exercisable*? Not completely; of the eight, only five are responsive to exercise. Physical activity is a useful adjunct, but *you can't outrun a bad diet*. In this book, I'll show you why.

The second key is the one that the *food industry doesn't want you to know*—all food is inherently good; it's what's been *done* to the food that's bad. The problem is that in the course of food processing, poisons are either added (stuffing the liver) or antidotes have been removed (starving the gut), or both. Minimally processed food (e.g., white rice, fruit juice) interferes with one or the other; while ultra-processed food (e.g., Cheetos) interferes with both. Now our livers are stuffed (from the sugar our bodies turn into fat) and we've literally turned ourselves into foie gras. Our guts used to be full of beneficial intestinal bacteria that munched on fiber and kept everything in our bodies copacetic. Now, that food has been stripped of its fiber, and those bacteria get so hungry they eat the mucin barrier off our intestinal cells, setting us up for inflammation and leaky gut.

The science also shows that ultra-processed food is the cause of other chronic diseases on the upswing, such as addiction, depression, obstructive sleep apnea, and autoimmune disease. While these diseases have always existed, their prevalence, severity, and death tolls are rising exponentially, especially in the Western world. And when we look for the source, it's traced back to what we eat. Or really, what *they did* with what we eat.

Michael Pollan (full disclosure, he's a friend), in his now-famous *New York Times Magazine* article, espoused seven simple words: *Eat food, not too much, mostly plants.* Three separate clauses, but I think that each clause is misleading. *Eat food* doesn't take into account that some people may do better on a low-fat diet, while others may do better on a high-fat diet. *Not too much* doesn't say how you are supposed to moderate that, as it doesn't take into account food addiction or what generates satiety. And *mostly plants* doesn't take into account that Coke, French fries, and Doritos are all plant-based. If you buy your organic, all-natural, GMO-free tortilla chips at Whole Foods, you're still stuffing your liver and starving your gut—you're just paying more for the privilege.

Similarly, Andrew Weil espouses the so-called anti-inflammatory diet, which is mostly plants. Seed oils are high in omega-6 fatty acids, which are highly pro-inflammatory; yet omega-3s, found in fish, are anti-inflammatory. It's not the plants that are important. Furthermore, the low-fat diet, a bastardized version of the plant-based diet, has been a dismal failure, killing more people than cigarettes.

And now we have a new controversy—vegan vs. keto (Chapter 14). Movies like *What the Health* (2017) and *The Game Changers* (2018) argue that animal products kill people. Vegan proponents argue that meat is killing people and the planet. Are these arguments based in science? It seems like everyone, from the Lancet Commission to the Intergovernmental Panel on Climate Change, is advocating a plant-based diet for both our health and for the environment. If this were the easy answer, India, which in large part eschews beef, would be healthier. But its diabetes rate is 8.8 percent and growing—the rate in the US is 9.4 percent. By the same token Argentina and New Zealand, which both eat double the meat per capita that the US does, would be fat and sick—but their heart disease, diabetes, and cancer burden are lower than ours.

Conversely, keto devotees argue that carbohydrate is the root of disease, some saying that eating nothing but meat is the healthiest diet and can even reverse most diseases. Is this true for everyone, or is this just spin? Keto adherents can't stomach the thought that there's a difference between grass-fed and corn-fed animal products, and they pooh-pooh the data that demonstrates that processed meats are not just correlated with, but causative of diabetes and cancer.

This meat versus no-meat controversy has caused the public to take their eyes off the ball, much to the food industry's delight. In fact, the vegan vs. keto battle is based on a false premise of metabolic health, and both diets can be abused, as the food industry peddles both processed carbs *and* processed meat. One of the goals of this book is to help bury the hatchet in this fake diet war by showing that real vegan and real keto can both work, as they have more in common than they realize. As I was writing this book, I thought, "Either I'll be embraced by both sides because I'll have validated their view, or I'll be shunned by both sides because I'll have validated the opposite view." I'm not the enemy. Both factions should be allied with me against the real enemy—processed food.

Then there's the environmental burden. While cows and sheep are indeed methane producers, the methane emissions from the animals (5 percent) turns out to be a pittance compared to the rest of agriculture (10 percent), and compared to industrial methane production (35 percent) and the transportation industry (50 percent). And the climate change impact of the animals is completely dwarfed by the nitrous oxide production resulting from synthetic fertilizer sprayed on all those plant-based products throughout the Midwest grain belt (see Chapter 25). I'm not against plants—plants can be Real Food. But they can also be processed food. Just like animals can be Real Food or processed food. Therefore, I propose that Michael Pollan's seven words for healthy eating can be re-stipulated into these six words: *1) protect the liver, 2) feed the gut.* This includes animals.

As I began in 2007 to debunk the nutritional mythology that has beset the field, it became apparent that the political mythology was even more egregious; in particular who stands to make a profit. The health-care field has been plagued for decades by a philosophical concept known as *moral hazard*, which denotes a situation where the perpetrator knowingly profits off the victim's suffering—an economic version of schadenfreude. An example of this is the health insurance industry. It didn't create your disease, but it clearly profits from it, as it denies coverage and jacks up your rates. It operates on the casino model—pay to play, and set the rates. The industry was happy when you got sick— they could raise your rates and still say no to coverage. They cleaned up; and until very recently, the industry had no reason to change.

The deeper I dug, the more I realized that the problem was much bigger; in fact, I am coining a new term—*immoral hazard*—to denote when the perpetrator specifically rigs the game to create its profit, knowing full well the victim will suffer. One example is how Big Tobacco lied under oath about the addictive nature of its products; a second is the petroleum industry deep-sixing the research on climate change in the 1980s to continue to heat the world to its boiling point; a third is our current opioid crisis—we now know that Purdue Pharma was behind the Marino bill (2016), which reduced the DEA's jurisdiction over opioids. But I will argue the subterfuge surrounding processed food is even worse, because no one ever said that tobacco or petroleum or opioids were supposed to be healthy, but you do have to eat and drink—and the food and beverage industries bait you with every box, bottle, can, and wrapper.

In this book, I will provide evidence for three separate, yet related *immoral hazards* perpetrated by Big Food, Big Pharma, and Big Government. As people get sicker, Big Pharma benefits from complicity, the food industry is protected from the costs of its actions, and the government profits from tariffs on processed food shipped to other unsuspecting countries. We've accepted this as normal. It's not, and we have the power to change it, for ourselves and for society at large—for health and healthcare, for economics, and for the environment. It's time to expose the maneuvers of the food industry and the pharma industry, and their influence on Congress to make us all fat, sick, and broke.

In the eight years since my first book, *Fat Chance* (2012), was released, the data on ultra-processed food has come in, and is absolutely damning. We now know the nature of the toxic metabolite of sugar in the liver, and the role it plays in cancer and dementia. We have the data to show that sugar is addictive and keeps us coming back for more. Conversely, we now know that dietary fat is not toxic (aside from *trans*-fat), and some fats can be therapeutic. We are beginning to understand the role of the gut and its microbiome in the development of autoimmune and psychiatric diseases. We have data on the side effects of diet sweeteners, and information on pesticides like glyphosate. The NOVA food classification system from Brazil categorizes the degree of processing, so we can determine what food industry practices are the most dangerous. I will show how and why this has occurred, and what each of us can do about it.

Now to the title. *Metabolical* is a portmanteau (a word blending two others) of "metabolic"—the workings of the body—and "diabolical"—the workings of food, pharma, and the Feds. All claim to be on your side, but they're on their own sides, and you're the victim of their propaganda.

This book will show you how what your doctor doesn't know can kill you. Each person can screen for and diagnose his or her own risk for chronic disease; how to treat, and in many cases reverse, those diseases so you can get off your medicines; and, most important, how to prevent these diseases and conditions from occurring in the first place (see Chapter 9).

While nutrition seems inordinately complex to most people, it's only become that way because of the competing messages, which unfortunately have also propagandized the medical, dental, and dietary professions. In fact, the education part of this book is very easy. I will battle the cacophony of conflicting information on food and chronic disease with these two easy precepts: *1) protect the liver, 2) feed the gut.* Every nutrient, every food, every food pattern, every food timing paradigm obeys these two precepts. However, implementing them is difficult and only possible with Real Food—even though that's not what Big Food is selling.

The answers you need, in simple terms, to change your food, your health, and your life are all within these pages. There's only one thing that's not—the bibliography! Because there are 1,054 references (more than most textbooks), an end-of-book paper bibliography would have grown the size of the book by seventy pages; such a book would be heavier, less environmentally friendly, and more expensive. Instead, the bibliography, with all the hyperlinks to the primary source material, exists at **www.metabolical.com**, for anyone to access. The science is here, the politics are exposed, and the public is finally ready to discard the previous old, worn-out dogma. It's time for us to understand the *real story of food*, and the *story of Real Food*.

Part I

Debunking "Modern Medicine"

CHAPTER 1

"Treatment" Is Not "Cure"— It's Not Even Treatment

There's a wasp buzzing around your attic. What do you do? Kill the wasp? Or get rid of the wasp's nest? You have to work *upstream* of the problem if you're going to fix the *cause*. Working downstream only fixes the *result*. And that's what we've been doing with healthcare for the past eight decades. Well, the wasps have come home to roost.

We're Number 1!—in Morbidity, Mortality, and Expense

The US has the best doctors, hospitals, and medical technologies, the most innovative surgeries, the best and newest drugs, and spends the most per capita on healthcare of all the countries on the globe.

Are Americans healthier? Do we enjoy better healthcare? Do we live longer? The answer to each of these questions is an unequivocal and emphatic no. In fact, it's quite the opposite; Americans have the worst health outcomes of any country in the Organisation for Economic

Co-operation and Development (OECD; the thirty-seven richest countries). In several of the most lethal chronic diseases, Americans rank
among the worst of the developed countries in the world: #1 in diabetes, #2 in Alzheimer's disease, #5 in cancer, and #6 in cardiovascular
disease (CVD).

No doubt, of all the OECD countries, the US is the sickest. We have
the most expensive drugs—double that of Europe—plus the most expensive doctors. We spend the most on hospitals and inpatient care.
And what do we get for it? Just take a look at this graph (**Fig. 1-1**).

There are two main takeaways from this graph: 1) the more money
we throw at the problem, the worse it gets—which either means we
haven't addressed the problem at all, or maybe we're even making it
worse; and 2) it wasn't always this way. Although the US has never been
particularly efficient with our healthcare dollars, we at least used to
keep up with the rest of the pack. We started going off the rails in 1970,
and even now we haven't come close to identifying the problem, much
less solving it. There's still no magic pill.

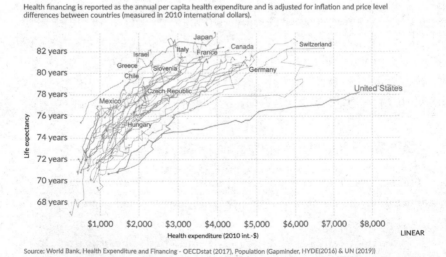

Health financing is reported as the annual per capita health expenditure and is adjusted for inflation and price level differences between countries (measured in 2010 international dollars).

Source: World Bank, Health Expenditure and Financing - OECDstat (2017), Population (Gapminder, HYDE(2016) & UN (2019))

Figure 1–1: Comparison between healthcare expenditures versus life expectancy for Organisation for Economic Co-operation and Development (OECD) countries over forty-five years, 1970–2015. The US spends the most but gets the least.

So what started in 1970? And why is it bankrupting healthcare? And why is our problem now a problem everywhere, and for everyone?

Infections Are Passé—or Are They?

Metabolic syndrome started rearing its head in the 1980s to become the scourge of the twenty-first century. Think about diseases that killed large numbers quickly in ancient and modern societies—leprosy, bubonic plague, syphilis, tuberculosis, influenza, malaria, HIV. All of them are infections. You'd think the diseases of metabolic syndrome have nothing to do with infection. After all, anyone can die from infection, as rapidly demonstrated by the coronavirus pandemic. But if you have metabolic syndrome, your risk of death goes up twenty-fold—and it's *your fault—because you're a glutton and a sloth. Wrong* on both counts. The simple fact is that, just like coronavirus, anyone can get metabolic syndrome—even those who are normal weight. Everyone is at risk—both ways.

As this book will explain, each of the chronic, noncommunicable diseases (NCDs) associated with metabolic syndrome—including diabetes, hypertension, and heart disease—are due to abnormal metabolism (burning of energy) in different cells in different organs of the body. To make the point more clearly, let's pick just one disease to examine—diabetes. When I went to medical school in 1976, diabetes was rare; only 5 percent of people in the US over age sixty-five had it, and the prevalence in the general population was 2.5 percent. And I would know, because my maternal grandfather was one of them. He wasn't overweight—I guess he was just "lucky." However, because of his diabetes he had four successive heart attacks before the final one that killed him at age seventy-two. Diabetes was a cloud that hung over my family—would I get it, too?

In 2000, it was estimated that there were 151 million diabetics walking the planet, and the prediction was, by 2010, there would be 221 million, for an amortized inflation rate of 3.88 percent. That's not what we saw—in fact there were 285 million, for an amortized inflation rate of

6.55 percent—double what was predicted. But despite all of the doctors, all of the knowledge, all the pills, and all the gym memberships—by 2014 there were 422 million diabetics, for an amortized inflation rate of 10.30 percent. That's triple the predicted rate! And in 2019, we're up to 463 million. And statistical modeling says there will be 568 million by 2030. No slowdown, despite all the global hand-wringing.

This epidemic affects all ages, races, and creeds, but that hasn't stopped people from making a buck on it. Almost one in ten Americans now has diabetes requiring some form of drug therapy (metformin or insulin)—yet despite the need and the urgency, the price of insulin has tripled in just one decade. Many patients have to choose between paying for their medicine or their food or their electricity. Some are rationing their insulin, which can lead to death.

While you could argue that this is akin to price gouging—what happens at the gas pump whenever there's a shortage—this is going on across the entire medical landscape. Currently sixty-four million people—35 percent of the adult US population—can't pay their medical debts. Of course, the US government and the insurance industry blame it on the patient—but what if Modern Medicine actually *made you sick*? What if seeing a doctor was actually the cause of these chronic diseases? I know this sounds preposterous—but there's actually data to support it. Medical economist Dr. Jay Bhattacharya at Stanford Medicine analyzed millions of medical records, and the factor that most correlated with increasing weight gain in the population was the number of visits to an HMO doctor. Now, that's correlation, not causation, but you have to wonder. Back in 1970 we spent 6 percent of our GDP on healthcare, and now fifty years later we spend 17.9 percent. Yet the average American's weight is up, health is down, and wallet is underwater.

Finally, in life expectancy, the US ranks only twenty-eighth among the most developed countries in the world, *and for the last four years our life expectancy has declined*. We're the only country in the OECD where this is true. Obamacare—increasing access to healthcare and covering preexisting conditions—hasn't solved any of these issues, because it isn't addressing the root cause of the problem. Then there was

Trump's response, which hoped to solve the problem by letting sick people die. Even the idea of Medicare for All that overtook the Democratic party in the 2020 election would just amplify the problem by increasing the costs going out the door (to the tune of $30 trillion) and still not address its root cause. Each of these amount to rearranging the deck chairs on the *Titanic.*

Modern Medicine Is Not the Solution to the Problem, Modern Medicine *Is* the Problem

It's an axiom that Modern Medicine works to keep people healthy. The thought process goes—people live longer today than a hundred years ago, and healthy people live longer, so people today must be healthy. But is that really the case?

Academics and clinicians nationwide stand by both Modern Medicine and our healthcare system. They feel that investing in areas and "personalized medicine" technologies that "cure" people diagnosed with cancer, cardiovascular diseases, or neurological diseases will ultimately yield better long-term results than focusing on public health measures. This conclusion is wrong, both at the individual and societal levels, and shows at best the misconception of what the real problems are, and at worst a perverse desire of various stakeholders to maintain the status quo at the expense of both lives and dollars. We spend 97.5 percent of our healthcare budget on individual treatment, and only 2.5 percent on prevention. Not a very good bang for the buck. Here are six clear reasons why we need to rethink Modern Medicine. Let's use cancer as an example.

First, ask yourself which is better: to be cured of cancer or to not get cancer in the first place? The fact is that only 33 percent of the people treated for cancer are "cured" (five-year event-free survival), and only 7 percent of them don't develop another cancer in the next twenty years.

Second, these meager results in curing cancer are matched by a very hefty bill. In the last two decades, the National Cancer Institute has spent over $60 billion on research and treatment. Given that this is public money, one could hope that some of it was used to make cancer treatment more affordable for the public. Alas, most cancer drugs launched in the last ten years were priced at more than $100,000 per patient for one year of treatment. The new personalized CAR-T cell treatments cost between $300,000 and $500,000 a year.

Third, those that advocate for Modern Medicine argue that the investment in curing chronic diseases like cancer allows for a better understanding of its causes. I'm not so sure. In the case of cancer, there remains a colossal debate on whether cancer is due to genetics or environment, and whether cancer is in fact a metabolic disease, a by-product of the conversion of food into energy. Similarly, in the case of Alzheimer's disease, in the last decade we've blown through $2.3 billion per year on research and over one hundred drugs have been tested and discarded. We're as close to finding the cause of Alzheimer's as we are to landing a man on Mars. And don't even get me started on heart disease. There are at least four theories that try to explain its causes. And please don't mention "good" and "bad" cholesterol. That's *so* twentieth century (see Chapter 2).

Fourth, one would expect that new generations would reap the benefits of the huge advances in Modern Medicine, our supposed ability to diagnose and better understand the causes behind several chronic diseases. Yet, the opposite is true. Only 13 percent of baby boomers—now fifty-four years old—report that they're in excellent health, compared to 32 percent of people who were fifty-four in 1988 to 1994. Fewer people today actually die from heart attacks, yet more people have suffered at least one.

Fifth, our healthcare system is collapsing because we have more people to treat, and the percentage of the population with multiple chronic diseases is growing since treatment often doesn't result in cure (that is, permanent resolution of disease). In 1980, 30 percent of the adult US population, or fifty-two million people, were affected by at least one chronic condition. Today it's 60 percent, or 145 million people. The percentage of those affected by two or more chronic diseases has grown from 16 percent to 42 percent. More baby boomers have combinations of hypertension, diabetes, and cancer, and they're developing these conditions sooner, not later, leading to earlier disability and more years of morbidity. The RAND Corporation estimates that 12 percent of the adult population is affected by five or more chronic diseases, and accounts for 41 percent of all healthcare spending. On average, patients with five or more chronic conditions spend fourteen times more on health services than people with no chronic conditions. Yet here we are, debating the merits of Medicare for All.

One recent study looked at the rates of cancer incidence (number of new cases per year). As we would expect, the incidence of smoke-related cancer declined, and the incidence of cancers detectable by better and more frequent screenings (e.g., colon, prostate, breast) increased because we're catching them earlier. However, the incidence of all other cancers—leukemia, melanoma, brain cancer, non-Hodgkin lymphoma, etc.—rose by 23 to 34 percent across gender and race. It's not just more people living with cancer, *it's more cancer every year.* And while genetics contribute 10 to 30 percent to cancer development, smoking and diet are the leading factors in 50 percent of cancers.

When Children Get Adult Diseases

Our decline in health and sharp increase in morbidity underlies the havoc we now see in our healthcare system. My Cornell med school colleague and Stanford pediatrician Paul Wise says, "Pediatricians are the ultimate witnesses to failed social policy." As a practicing pediatrician for four decades, I was supposed to be spared the ravages of treating chronic disease, yet that was what ended up populating my entire clinic. When you look in a teenager's eyes who complains of a headache, and see their retinas are detaching due to increased intracranial pressure from severe metabolic syndrome, you know kids are the canaries in the coal mine. For Medicare and Social Security to work, young, healthy working taxpayers have to pay into the system, from which they'll benefit in their later years. But those healthy taxpayers are getting sicker, are on disability, and, instead of paying in, they're mostly taking out. The Social Security gap must be bridged by debt—leaving a poison-pill inheritance for subsequent generations, our children and grandchildren. Currently, the Office of Management and Budget predicts a complete Social Security collapse by 2035.

To make things worse, the leading causes of death and morbidity (loss of function or income) in the US are the most expensive for the system: cancer, neurodegenerative diseases (Alzheimer's and vascular dementia), cardiovascular diseases, and type 2 diabetes—all noncommunicable disease (NCDs). Right now, America is clocking about fifteen years of morbidity per person from these diseases. That's $1.9 trillion (60 percent of our healthcare budget) wasted on diseases that should never have occurred, and that money is coming *out* of Social Security, rather than workers paying into it.

If doctors and medical professionals made their money with the expectation that they were actually treating or mitigating our chronic disease while disavowing all culpability, that would be prototypical *moral hazard*—like the insurance industry. But what if they treat us and take our money, knowing full well that they're not even remotely coming close to addressing the problem? That is *immoral hazard*—knowing that what they're doing is nonproductive, generating charges at their and society's expense, price gouging off the sick, all in direct violation of the Hippocratic Oath.

Yet the solution to this metabolic, economic, and environmental Armageddon is *safe, simple, cheap*, and *green*. It's called Real Food. This book will show you why, and why there's no other choice.

The "Kicking the Bucket" List

It's easy to imagine type 2 diabetes, heart disease, and hypertension as diet-related; after all, they're all associated with obesity. Yet there's another collection of chronic diseases that is also increasing in incidence and prevalence, but which the public hasn't yet associated with food. People don't normally think of cancer, autoimmune disease, dementia, and psychiatric disease as food-related. In fact, they are processed food–related. All of them are increasing in prevalence, and in the same fifty-year time span as our diet has gone to hell.

Cancer is being diagnosed at earlier ages than has occurred in previous generations. Cancer is thought to have a genetic basis, or perhaps is a result of environmental exposures causing mutations in DNA. And that's likely true for cancer *initiation*, which likely occurs in each of our bodies every day (but the immune system clears those mutations out before they cause havoc). However, cancer *promotion* is the real issue because that's how it spreads and grows. And processed food is feeding those mutated cells exactly what they need.

In the last few decades, as we've eschewed proper nutrition in favor of processed food, the incidence of obesity-related cancers (e.g., colon, liver, pancreas, kidney) has continued to grow at annual rates of 2 to 6 percent a year for people in the thirty to fifty age bracket. Processed food (e.g., Doritos and Kit Kats) uniquely feeds cancer growth. Specifically, sugar supplies the backbone for the structural elements that allow the cancer cell to divide and multiply (e.g., lipids, ribose, amino acids) that allow cancer cells to multiply.

Autoimmune diseases (like Crohn's disease) are thought to attack randomly, but we now know that intestinal bacterial pathogens are frequently the target of a disordered immune response to the consumption of processed foods. As I said in the introduction, the key to your health is to *protect the liver and feed the gut*. Before the advent of packaged and microwavable food, gut bacteria were used to getting what they wanted to eat—fiber (see Chapters 12 and 19). But now those same bacteria are starving, and they're not happy. They are causing the normally impervious intestinal barrier to become "leaky," leading to inappropriate immune system activation and chronic inflammation (see Chapter 7). Worse yet, the antibiotics we give animals raised for food kill off the good bacteria in our intestines, allowing the bad bacteria even more access, and thus driving even more chronic disease (see Chapter 20).

The brain is also not immune to the effects of processed foods. *Dementia* used to be a relatively rare occurrence when I was in medical school. In 1978, my four-person dissection group in pathology class had the only cadaver with Alzheimer's disease, a man who died at age eighty-five. Back then about 10 to 15 percent of eighty-five-year-olds would go on to get Alzheimer's, and it wasn't even remotely thought to have a nutritional component. However, between 1970 and 2014 (the years of processed food being introduced so broadly into our diets), the prevalence of Alzheimer's has doubled throughout the world. Interestingly, in high-income countries like the US, prevalence is at 6.5 percent and steady for the past decade, while in developing countries it's increased by 50 percent in that interval. Exploring the link between food and Alzheimer's is in its infancy, but new data are generated every day.

Finally, we have *psychiatric disease*. It's easy to blow this off as an individual, or even a country-specific, issue. But the World Health Organization (WHO) documents a 20 percent increase in depression and schizophrenia worldwide in one decade. These are the brain manifestations of chronic metabolic disease. And I will show you that, while clearly not the only causal factor, processed food makes cognitive dysfunction much worse (Chapters 15 and 19).

Clear and Present Danger

While some of the other advanced world economies have fared slightly better than the US, the truth is that longevity and health are beginning to stall throughout the developed world. As globalization has spread, so has the consumption of palatable industrial foods; thus, chronic diseases and morbidity have expanded almost everywhere in the developed and developing world. Rising global NCD rates yield an annual mortality of thirty-five million people, with a disproportionate 80 percent of these deaths occurring in low- and middle-income countries, wasting precious medical resources. In 2011, the UN Secretary-General announced that NCDs are a bigger threat to poor countries than infectious diseases, including HIV. American corporations and our government don't just export bad reruns of *Baywatch*, we also export our lifestyle, our food, and its subsequent diseases. Our first-world problem has become their third-world problem.

The holy grail of Modern Medicine is you can't fix healthcare until you fix health; and you can't fix health until you fix the food. Everyone is talking about healthcare, few people are talking about health, and nobody is talking about the food.

Medical Incompetence

To be clear, better screening, diagnostics, and treatment is what Modern Medicine *does*; but preventing or reversing NCDs is what Modern Medicine *doesn't* do. The net effect of these two trends is a decrease in overall health—matched by an increase in number of people with morbidity who stay alive longer but not healthier—and an acceleration of US healthcare expenditures. We now have a decline in life span for four years running to prove it.

Better screening or diagnostics or treatment is missing the point. Improving medical resource allocation or efficiency is missing the point. Treatment is after-the-fact; it's like going into the wasp-infested attic armed with a flyswatter. By the time you've killed one, the swarm has stung you into submission.

CHAPTER 2

====

"Modern Medicine" Treats Symptoms, Not Disease

When Was the "Golden Age" of Modern Medicine?

From the beginning of recorded time through the first half of the twentieth century, people got sick and died. Quickly—too quickly to cost too much money. And young—too young to need chronic care. Sure, some people had chronic infections like tuberculosis or leprosy or syphilis or trichinosis, and they hung around a little longer, but they didn't bankrupt any healthcare system. There were enough leeches and laxatives to go around. Aside from kashruth (Leviticus 11:3), prevention was unheard of; and aside from Jesus (Matthew 8:2–3) and Lourdes, cures were rare. In the Middle Ages, you'd go to your corner barber surgeon to gossip about the neighbors, have your hair trimmed, and your veins cut open to bleed out your various afflictions. Sanitaria were the first chronic care facilities, and madhouses were the first mental health facilities. Quarantine the afflicted, pray a lot, and save money.

The first bona fide win for rational prevention started in the 1790s, when Edward Jenner figured out that vaccination of humans with cowpox also immunized them against smallpox. The second win was in 1854 in response to the London cholera epidemic. John Snow (not the one from *Game of Thrones* but an anesthesiologist) used the concept of triangulation to isolate the Broad Street pump as the source of the epidemic. In the process, Snow invented the field of epidemiology. He didn't know what bacteria were, but he knew that the water supply was the source of the illness. Knowing that tainted water carried disease, surgeon Joseph Lister in 1883 argued for sterilization of surgical instruments and handwashing. Back in the "bad old days" of medicine, prevention was all we had, and we didn't even know what we were preventing. Yet the results spoke for themselves. Preventing infections at a public health level was on a roll and people stopped throwing buckets of feces out the fifth-floor window. Hygiene, quarantine, sanitation, and immunization were the first major wins for public health. Tuberculosis and typhus were both battled back by changes in societal hygiene. And government had to intercede, both as a regulatory and funding agency, in order for "public" health to reach the populace.

Then came the Industrial Revolution, and with it the advent of sweatshops, accidents, sickness, and nutritional deficiencies. The public outcry was muffled by the roar of the machinery. Health didn't improve until the workers rose up and demanded it, and still it took government to institute it. But by the second half of the nineteenth century, canning of food was all the rage, and so was lead poisoning, with attendant lead encephalopathy (brain dysfunction and swelling) causing the rage. Government didn't get involved for decades, because it's harder to remove a chronic exposure than it is to prevent an acute one; especially when Big Business stands to make a profit. Lead toxicity was first described in 1892, but the US government didn't get the lead out of paint and gasoline until 1982—a ninety-year on-ramp.

Other chronic toxic heavy metal exposures, like arsenic, mercury, and cadmium, were also slow to the party, and barely made the Hit Parade.

The bottom line is if there's going to be effective change in curtailing various acute and chronic diseases, public health supported by government regulation will ultimately be required. In each previous case, it's proven successful. And of course, when government doesn't assume responsibility, you get what happened in Flint, Michigan.

Then, in what amounted to a complete turnaround, the paradigm of government being the guardian of public health shifted. In 1940, Albert Alexander, a London constable, was the first human to receive a dose of penicillin for an acute facial infection that had spread to multiple abscesses and claimed his eye. Left untreated, it would have been fatal. His response to the medication was "remarkable." But it didn't last—the infection relapsed within six months, and Alexander died a year later. Nonetheless, the "Golden Age" of Modern Medicine was launched. Therapy targeted to the pathology. The right antibiotic could kill the right bacteria, and people got better. Screw prevention, which takes time, infrastructure, and investment. Now, you could achieve cure. There's a pill for that. Targeted therapy via personal intervention became the unyielding goal of Modern Medicine.

That first Golden Age of Modern Medicine didn't last even a decade. In 1947, four years after mass production of penicillin, the first bacterial species to develop resistance to the antibiotic reared its ugly head. And so the race was on to develop the next antibiotic—methicillin. And on and on.

Since then, we've continued to chase the concept of targeted therapy, we think we have it within our sites, and yet cures continue to elude us. We've now reached critical mass—of drug-resistant bacteria, that is. There are so many resistant species that they now can share intelligence; that is, they can transfer resistance genes between species; a Rise of the Resistance that would terrify all minions of the Empire. Our current crop of antibiotics is coming close to being useless. Add to that the fact that viral diseases are now even more dangerous and harder to control than bacteria ever were, as exemplified first by HIV in 1979, hantavirus in 1993, Ebola in 2014, and coronavirus in 2020. Even so, these aren't even the biggest problems with Modern Medicine.

Golden Age 2.0?

We believe we're in a new Golden Age of Modern Medicine, as we now use high-tech screening of drugs, Big Data informatics, and genetic editing like CRISPR-Cas9 in an attempt to target therapy to the individual and the pathology. For certain genetic diseases, such as severe combined immunodeficiency disease ("bubble boy" disease), and maybe for sickle cell disease, or Tay-Sachs, such therapies that are targeted to the pathology will likely result in "cure." And that's great—for these one in ten thousand to one hundred thousand diseases. We're even looking to use viruses to program an individual's own immune cells to kill cancers in that same individual—the ultimate targeted therapy. We're using robotics and cyberknives to reach surgical outcomes previously unimagined. At UCSF, my colleagues are harvesting stem cells from individuals with type 1 diabetes, using growth factors to differentiate them into pancreatic beta-cells in a petri dish, and then injecting them back into the patient to attempt to cure their diabetes. It's true that patients who previously had no hope now have hope. Which is absolutely great—for those patients, and only if they can afford these treatments.

But these targeted cures are not even remotely close to addressing what is reducing life span and health worldwide. This scourge has no targeted cure despite what doctors may tell you, and is increasing morbidity, costing big dollars, and breaking healthcare in every country on the planet. Because today, for the chronic diseases that affect society the most, the cluster of NCDs folded in under the umbrella term *metabolic syndrome* (that cost 75 percent of healthcare dollars in the US and half of healthcare dollars around the world) are diseases that do not have one gene, or one pathway to target. These are multifactorial diseases with multiple morbidities. And while each existed before 1970, each has exponentially skyrocketed in prevalence and severity during the modern era, and all for the same reason.

Insulin 101

Before we go any further, I want to do a brief discussion of insulin and its role in NCDs (more in Chapter 7). We all need insulin—it's the hormone that allows glucose (your body's primary source of fuel) to enter the cells of your body so it can be burned. But insulin resistance occurs when the cells in your muscles, fat, and liver no longer respond to the insulin signal. The glucose can't get in—the cells are starving—so they send signals to the pancreas to crank out even more, but to no avail. The glucose builds up in your blood at the same time that your cells are starving, adding insult to injury. You'll see that it's this condition that is the underlying cause of most of our troubles.

Insulin resistance is the primary defect in metabolic syndrome, the cluster of NCDs. Insulin resistance manifests itself in a myriad of tissues and ways, which may vary from person to person. You may be overweight, or not. You might have high cholesterol, but maybe it's normal. You might have high blood pressure, although it could be low. All of these are tissue-specific symptoms of metabolic dysfunction. Previously, doctors only diagnosed metabolic syndrome if you were obese. Now we know better. Even people who aren't overweight develop metabolic syndrome. The issue is that doctors are still targeting obesity, which they think is the disease. Rather, it's just another symptom.

Two other hormones also play a role in the hunger-satiety system. Leptin is a satiety hormone released from your adipocytes that tells your brain, "I have enough energy on board; I can stop eating." Ghrelin is a hunger hormone released from your stomach that tells your brain, "I'm empty—feed me!" Normally, insulin does double duty—it tells your body to "store," while it tells your brain to "stop eating." When insulin is low and working right, both insulin and leptin counterbalance ghrelin and keep you weight-stable. But when you become insulin resistant, the leptin signal is blocked—now the ghrelin runs things, so you're hungrier and storing like crazy. Therefore, the prime directive of metabolic therapy is "get the insulin down." And that's true, regardless of your weight.

1. Obesity Is a "Red Herring"

Red herring refers to a clue that's meant to be distracting. And that's what obesity is—distracting. Everyone thinks that first you gain weight, and then you get sick. Yet, 80 percent of the time, it's actually the other way around. First you get sick, then you gain weight. How do we know this? Because only 80 percent of obese people are metabolically ill. The other 20 percent of obese people are metabolically healthy. We even have a name for them—*metabolically healthy obese* (MHO). They will live a completely normal life, die at a completely normal age, have normal-length telomeres (the ends of the chromosomes that determine how sick you are and when you'll die), and they won't have exorbitant health insurance claims. The key is that these people have lots of subcutaneous fat, very little *ectopic* fat (fat in cells that shouldn't have fat), normal metabolic function, and low insulin levels.

Metabolic syndrome is the inappropriate storage of energy in the wrong form in cells that shouldn't store it. There are only three types of cells in the body that should store energy: subcutaneous (i.e., stored in the butt) and visceral (i.e., stored in the belly) adipose tissue is supposed to store excess energy as fat; muscle tissue and liver tissue are supposed to store excess energy as glycogen (starch). That's it. Fat stored anywhere else in the body is called *ectopic* fat. If the muscle or liver or any other body tissue store any amount of ectopic fat, then that tissue will develop metabolic dysfunction, and promote some clinical manifestation of metabolic syndrome. The pathways of metabolic dysfunction within each organ are pretty complicated, but if you really want to see the science, my friend and colleague Dr. Alejandro Gugliucci of Touro University and I constructed a poster to illustrate it (see metabolical.com).

How about the other 80 percent who are overweight and sick? They were sick first—they had metabolic syndrome—and that caused insulin resistance, which led to high insulin levels. But because their fat cells still responded to insulin, and that extra insulin allowed the fat cells to accumulate more energy, they got bigger. Therefore, their weight is a *biomarker* for their metabolic dysfunction.

When you look at the normal weight population, approximately 40 percent of those people also have metabolic syndrome—meaning they have metabolic dysfunction, insulin resistance, and high insulin levels (see Chapter 7). But for whatever reason, they're just not obese. In some of them, their fat cells are insulin resistant, too, so energy doesn't accumulate in the subcutaneous tissue. Instead they put it in other organs that shouldn't have fat, such as muscle and the liver. This has spawned a new medical term with 1,500 citations in the literature called TOFI, or *thin on the outside, fat on the inside.*

And then there are the 20 percent of people who are overweight but *not* sick. Because the subcutaneous fat tissue can actually be protective, giving excess energy a nontoxic place to go. Just because they're obese does not automatically mean that they harbor the egregious and deadly forms of fat in other organs where it shouldn't be. Rather, it's the *ectopic* fat that determines if they'll develop diabetes or heart disease. In fact, my group at UCSF and others have shown that fat in the liver is the most predictive of whether someone will get diabetes in the future— which is why one mantra of this book is *protect the liver.* Furthermore, nonalcoholic fatty liver disease can lead to cirrhosis (scarring of the liver, which is lethal), just as can happen in chronic alcoholics. I've had to send two fifteen-year-old, four-hundred-pound boys for liver transplants, due to cirrhosis from soda consumption. We've even shown that kids with fatty liver disease also have fatty pancreas disease—and if your pancreas has fat in it, no wonder you can't make enough insulin for your body's needs.

Each of these conditions occurs in normal weight people, too! Obesity is just another *symptom* of the problem, not the problem itself. But Modern Medicine treats the biomarker (the weight) rather than the actual underlying pathology—and does a really crappy job of it.

OK, now you're going to tell me about your Uncle Marvin, who went on a strict diet, started exercising, and his diabetes disappeared. And while this can absolutely work at the individual level, it doesn't work at the societal level. Yes, the relative risk (RR) for lifestyle interventions in preventing diabetes is 0.61—that means, if you can carry out those interventions, your risk for diabetes goes down 39 percent. Sounds good, right? And if you're one of the people for whom it works, fantastic. But the RR is not the important factor. The number needed to treat (NNT)—the number of people who have to go on a diet and lose weight to prevent one case of diabetes—is twenty-five. That's right, twenty-five people have to diet and exercise insanely to prevent one of them from progressing on to developing diabetes.

No doubt, you've also watched some TV-doctor show where the guest dropped weight, their diabetes got better, their insulin went down, and they got a makeover. Cue studio applause. But it's actually the other way around. Their insulin didn't go down because their weight went down—their weight went down because their insulin went down. How do we know this? Because at UCSF, we got children's insulins to go down without losing any weight, simply by getting them off dietary sugar. What they lost as a result was liver fat, which then made them insulin sensitive.

Again, obesity is a red herring. Forget the obesity. Fix the metabolic problem. And Modern Medicine doesn't.

2. Roto-rooting LDL

We all need cholesterol to survive; it's an integral part of membranes and the precursor of steroid hormones. If you don't consume cholesterol, your body makes it—it's that important. You've probably heard that there's "good" cholesterol and "bad" cholesterol. Doctors measure the bad stuff and tell you to lower it.

Let's start with low-density lipoprotein cholesterol (LDL-C), the ostensible villain, the "classic" biomarker of risk for a future heart attack. Clinicians are taught to treat LDL-C with statins; but do statins actually work to reduce heart attacks?

Cholesterol (and more specifically LDL-C) emerged as a risk factor from the Framingham Heart Study, an observational study in Massachusetts that started after World War II and continues today. The takeaway was that if you had very high LDL-C you were more likely to suffer a heart attack. But when the data were analyzed, unless LDL-C was very high (over 200), it wasn't a risk factor. In fact, patients with really high LDL-C levels often have a genetic disorder (I'm one of the lucky carriers). Your LDL-C level is for the most part genetically determined. Conversely, those with LDL-C levels less than 70 develop relatively little heart disease. Yes, there seems to be a genetic protection at the low end, and risk at the high end.

But for the rest of the population, LDL-C is not a great predictor of who will suffer a heart attack. It's true that the HR ratio (hazard risk ratio; a measure of difference in risk versus the general population) of LDL-C is 1.3, which means that if your LDL-C is high, you have a 30 percent increase in risk for a heart attack. But correlation doesn't mean causation. For example, if LDL-C is truly the bad boy of heart disease, as the Medical Establishment says, then why, when you remove younger people from the analysis and just look at older people (greater than sixty years), do high LDL-C levels correlate with longevity? Maybe, once you factor out the people with genetic reasons for high LDL-C (like those with genetic disorders), then LDL-C isn't really so bad. Or maybe we're measuring the wrong biomarker.

Let's say you go see your provider, who tells you that you have high LDL-C. Nine times out of ten you're going to walk out of that office with a prescription for a statin, which inhibits cholesterol synthesis. The current mindset among clinicians is to downshift everyone's LDL-C through low-fat diet and drugs. Because that's what they're trained to do. I would know. I'm one of them. But really how beneficial are statins, and for what? Despite governmental recommendations to eat low-fat and despite a high prescription rate of statins, at a population level LDL-C levels haven't change appreciably. It isn't just the pill that's the problem. The recommendation of a low-fat diet is just as bad (see Chapter 12).

It's true that fewer people are actually dying of heart attacks in the US and other high-income countries (although low-income countries still have high mortality rates). But that statistic belies the truth. While fewer are *dying* of heart attacks, more people are suffering them. Of course rising numbers could be due to improved recognition, ambulance response time, emergency room functioning, the clot-buster tissue plasminogen activator (tPA), and heart attack post-care.

But the real story is that more people are suffering heart attacks with lower LDL-Cs than before, because the standard fasting lipid profile—the blood test ordered by your practitioner to test your cholesterol—assumes that all LDL particles are the same. There are two different LDLs, but the lipid profile test measures them together. The majority (80 percent) of circulating LDL species are called *large buoyant* or type A LDL, which are increased by dietary fat consumption. This is the species reduced by eating low-fat or by taking statins. However, large buoyant LDL is cardiovascularly neutral—meaning it's not the particle driving the accumulation of plaque in the arteries leading to heart disease. Then there's a second, less common (only 20 percent) LDL species called *small dense* or type B LDL. There is some debate as to whether or not it's the actual perpetrator of the plaque, but it doesn't matter; small dense LDL is predictive of risk for a heart attack. The problem is that statins will lower your LDL-C because they're lowering the type A LDL, which is 80 percent of the total; but they're not doing anything to the type B LDL, which is the problematic particle.

Over the years, medical guidelines have continually expanded the number of individuals for whom statin therapy is recommended. Proponents argue that statins are "life-savers" and that "people will die" if they discontinue their medicine. Prominent researchers from reputable universities have declared that "everyone over fifty" should be on a statin to reduce their risk of CVD. Without a doubt they lower LDL-C. No argument, if the goal is reducing LDL-C, statins are a simple way to do it. And if you have a genetic disorder, they're a necessary way to do it. But do they reduce the risk of heart attack across the board? Without a doubt they don't!

Almost assuredly, statins are reducing the large buoyant LDL but not doing anything about the small dense LDL—therefore the risk of a first heart attack remains unchanged. Conversely, up to 20 percent of statin users demonstrate some form of side effect, often quite serious. There's now a burgeoning literature that statins increase glucose intolerance and risk for both diabetes and weight gain. Is it that, by acting on the liver, statins worsen insulin resistance? Or could it be the inverse—that statin use makes people think they can eat whatever they want because they are now impervious to any cardiovascular risk? It could be both.

So, are statins good or bad? If you don't *need* to take statins, then why would you incur risk of a side effect, which could include muscle breakdown, kidney failure, and type 2 diabetes? The real question is, good or bad for *whom*? For you? Your provider needs to know, but nine times out of ten, they don't. But are they good or bad for the insurance company, which gets to increase your rates for a preexisting condition (still true, even with the advent of Obamacare)? And good or bad for the drug manufacturer, who makes a fortune peddling their "cures"? And good or bad for the government, who are influenced by Big Pharma (see Chapter 6), and who follows the dictum that their voting contingencies will live longer?

Recognizing that the data on statins and heart attack are industry-generated (and likely best-case scenario), the increase of median life expectancy in those with heart disease thought to be the best candidates for statins over a five-year period is a meager four days. Four days? *Really?* And that's a reason for the whole world to be taking them?

What we've learned in this futile exercise is that reducing LDL-C with statins is targeting the wrong pathology. It reduces the benign type A large buoyant LDL but the type B small dense LDL is unaffected. This is important because the problematic small dense LDL-C is a sign of insulin resistance and metabolic dysfunction. Yet the LDL-C level has become so important to Modern Medicine (i.e., the statin manufacturers) that the American Heart Association has advocated to reduce the LDL-C even lower. Indeed, the AHA has developed definitive criteria as to who needs treatment. Meanwhile, pharma companies sold patients and doctors globally close to $1 trillion worth of statins; close to $400 billion in the US alone. That is a pretty hefty haul for a four-day improvement in morbidity and mortality in otherwise healthy people.

Even the American Academy of Pediatrics says that eight-year-olds with high LDL-C need to be treated with statin therapy. I practiced pediatrics for forty years, twenty-four of them focused on obesity, diabetes, and lipid problems. Want to guess how many children I treated with statins? Five—in twenty-four years. Not because I'm a therapeutic nihilist. Not because I didn't know what LDL was. In fact, I didn't give them statins because I *did* know what LDL was. It was a marker of the problem, not the problem itself. And when I got my patients' insulin down by getting them off processed food, their LDL and their triglycerides both came down as well.

What about other drugs that lower LDL? There are other newer drugs on the market, for instance ezetimibe (Zetia), which reduces intestinal cholesterol absorption, and evolocumab (Repatha), an inhibitor of an enzyme, which when blocked helps the liver clear more LDL. These drugs definitely reduce LDL-C, but thus far there are no data for either drug on cardiovascular risk reduction. Because the real problem is metabolic dysfunction due to insulin resistance—and statins do nothing to fix that. Processed food is the true upstream cause, but we refuse to own up to it. In Chapter 9, I'll show you what you *should* look for in your lab data to diagnose your own metabolic disease, how to interpret it, and what to do about it.

If you have a high LDL-C level, your provider is likely to tell you to eat a low-fat diet. Similar to statins, while your LDL will go down, it's only affecting the large buoyant LDL and not the small dense LDL, which is the actual problem. In fact, small dense LDL rises because they are responsive to dietary refined carbohydrate (i.e., fiberless food) and especially sugar consumption, which is what is substituted in lieu of the dietary fat. One of the most compelling arguments against LDL-C as the primary target of CVD prevention or treatment is the Lyon Diet Heart Study. The adoption of a Mediterranean diet for secondary prevention (after you've already had a heart attack) reduced the risk for recurrence. It's clear that eating a Real Food diet, devoid of processed food (how they eat in Lyon) delivered far more impressive results when compared with statins—without the side effects and at a much lower cost. And this diet is decidedly not low-fat. Given that statins can give the illusion of CVD protection yet cause serious side effects, stopping statins and eating Real Food may paradoxically save more lives and improve quality of life.

Your fasting lipid profile test also measures another particle, which is much more egregious than LDL—triglycerides. The level of these particles tells you how your liver is doing. The HR ratio for triglycerides and heart disease is 1.8 (meaning that if they're high, you have an 80 percent increased risk for heart attack) compared to LDL-C at 1.3. Further, the main reason for high triglycerides has nothing to do with LDL-C; rather, it's the refined carbohydrates and sugars in your diet. Again, the #1 risk factor for heart disease isn't LDL-C; it's the insulin resistance of metabolic syndrome, of which triglyceride is a much better biomarker than LDL-C. In fact, the largest study of heart attacks in the US revealed that 66 percent of the victims had metabolic syndrome. And the primary driver? Insulin resistance. And its primary driver? Our out-of-control sugar consumption. Insulin resistance can be in part measured by your triglyceride level (see Chapter 9), which is a better predictor of death by heart attack than high LDL-C ever was.

3. The Blood Pressure Blow-out

Everyone agrees that hypertension (high blood pressure) is bad for you. When they strap on the blood pressure cuff in the doctor's office, what they're measuring is how well your heart is working, and how well it's perfusing the rest of your body with blood. There are two numbers that convey this information: systolic blood pressure (the first number), which indicates how much pressure your blood is exerting against your artery walls when the heart beats; and diastolic blood pressure (the second number), which indicates how much pressure your blood is exerting against your artery walls while the heart is resting between beats.

In 1974, fifty-three million Americans had hypertension; that number has now doubled to one hundred million Americans. In the years between 1988 and 2017, the percentage of hypertensive patients taking medication quadrupled from 7 percent to 31 percent. This isn't just diagnosis creep (even though the AHA recently lowered the systolic blood pressure threshold from 130 to 125). Once upon a time, fifty years ago, the diagnosis of hypertension was made when the systolic blood pressure was 100 plus the patient's age. So hypertension in a forty-year-old was a systolic of 140. But this dropped to 130 in the 1980s as hypertension treatments started flooding the market, and Big Pharma advocated putting more people on more drugs. And now, hypertension is the #1 risk factor for death globally. Each 5-point rise in blood pressure increases your risk for death by 10 percent.

First problem of tackling hypertension: you can lower blood pressure in anybody with enough medicine. But what about side effects? You could experience weakness, dizziness, fainting, muscle cramps, or vomiting, or develop electrolyte imbalances. In general, lowering blood pressure is a good idea, but there's still a 1 to 2 percent risk for death. For example, older people on blood pressure medicines could faint and break their hips—and falls are the leading cause of fatal and nonfatal injuries in older adults. Not a good look when the treatment is worse than the disease. There's an increased mortality in older adults whose blood pressure is less than 130 as a result of the medication.

But is it the blood pressure, or the stuff that comes along with the blood pressure? Most people in the US who are being treated for mild hypertension (140 to 160, or 90 to 110) are taking some medication. However, patients with mild hypertension show no benefit from blood pressure reduction whatsoever in terms of cardiovascular disease, stroke, and death. Fixing the numbers doesn't fix the patient. Furthermore, patients need to know these statistics before they're placed on any blood pressure medications. Their doctors won't tell them because they don't know; they're taught to push the pill. Which is where this book comes in—to explain that changing your diet can reverse metabolic syndrome more effectively and without side effects.

And why is so much of the population hypertensive *now?* Why is its prevalence rising? Does the whole country actually need to be taking a blood pressure pill? The UK documented a 40 percent reduction in stroke between 2006 and 2012 via the simple public health maneuver of forcing the food companies to reduce the amount of salt allowed in processed foods. This strategy worked because the government targeted the pathology, recognizing that a primary cause was processed food, rather than just the symptom of being hypertensive. Reducing salt in the UK cost nothing, while the overall cost of pills for the whole population with high blood pressure was north of $3.3 billion in 2006.

So, is salt really the villain we make it out to be? Currently, the FDA suggests that we consume a maximum of 2.3 grams per day, and only 1.5 grams for those with hypertension. This admonishment exists despite our current median salt consumption of 6.9 grams per day, a tripling over what we actually need. Then again, our recent ancestors, prior to refrigerators, would consume over 15 grams of salt per day! In the bad old days of clipper ship fishing without engines or refrigeration, the fish would have to be salt-cured to protect them from bacterial infestation and contamination. You survived in the winter because you salt-cured your meat and fish in the spring.

So why didn't 15 grams of salt a day cause our ancestors to stroke out routinely? The reason is because the kidney is very adept at excreting excess sodium. But there's one thing that inhibits sodium excretion by the kidney—insulin resistance. High insulin levels increase blood pressure, even with relatively low sodium intake. And many people are insulin resistant—and those people do need to lower their salt as a treatment of the disease. It isn't just the salt—it's also our processed food.

Just a Spoonful of Sugar Helps the Blood Pressure Go Up

What dietary maneuver can fix blood pressure even faster? How about sugar restriction? See **Fig. 2-1a,b** to see how sugar raises your blood pressure more than salt. Sugar also causes liver fat accumulation, insulin

Metabolical

resistance, and increased diastolic blood pressure. Sugar restriction quite rapidly reduces both systolic and diastolic blood pressure, as long as the patient in question doesn't have preexisting kidney disease.

So what's the most effective method of treatment: lowering salt, getting rid of sugar, or taking blood pressure medication? If you take processed food out, you've lowered salt *and* sugar, and you wouldn't need the medicine.

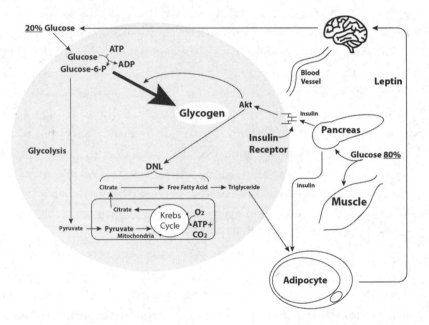

Figure 2–1: a) Pathway of liver glucose metabolism. More information can be found in Chapter 7, under "Cell Bio 101." Only 20 percent of a glucose load enters the liver, and the majority is turned into glycogen (liver starch) for storage. A small amount of glucose will undergo glycolysis (the first step of glucose metabolism, which doesn't need oxygen) to the breakdown product pyruvate. Pyruvate can then enter the mitochondria to be burned via the Krebs cycle all the way to carbon dioxide and water, capturing energy in the form of the chemical adenosine triphosphate (ATP)—the energy is in the phosphates. b) Pathway of liver fructose metabolism. 100 percent of a fructose load enters the liver. Fructose leads to loss of phosphates from ATP, generating of uric acid, which reduces nitric oxide, your blood vessels' relaxing agent, which leads to hypertension. Most of the fructose is turned into pyruvate, the mitochondria become overwhelmed, and the excess generates liver fat, which causes insulin resistance. High insulin interferes with satiety, driving further consumption.

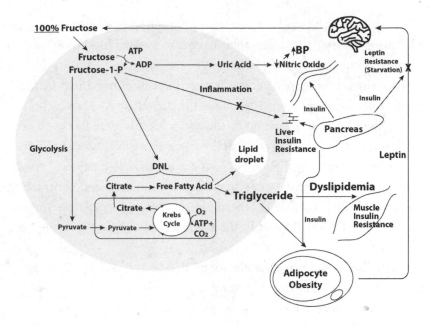

4. Blood Glucose—Dude, Are You *High*?

Let's talk about hyperglycemia (high blood glucose)—the classic symptom of diabetes. First of all, there are two kinds of diabetes: type 1 is due to insulin deficiency (an autoimmune destruction of the pancreas) and is usually associated with children (although some adults can get it); type 2 is due to insulin resistance (see above), the key driver of metabolic syndrome and usually associated with adults (although some children, especially ones I see in my clinic, can get it).

A fasting blood glucose level is the common test ordered by your doctor in addition to testing your cholesterol. This test administered on type 2 diabetics will reflect high and fluctuating glucose levels. Another blood test for chronically high blood glucose levels is the diabetes biomarker hemoglobin A_{1c}. If you have type 2 diabetes and run high blood glucose levels, you're at increased risk for disease in several organs, such as retinopathy (eye), neuropathy (peripheral nerves), and nephropathy (kidney). And when diagnosed, your clinician is likely to prescribe medications such as oral hypoglycemics (glucose-lowering agents) and injectable insulin to lower blood glucose and hemoglobin A_{1c}.

So why do these medications lead to increased mortality? Initially, it looked like these medicines made things better. There was an initial reduction in amputations in dialysis with intensive blood glucose control. But the rates of type 2 diabetes continue to climb, and the potential side effects of these meds, which can include dizziness, drowsiness, heartburn, gastrointestinal distress, and seizures, continue to accrue. In fact, the side effects of glucose-lowering meds are responsible for 100,000 ER visits in the US per year. Again, these meds are treating the symptom, not the cause.

The fact of the matter is it's not really about blood glucose. Blood glucose is just the indirect measurable proxy for the real culprit—which is the blood insulin level. Insulin is the real bad guy in this story—it is its own risk factor, and while high blood glucose can trigger an insulin response, most of the time your blood insulin is *unrelated* to blood glucose. We know this at a basic molecular level, because of seminal mouse studies done by Dr. C. Ron Kahn's lab at Joslin Diabetes Center in Boston.

Kahn's lab constructed eight separate tissue-specific insulin receptor knockout (IRKO) models. Each mouse was genetically engineered to be missing their insulin receptor in a different organ (normally, both mice and humans have insulin receptors in every organ), and therefore insulin has different effects in each mouse. The scientists took the insulin receptor out of the liver, brain, fat cells, brown adipose tissue, muscle, beta-cells, vascular smooth muscle, or kidney. Each mouse developed some form of pathology, none were healthy. But the pathologies were all different from each other. Interestingly, only the liver and the brain IRKO mice developed high blood glucose, and only the brain IRKO mouse became obese and developed metabolic syndrome. And even more interestingly, the kidney IRKO mouse had normal blood glucose, but developed diabetic kidney disease anyway. These various mice show that the cause of the disease is not the high blood glucose—it's the insulin! And this isn't just in mice—we know this is true in humans as well. Because when people with type 1 diabetes (insulin deficiency) are diagnosed, they have normal kidneys, and it takes about ten to twenty years of bad glucose control before they develop kidney disease. Yet, people with metabolic syndrome (insulin resistant) already have kidney disease even before their glucose levels start to rise.

The reason for this dichotomy is because insulin is both *good* for you—because it lowers blood glucose to prevent microvascular disease—and *bad* for you in that it increases the smooth muscle around the coronary arteries or in the kidney, leading to narrowing, and more risk for a heart attack or kidney failure. Let me explain why. Insulin has two actions in cells: 1) metabolic (lowers glucose, stores energy); and 2) cell proliferation (meaning growth and division). Every insulin molecule your pancreas makes is both good *and* bad for you, all at the same time—short-term gain (blood-glucose lowering) for long-term pain (vascular dysfunction and cancer). This dichotomous effect of insulin has been seen in every intensive blood glucose control study, such as the UK Prospective Diabetes Study (UKPDS), the Action to Control Cardiovascular Risk in Diabetes Study (ACCORD) on the effects of rosiglitazone, the Veterans Affairs Diabetes Trial (VADT), and the Action in Diabetes and Vascular Controlled Evaluation (ADVANCE), which actually had to be stopped midstream because of the increase in patient mortality from large vessel disease (heart disease). We need insulin to survive, but if we are insulin resistant, adding extra insulin lowers glucose only at the expense of contributing to chronic disease. Short-term gain for long-term pain.

The point is that high blood glucose is the *symptom* of the disease, not the disease itself (see Chapter 7). Yet blood glucose has become so important to Modern Medicine (because we can measure it!) that even some nondiabetics are now walking around with continuous glucose monitors (CGMs) attached to their arms, in an effort to lower their glucose excursions and therefore improve their metabolic control.

Glucose levels are a poor man's proxy for insulin levels, and not a very good one. The costs to the system of worrying about high blood glucose instead of high blood insulin aren't insignificant. In the US, the total expenditure in diabetic drugs, monitors, and treatment reached $350 billion last year—that's 10 percent of the overall healthcare expenditure. That's a problem that Medicare for All, or any insurance paradigm for that matter, can't fix. The system is broken not because of healthcare, but because of health. And treating the symptoms isn't enough. We have to treat the root cause.

Treat the Symptoms, or Reverse the Disease?

Debates over treatment of symptoms versus reversal of disease are rampant throughout the medical literature. What these arguments demonstrate is that treatment can be targeted and individualized (thus preserving "personal liberty"), but it can exact a hefty cost—not just to the patient, but also to society.

Conversely, prevention doesn't need to be targeted—it can be global, across the board, therefore saving money and lives. Managing metabolic syndrome disease is 75 percent of the total healthcare budget; and we're not really treating it—we're papering it over, which means that the costs are cumulative. Morbidity keeps costing until you die, and people are dying earlier, not paying into the system, and therefore costing more.

Modern Medicine works downstream of the problem by treating the symptoms, rather than working upstream to treat the cause. Doctors continue to fill the wrong prescription over and over. And it's breaking the bank and costing us our lives.

CHAPTER 3

Doctors Need to "Unlearn" Nutrition

Mark Twain said, "Education is mainly what we have unlearned." Yoda implored, "You must unlearn what you have learned." If the last fifty years of medicine has taught us anything, it's that we physicians have a whole lot to unlearn—except when it comes to nutrition, in which case you can't unlearn what you were never taught in the first place.

Modern Medicine is a racket. Full disclosure—I was part of that racket through my forty years of practice, although when it came to money, I was the lowest (academic) of the lowest (pediatric) of the low (endocrinologist). I learned nutrition in college, and then unlearned it in a medical school curriculum influenced by Big Pharma (see Chapter 6).

I had to relearn everything I know about nutrition and NCDs on my own, through my own research and experience, even though I had a whole lot of people telling me that I was shooting myself in the foot. In one ignominious episode in 2009, I was even thrown out of the UCSF Pediatric Diabetes Clinic, which focused on kids with type 1 diabetes. And this ouster was led by, of all people, the clinic dietitian. At that point I'd been an endocrinologist for twenty-six years, fourteen of them spent specifically on insulin and its role in obesity and chronic disease, as the director of the Weight Assessment for Teen and Child Health (WATCH) Clinic, a separate entity from the diabetes clinic. We saw those kids with type 2 diabetes resulting from insulin resistance and metabolic syndrome—and as we know, there are no patients more at risk for chronic disease than those with type 2 diabetes due to insulin resistance.

What about type 1 diabetes, due to insulin deficiency? They get diabetic complications in part due to their overinsulinization over time. Both forms of diabetes (type 1 and type 2) are extreme carbohydrate intolerance, so I thought, what if we tried to reduce the insulin requirements of type 1 diabetic kids by getting the refined carbohydrates and sugar out of their diets? Would their blood glucose swings be easier to control?

Even ten years later, in 2019, this concept was still considered alternative, yet is becoming slowly accepted practice and with lots of data supporting it. But in 2009 cutting back on insulin dosage was heresy. For decades the American Diabetes Association said that both type 1 and type 2 diabetics could "eat all the carbs you want, just take enough insulin to cover it" (to their credit, the 2019 ADA guidelines for the first time mentioned carbohydrate restriction).

In my opinion, this was among the most dangerous medical guidance ever given. Despite my working in the UCSF Pediatric Diabetes Clinic for eight years, the clinic's dietitian toed that party line against me, telling kids and their parents to eat as many carbs as they wanted but to inject enough insulin to counteract the effects. She admonished me with, "Well, I wrote a book." Her flippancy prompted me to deliver a lecture for the University of California Mini Medical School for the Public, entitled "Sugar: The Bitter Truth," which has now received twelve million views and counting. And then *I* wrote a book, *Fat*

Chance, as my rebuttal. The fact is, increased refined carbs in kids and adults with both type 1 and type 2 diabetes can have serious long-term health effects.

Does Science Advance "One Funeral at a Time"?

This offhand comment made by German physicist Max Planck at the turn of the twentieth century was based on his observation that scientists are like mafiosi—they exert a stranglehold on their fields, preventing new ideas from percolating to the surface and, like Don Corleone, you had to wait for them to die in order for science to move forward.

The National Bureau of Economic Research put it to the test. They assembled the names and papers of all the members of the National Academy of Sciences for twenty years, and then assembled the names and papers of all of their coauthors. They looked to see who passed away in that twenty-year interval and assessed the coauthors' research productivity after their leader died. Not surprisingly, the collaborators fell off the academic cliff without their Godfather. Then they used medical subject heading (MeSH) terms to see who was publishing in that area afterward. Turns out it was an entirely new crop of scientists with completely new ideas. Indeed, the big bosses squelched any dissent in order to maintain their influence.

Well, the nutritional gurus of the 1970s, with their mantra of "low-fat, high sugar" are now dropping off, so it's not surprising that the field is finally starting to move forward again. And everyone, doctors and patients alike, needs to take heed of the "new nutrition."

Academic Arrogance

The octopus-like grip academic gurus maintain on their respective fields involves many tentacles. One big motivation is grant funding—after all, if an authority is proven wrong, the funding will dry up. Second, and even more pernicious, is the ephemeral currency of academia. In Washington, it's power. On Wall Street, it's money. In the ivory tower, it's credit. Credit—*really*? It's true; credit is the green-eyed monster of academia. It's all about how many papers you've published in what journal and whether your name is listed first or last (if neither, your contribution is seen as second-rate). The motto really should be "publish *and* perish." Academic medicine is the worst, because never has so much been fought over for so little.

And then, finally, there's the most ridiculous monster of all: skepticism. Now, it's good for academicians to be skeptical—after all, they're supposed to apply the scientific method to their deliberations, and keep their own personal biases separate. But what if that skepticism is misplaced? What if it's being driven by personal hubris rather than good scientific suspicion?

Here is my own very recent example of how this kind of skepticism works to everyone's detriment, except the academician. I first aired the "sugar is toxic" message in public in 2009. In 2011, Gary Taubes wrote his *New York Times* article "Is Sugar Toxic?," followed by my 2012 *Nature* comment (written with UCSF colleagues Laura Schmidt and Claire Brindis), "The Toxic Truth about Sugar." We then published our landmark fructose restriction study (see Chapter 20) in the journal *Obesity* in 2016, which demonstrated causation between sugar consumption and metabolic syndrome. Despite all the information and science gleaned by myself and others, an incredulous WebMD video appeared online asking Joslin Diabetes Center CEO Ron Kahn the question, "Can eating a lot of sugar cause my diabetes?" Kahn responded (and I quote): "Eating a lot of sugar definitely does not cause diabetes if you don't eat so much sugar that you gain weight. And in fact, sugar to a certain extent is OK because it stimulates the pancreas to make more insulin, which actually helps to control the blood sugar . . ."

This is the head of the Joslin Diabetes Center, saying in 2015, "a calorie is a calorie," "it's about obesity," and "insulin is good." With all we knew at that point, to be that unabashed about one's stance on a seminal point that has such important clinical implications—think about that.

To Kahn's credit, he has finally come around—in part, because he senior-authored a 2019 article in *Cell Metabolism* showing in mice that fructose decreases mitochondrial function, while glucose stimulates it. He issued this statement to *Science Daily* about his paper: "The most important takeaway of this study is that high-fructose in the diet is bad. It's not bad because it's more calories, but because it has effects on liver metabolism to make it worse at burning fat. As a result, adding fructose to the diet makes the liver store more fat, and this is bad for the liver and bad for whole body metabolism."

OK, Kahn finally accepts that *a calorie is not a calorie*, and that *sugar is toxic*. Hooray. But why? And why now? The answer is simple: he had to do it himself. That way, he looks like the consummate critical investigator, being appropriately cautious. But it also gives him the opportunity to ignore what came before, dissing other scientists, and allows him to take credit for a new paradigm shift. And remember, in academia, it's all about the credit.

Conflict or Confluence of Interest?

There are some scientists who aren't just cautious or contrary—they're plain calcified. They won't ever flip—not even when presented with new data or hypotheses. Sure, everyone has a belief system; that's how we make sense of the world. Some people will allow for rational challenge of their beliefs when they are debunked—we call them moderates—while others defend against it to maintain their worldview at any costs and are called zealots.

But then there's another class of thinkers who are intransigent because they make money to keep it that way. And in the nutrition field, this seems to be the case more often than not. Credit is the end game of most medical academicians, and clinicians are taught to respect the medical literature. But many docs also rely on the lay press, which often gets it wrong, depending on who is funding the message. They still follow the advice of their big-name colleagues, but are often unaware of who is paying them.

A recent example of zealotry became evident during the 2019 skirmish over whether red meat is good for you or not. A nonprofit scientific group calling itself NutriRECS, headed by Gordon Guyatt (originator of the GRADE system of evidence-based medicine), published a meta-analysis in the *Annals of Internal Medicine* that couldn't conclude that red meat was bad for health. They didn't conclude it was *good* for health either, just *not bad*.

This article set off a firestorm in the nutrition community—and most worrisome, before it was even published. A nonprofit nutritional education organization called True Health Initiative (THI), headed by self-proclaimed nutritional entrepreneur and anti-meat advocate David Katz, upon reading the embargoed press release, launched an all-out attack on the *Annals* office in Philadelphia. This included an email bot campaign on the editor, spamming, and an unheard of request for formal pre-publication retraction. Katz, in conjunction with Neal Barnard of the Physicians Committee for Responsible Medicine (PCRM, another anti-meat advocacy group), petitioned the Philadelphia district attorney to open a case against *Annals* "to investigate potential reckless endangerment," and a separate petition to the Federal Trade Commission. All this about a paper that hadn't even been published yet. Katz himself called *Annals* a vehicle for "information terrorism."

Katz and THI don't dispute the science in this meta-analysis; rather, they call into question the first author, Bradley Johnston, who three years prior had taken money from the International Life Sciences Institute (ILSI; see Chapter 23), a front group for the food industry. They accused another coauthor, Patrick Stover, of having an undisclosed conflict of interest because he is vice chancellor and dean of Texas A&M College of Agriculture and Life Sciences, which had received an endowment to support the International Beef Cattle Academy.

What THI leaves out is that they're equally if not more conflicted, with a web of cash receipts or endorsements from the likes of #NoBeef, the Olive Wellness Institute, the Plantrician Project, Wholesome Goodness, Quorn, and the California Walnut Commission. Other THI board members, including former U.S. Surgeon General Richard Carmona, served on the board of Herbalife Nutrition Foundation; and David Jenkins, who penned an article about resisting corporate interests, takes money from Pulse Research Network, the Almond Board of California, the International Nut and Dried Fruit Council, Soyfoods Association of North America, the Peanut Institute, Kellogg's Canada, and Quaker Oats Canada. Calling the kettle black.

Katz for his part stated, "I think there's a big difference between *conflict of interest* . . . versus a *confluence of interest*. The work you do is what you care about. . . . No one's ever paid me to say anything I don't believe. . . . There's nothing fundamentally wrong [with] industry funding." Is he right?

Academic Societies Have Their Own Agendas

The US has many academic medical societies. Many of them overlap, and all are political. For instance, who is in charge of diabetes? Those organizations laying claim include the Endocrine Society, Pediatric Endocrine Society, Juvenile Diabetes Research Foundation, American Association of Clinical Endocrinology, Diabetes Technology Society, and the omnipresent and ubiquitous two-thousand-pound gorilla in the room, American Diabetes Association (ADA). Many of these societies say that they issue clinical guidelines for clinicians, in order to promulgate and maintain "standards of care" within the profession. But is it more to promulgate and maintain a choke hold over thought and discourse?

The ADA has been particularly egregious in its ignorance of the science involved in the issuance of its guidelines. Full disclosure—I don't belong and have never belonged to the ADA, in part because of their head in the sand approach to diabetes care.

I got into the obesity field in 1995, and went to my first ADA meeting in 2002. I was dumbfounded. First, there was not one talk on prevention of type 2 diabetes, only on treatment. Second, here is the society that presumably knows the most about the role of insulin in disease—and they're promoting the message that obese people are at fault for eating too damn much. Then, they tell people with diabetes to eat whatever they want, just so long as they count their carbs and take enough insulin to cover it. Given what we know about glucose and insulin excursions causing chronic metabolic disease, why would they advocate for that? Nonetheless, the ADA guidelines advised this through 2018.

I saw plenty of kids with type 1 diabetes over the years, and the best way to get their hemoglobin A_{1c} down was to get their carbohydrate consumption down, although not every study has been able to get kids to do this effectively. I never understood the ADA's stance against carbohydrate restriction, and I've spoken out against it on many occasions.

The lightbulb of just how conflicted the ADA is went off for me on April 28, 2017, when Stephen Dubner, host of the podcast *Freakonomics* and a personal hero, released his report: "There's a War on Sugar: Is It Justified?" Three people were interviewed: Dr. Margaret Hamburg (an MD and former head of the FDA), Dr. Richard Kahn (a PhD and former chief science officer of the ADA until 2009; no relation to C. Ronald Kahn), and myself.

Richard Kahn is a true case study. In 2014, he coauthored an editorial in *Diabetes Care* exonerating sugar as a cause of obesity and diabetes. In this *Freakonomics* episode, when Dubner asked Kahn about the cause of obesity, he said, "There's been some evidence, that with the increased use of psychotropic drugs, anti-depressive drugs, drugs for schizophrenia and other mental disorders, those drugs tend to promote weight gain . . . and when people stop smoking, that's usually been associated with weight gain . . . many people do believe that sugar consumption has been the cause . . . of our obesity epidemic, and subsequently diabetes. But I believe the evidence for this is pretty weak." In 2017, San Francisco was debating adding warning labels to cans of soda akin to packs of cigarettes, a campaign in which I was the scientific expert and reviewer of promotional materials. Richard Kahn, in opposition, coauthored an expert report on behalf of the American Beverage Association. In that report he wrote, "There is no scientific consensus that added sugar, including added sugar in beverages, plays a unique role in the development of obesity and diabetes." Could it be because Kahn, during his tenure at the ADA, signed a three-year $1.5 million sponsorship deal with Cadbury-Schweppes, the world's largest confectioner? In the end, bowing to political pressure from Big Food, California put the kibosh on the campaign before implementation.

Interestingly, my UCSF colleague Dean Schillinger looked at the same datasets Kahn did (sixty studies in all; see Chapter 23) and when taken *in toto*, Kahn is correct—there's no clear consensus. But Schillinger added one variable—food company sponsorship. Lo and behold, of the twenty-six studies sponsored by food companies, all twenty-six showed no effect. Of the thirty-four studies that were independently funded, thirty-three showed a clear relationship between sugar consumption, obesity, and diabetes—meaning the food industry has polluted the data (see Chapter 23), and Kahn toes the same line, polluting it further. He ultimately was replaced by a true National Institutes of Health (NIH)-trained MD diabetes researcher, William Cefalu, and for the first time, the 2019 ADA guidelines mention that carbohydrate restriction could be a viable option for some diabetics. Yet they still haven't acknowledged sugar as a cause of diabetes. And they're not the only ones. On its website, Diabetes UK says, "With type 2 diabetes, we know sugar doesn't directly cause it, but you are more likely to get type 2 diabetes if you are overweight." Maybe this assertion has something to do with the fact that Diabetes UK received a 500,000 pound contribution from Britvic, the company that is licensed to sell PepsiCo in the UK. This, at the exact same time that the International Diabetes Federation (IDF; which represents 198 countries, just not the US, UK, and Australia) told the Group of Twenty (G20; an international forum of central banks) that taxing sugar could save lives and money.

Why does the ADA and Diabetes UK say sugar doesn't cause diabetes, while the IDF says taxing sugar could prevent type 2 diabetes? Because many of the IDF's member countries are poor—they can't afford the refrigerators to store the insulin, never mind the insulin itself. As a result, they have to prevent disease—and that means changing the food. But to implement the same changes, the US, UK, and Australian diabetes societies would have to admit that they were wrong, and have continued to be wrong for decades now. When given the choice, it's easier to throw meds at the problem and throw shade at the critics.

Academic societies often blur the facts. What would happen to the ADA if people knew they could prevent diabetes without medicine? What would happen to all the Big Pharma money coming in to support the ADA budget? In the "bad old days," many academic organizations sold their name to corporations; for instance, the American Medical Association to Sunbeam, and the ADA to SnackWell's. But that practice is now frowned upon. The ADA is #100 in profitable charities, with $182 million in annual revenues, of which 40 percent come from pharmaceutical corporate donations. In the decade 2002–2013, while the ADA declared diabetes a treatable disease with meds, thereby increasing the market, the cost of insulin tripled.

After all, why would a private nonprofit society dedicated to eradicating a disease want the disease eradicated? Most medical/professional societies eschew nutritional information and policy because appropriate nutrition *can both treat and prevent* disease—while most organizations are in the business of only *treating* disease with medications. For example, we know that sugar consumption drives the development of type 2 diabetes, but the US, UK, and Australian diabetes associations refuse to acknowledge that we could prevent and treat type 2 diabetes through sugar restriction. They much prefer issuing prescriptions. Why? The answer is simple: because if we prevented diabetes, they'd go out of business.

And after all, medical societies are run by people, who've got their own skins, or wallets, in the game. There's more money at stake than you might think. A recent analysis of the ten US societies with the costliest disease expenditures shows that 72 percent of board members have extensive ties with industry, receiving a median honorarium of $32,000, with an upper range of over $500,000 for the oncologists. No wonder drugs rule medicine (see Chapter 6).

The Clinician's Conundrum

Ivory tower academicians are supposed to advance scientific discourse, but they frequently hold it back, especially when they're subordinated by their guru, organization or university, or academic society. But what is holding clinicians back from doing right by their patients when they know the truth?

The first thing we've learned over the last forty years is that doctors are parochial. We only get information from other doctors, in the form of journal articles, clinical meetings, and webinars. Most of these venues are sponsored by Big Pharma to push their products—you can check for yourself who funds the satellite events at the ADA, for example.

The second thing we've learned is that doctors are sheep, meaning doctors follow the herd of other doctors. And there's good reason. If you don't follow the medical guidelines, you get a lousy evaluation on Healthgrades—the online company that evaluates physicians and gives them a number score—and the hospital medical board will then investigate you and can revoke your privileges.

The third thing we've learned is that most of us doctors don't listen to our patients. We talk. In part, because insurance companies tightened the screws, so we only have ten minutes with you. Once we have your set of symptoms and arrive at a provisional diagnosis, we're on to the quickest and easiest form of treatment, whether it's the most efficacious or not, and our hand is on the doorknob. Next time you go to the doctor, time your visit. Talking about lifestyle changes takes time that we don't have—because that's how we've been trained and how we get paid.

Nutritional "Know-Nothings"

Nowhere in medicine are the principles more challenged than in the field of nutrition. Nothing is more important than nutrition for correct and optimal bodily and mental functioning, yet nothing in medicine generates more heat and less light.

Only 28 percent of medical schools have a formal nutrition curriculum; even fewer than in 1977 when Congress passed the law that created the Dietary Guidelines and called for more nutrition science in the medical classroom. Now, medical students receive on average 19.6 contact hours of nutrition instruction during their four-year medical school careers, about 0.27 percent of the time spent in class. How is your doctor supposed to provide nutrition advice if they never learned it in the first place?

Apart from rare specialized symposia (e.g., the University of Arizona's Integrative Nutrition annual symposium, or Tulane University's Health Meets Food symposium), there are virtually no continuing medical education programs on nutrition that aren't corrupted by industry influence. This includes nutraceutical companies peddling dietary supplements, as they're trying to insert themselves between food and medicine. Even more concerning is that this isn't an exclusively American problem; nutrition is poorly taught around the globe.

Predictably, the focus of medical school education is on treatment—drugs, devices, and digging (surgery)—because they make money for the physician, Big Pharma, and Med-Tech. This is why medical school operating costs are underwritten by pharma companies (see Chapter 6). After all, why would your doctor recommend a $0.10/day dietary supplement or a $0.50 vegetable/day that doesn't need a prescription, over a $10.00/day pharmaceutical that needs their signature and continued follow-ups?

Nutritional epidemiology is fraught with controversy. Recently, there have been calls to curtail nutritional research because it is hard to do properly. For most nutrients, patient recall is the only method for estimating consumption, and people forget, especially about items that they think aren't good for them. Furthermore, analysis of data is always suspect since correlation is not causation. In order to determine causation in research, you need one of two kinds of studies. The first is called randomized controlled trials (RCTs; this is the gold standard for drug evaluation), but nutritional studies can't be controlled very easily, because with prospective (following patients over time) studies it's hard to alter people's diets for any length of time. When one nutrient goes up (e.g., carbohydrate), another goes down (e.g., fat). The other kind of study is known as econometric analysis, in which natural history studies of changes in disease rates over time are analyzed, taking into account all other co-occurring factors. This is how we determined that tobacco causes lung cancer—because doing an RCT would get you thrown in jail. Econometric analysis is more conducive to nutritional research, and is how we proved that sugar is causative for type 2 diabetes.

Of course both kinds of studies are complicated to perform, require appropriate statistical analysis, and drive the cost of such projects up. Another reason, as discussed above, is that the food industry has put the thumb on the scale of many nutritional studies, polluting the literature. Last, you have to measure the correct metric, which is difficult, expensive, and time-consuming. For example, biomarkers (e.g., LDL-C) are not the same as events (e.g., heart attacks) (see Chapter 2). Doctors figure, why bother to try?

Patients are notorious for ignoring medical advice, even as it relates to their own longevity. Most can't or won't change their diets, or miraculously start exercising just because their doctor tells them to. Stanford nutritionist Christopher Gardner showed in his A to Z study that all dietary interventions regress to the mean—meaning by two months on any specific diet, the subject will return to eating the same way they were before the intervention. Dieting is hard, and rarely works in the long term. You *can* alter your health, but you have to know why; your doctor does, too. They need to be able to explain the "why" back to you. One thing I've learned after forty years in medicine is that if you don't understand and tell people why something will work, they won't do it.

You really can't blame the public for their nutritional whiplash. We are exposed to a daily barrage of contradictory statements and straw man arguments about basic science (one day "fat is bad," the next day "fat is good") coming from physicians and dietitians, while nutritional biochemistry is ignored (i.e., how metabolism works versus calorie counting and body weight). The physicians don't understand it themselves. If there's no science or understanding, there's no imperative to change.

Another reason that patients can't or won't alter their diets is that they're abusing sugar—the food additive that's most addictive, induces metabolic disease, and reduces longevity. These patients need help from their doctors more than ever, but doctors understand addiction about as well as they understand nutrition—witness the doctors' response to our current opioid crisis where we have two million addicted people and only 5,500 physicians trained in addiction medicine.

Since there's been perennially so little money for nutrition research, Big Food has stepped in to fill the void. They conduct their own studies, which are 7.36 times more likely to support their own product than not. They pollute the professional journals with biased research, so they can point to their own studies and say that a nutritional principle is not "settled science." And they use their money to buy the loyalty of dietitians (see Chapter 4), and to co-opt and pay off scientists and critics alike.

Who's on the Hot Seat?

Doctors are kept honest by their medical organizations, who propose and codify state-of-the-art clinical guidelines. But doctors are also kept honest by their patients, as many of them won't improve by following those same guidelines. Astute clinicians are pattern recognizers; they know when they're seeing the same thing time and again—they know something's up; they might not know what it is exactly, but they know they need to change something. One such pattern recognizer was Robert Atkins, who rethought human nutrition and metabolism, realized refined carbohydrates were hurting himself and his patients, and wrote a book to explain his change in practice. Some called him a huckster and charlatan, some called him dangerous; but he was listening to what his patients were telling him, and ultimately he was proved right.

A most unseemly aspect of medicine is when professionals in the community turn such pattern recognizers into criminals, for daring to think outside the box. Three physicians—Dr. Tim Noakes in South Africa; Dr. Evelyne Bourdua-Roy in Quebec; and Dr. Gary Fettke in Australia—have been formally investigated by their countries' respective medical boards for promoting low-carbohydrate lifestyle advice. They're charged with giving "medical advice" on the radio or in lectures that could "mislead the public on low-carb, high-fat (LCHF)/ketogenic diets." In each case, the charges were brought to the medical board by the dietetics board of each country, without evidence in support of the claims, and without any alleged "victim" of that "dangerous" medical "advice" coming forward.

Noakes was referred to his medical governing board by Johannesburg dietitian Claire Julsing Strydom, president of the Association for Dietetics in South Africa, due to a single tweet he made to a breastfeeding mother. In it, he said that good first foods for infant weaning are LCHF. Thus, for infants, he was suggesting meat, fish, chicken, eggs, dairy, and vegetables. The ADSA views LCHF diets as fashionable and instead supports orthodox low-fat, high-carb diets (e.g., rice cereal, strained fruits). Noakes went on trial twice to have his medical license revoked, and despite being exonerated with testimony from international experts on metabolism and nutrition, has suffered through waves of negative publicity and censure.

Bourdua-Roy's investigation by Quebec's medical board is ongoing. The charges against her advocating a LCHF diet were levied by prominent dietitians who wrote an opinion piece in the *Le Soleil* newspaper. The letter's first signatory is Caroline Dubeau, regional director of the Dietitians of Canada (DoC) for Quebec; although Dubeau is careful to stress that neither she nor the DoC lodged the complaints against Bourdua-Roy, she wouldn't say whether the nutritionists who complained are DoC members. The DoC website says that *dietitian* and *nutritionist* are protected titles in Quebec. Just as with other sister dietitian associations globally, DoC is heavily conflicted. Like some medical societies, they accept sponsorship money from Big Food, Big Sugar, Big Soft Drinks (with Coca-Cola driving from the front), and

Big Pharma. Many of their members have industry links. Last year, over seven hundred doctors, dietitians, and nutritionists signed a letter to their government in support of Bourdua-Roy, calling for radical reform of nutrition guidelines to include low-carb, healthy-natural-fat diets. Bourdua-Roy herself posted a hard-hitting response to Dubeau's letter, in an article in the *HuffPost* that eighty other Canadian doctors signed. The headline: "Low-Carb, High-Fat Is What We Physicians Eat. You Should, Too." Dr. Bourdua-Roy has not yet been exonerated.

Fettke, an orthopedic surgeon by training, developed an aggressive pituitary tumor requiring surgery, chemotherapy, and radiotherapy, and through his own research, has been able to stave off its progression by adopting an extremely low-carbohydrate, high-fat diet, known universally as the ketogenic diet (see Chapter 12). This diet is now in trial around the world (at notable research institutions such as Memorial Sloan Kettering in New York and MD Anderson Cancer Center in Houston) to "starve" the tumor, and reverse its growth. Fettke, as a caregiver, prefers not to have to amputate limbs from diabetic patients as a consequence of their condition, so he tells his patients that a simple dietary change can save both life and limb. For informing his diabetic patients to reduce their sugar intake, Fettke was stripped of his ability to provide nutritional counseling or medical management of his patients. Fettke still doesn't know the names of the persons who reported him to the Australian Health Practitioner Regulation Agency (AHPRA), but he does know that the complainants are members of the Dietitians Association of Australia (DAA). They accused him of "inappropriately reversing a patient's diabetes." Really? The DAA has made its opposition to LCHF and ketogenic diets well known. And AHPRA slapped a lifetime ban on Fettke for his attempts to try to save diabetic patients' limbs from being sawed off and their lives from being snuffed out. The good news is that Dr. Fettke, with help from the international medical community, finally won his appeal in 2018.

It's clear that sugar and processed food drive obesity, heart disease, stroke, diabetes, and fatty liver disease (see Chapter 2), and there's emerging data that processed food is responsible for cancer and dementia as well. It's also clear that low-carbohydrate diets haven't worsened this trend, and in some cases have reversed these diseases. Yet the medical establishment refuses to be reeducated, and instead prosecutes the re-educators.

The New Wave of Health Professionals Leading the Charge

I didn't have an Obi-Wan Kenobi to urge me to "use the Force." I had no Deep Throat to prod me to "follow the money." But ultimately that's just what I did, and what the medical profession needs to do now. There are a few branches of Modern Medicine that have recognized both the problems and the importance of nutritional therapy; for instance, integrative and functional medicine and psychiatry. Their charge is to treat the upstream causes of disease, not the downstream symptoms. Many of these doctors and healthcare professionals eschew medications, rather opting to use food as medicine. And this makes sense, because as we will learn in Chapter 10, the cellular pathways that lead to chronic disease are not *druggable*, but they are *foodable*.

Unfortunately, such doctors are still few and far between. There are a few courageous practitioners who've spoken up, but most of them have been marginalized by the medical establishment for all the reasons stated above. However, this new wave of physicians has some guiding lights *and the data* to make inroads into the medical debacle we find ourselves in. It's about time.

CHAPTER 4

Dietitians Lost Their Mind

It's bad enough that doctors don't learn nutrition in medical school, but at least their diplomas say *medicine*, not *nutrition*. However, that's exactly what dietitians' certificates say they learned in their nutrition and dietetics training programs—but they didn't. Dentists used to learn nutrition in dental school until 1947, but then they left it behind—why? The entire gamut of the health services professions has been co-opted in one way or another around nutrition, to everyone's detriment. This is a nefarious tale of how religion can co-opt nutrition, both directly (through the professionals) and indirectly (through the public).

Dietitians and Math

Decades ago, the ability to dispense nutritional advice was "claimed" by dietitians. The field of modern dietetics was borne out of two concepts, both of which turned out to be false. The first is the idea that a "calorie is a calorie," which was espoused by the Atwater system, developed by agriculturist Wilbur Olin Atwater in 1916. His claim to fame was that he standardized how much *heat energy* (i.e., how many kilocalories, or kcal) three specific macronutrients would liberate when burned in a bomb calorimeter (a device that measures heat release of organic substances), and he calculated the ratios, which computes the number of kcal in a given food by its protein (4 kcal/gm), carbohydrate (4 kcal/gm), and fat (9 kcal/gm) content. As fat was the most calorie-dense, Atwater thought it was the most egregious in terms of weight gain.

Since then, dieticians have clung to the idea that a patient's food plate can be calculated using this arithmetic. The problem is that our bodies are a bit more complicated. The Atwater equation neglected to account for the intestinal microbiome and its inherent metabolism of approximately 25 to 30 percent of everything you eat, as well as the role of fiber in altering that percentage (see Chapter 12). Since fiber doesn't contribute any calories to your total but alters the percentage of the total that you absorb, the number of calories you eat versus how many you metabolize are completely disparate. Nowhere is this more true than for nuts such as almonds, where the amount of calories absorbed is a full 30 percent less than those generated from a bomb calorimeter; in fact, some manufacturers are now ratcheting down the labeling of caloric content of their products specifically to reflect this fact. But, of course, we didn't know the intestinal microbiome even existed back in 1916. We do now, but the dietitians have not changed their math, methodology, or message.

The modern dietetics movement began in 1917, with the founding of the American Dietetic Association, rebranded in 2012 as the Academy of Nutrition and Dietetics (AND). The AND has always argued that obesity, and indeed all of nutrition, can be determined with some simple math. Just add up what's in the food versus what you need, and you have all the evidence you need to determine nutrient deficiency or excess. They say that chronic disease is caused by excess calories, and therefore obesity—thus giving rise to the partnerships between the Big Food companies and the AND, as exemplified by their motto "Eat Right" and exercise. In the process, we were offered such subterfuges as Smart Choices (a food industry coalition), NuVal (David Katz), and the Global Energy Balance Network (both Coca-Cola); fortunately, all of these are debunked and relegated to the dustbin of history. Nonetheless, the beat goes on. Coca-Cola sponsors the nonprofit Exercise is Medicine, to get people to focus on exercise, not diet.

Corporate dietitians have continued to exonerate processed food over the decades, as has the AND. They do this for three reasons. The first is that they espouse calories, and virtually all food has calories, so what makes an individual food a problem? The Atwater system was, is, and always will be defective. Where those food calories come from determines where they go. It's not physics, it's nutritional biochemistry. My hope is that you will see past this fallacy, and that this book will finally *kill the calorie*, a stake right through the heart of the myth, once and for all. They also claim it's what's in the food that matters—this is clear from their support of the Nutrition Facts label. Except that it's not what's in the food, it's what's been *done* to the food, which doesn't appear on the food label (see Chapter 17). They've missed the mark on both counts.

And, last, 90 percent of their operating budget comes from Big Food, as documented by public health lawyer Michele Simon. They exonerate dietary sugar even to this day because they can't possibly kill the goose that lays the golden eggs. This was proven to me personally, when I was attacked by a Dallas dietitian, Neva Cochran, RD, while I was a guest on the *Diane Rehm Show* in 2013, for arguing that *a calorie is not a calorie*. Despite the evidence, Ms. Cochran later lashed out on YouTube, saying *a calorie IS a calorie*. Why was Ms. Cochran so vehement? Because she represents the processed food industry. Calories are the industry's shield; it's how they hide from culpability. It's Ms. Cochran's job to discredit me, and anyone else who gets in the way of processed food.

Dietitians Need a Schooling

It should be disturbing to all of us that public schools are now the biggest franchise food operation in the world. The School Nutrition Association is the biggest proponent of processed food—no surprise, just look at who sponsors them—so how do you expect to change the food in schools? In 2015 at the St. Louis Chapter of the AND, I was supposed to debate Courtney Gaine, PhD, RD, president of the Sugar Association (note, she's a dietitian paid to uphold sugar), but she canceled two days before. Instead I debated Connie Diekman, RD, who was the local spokesperson for the AND. Ms. Diekman upheld the Sugar Association's party line about Energy Balance. So who do you expect to change the food in schools?

Since dietitians (either actively or passively) took over nutritional counseling back in the 1960s, our health has steadily gotten worse. Maybe that's correlation rather than causation, but the one thing we can say is that despite the abject deterioration of American health, dieticians haven't altered their advice; they're still stuck on calories. Current modeling suggests that virtually half of all Americans will be obese by 2030. Patients remain ill, because processed foods are addictive, doctors are ambivalent, confused, or just plain ignorant, and dietitians are complicit with Big Food.

If you want further proof, just look at the quality of the food served in hospitals. There's a fast food concession in 28 percent of children's hospitals in America, and any food in the lobby, either for the patients, staff, or visitors, has to be approved by the hospital dietitians. How is that modeling for parents and kids? And in hospitals where doctors have suggested the removal of sugared beverages from the menu, the hospital dietitians revolted, claiming that this is "cruel and inhuman punishment" (yes, that's a direct quote). Even at UCSF, where we were able to remove all sodas from the campus and subsequently showed improvement in metabolic health in the employees (see Chapter 28), we still weren't able to remove fruit juice, because the dietitians would not yield.

Ultimately, you can be part of the problem, or you can be part of the solution. To be sure, many dietitians are attempting to change the profession from the inside, and they are to be applauded and supported. But the core of the profession must abide by the AND and its corporate sponsorship in order to receive and maintain certification.

How can you tell which side a dietitian is on? One question: ask them if you need sugar to live.

Dietetics Is a Protection Racket

Dietitians around the country are indemnified from lawsuits by an entity known as the Commission on Dietetic Registration (CDR). Their mission statement is: "To administer valid, reliable, and rigorous credentialing processes to protect the public and meet the needs of CDR credentialed practitioners, employers and consumers."

Currently, 104,000 dietitians and nutritionists are registered with the CDR. Legislation exists in forty-seven states (Arizona, Michigan, and New Jersey are not included) to protect dietitians registered with the CDR. This has created a monopoly position on giving out dietary advice. Their only responsibility: conform to the policies of the AND— including those about processed food. Well, where does the AND get its marching orders? Here is the list of funders and sponsors for 2019: Abbott; American Pistachio Growers; a2 Milk Company; BENEO Institute; Campbell Soup Company; Conagra Brands; DanoneWave; Egg Nutrition Center; Florida Department of Citrus; FMC (a chemical producer); Ingredion; Lentils.org; National Cattlemen's Beef Association; National Dairy Council; Nestlé USA; Premier Protein; Quaker Tropical Gatorade; Splenda sweetener; Sunsweet Growers; and The Wonderful Company. Some Real Food companies, to be sure, but a whole lot of processed ones as well.

Dietitians and the Battle for the "Soul" of the Profession

The second false concept of dietetics stems from a religious principle rather than a scientific one. Lenna Cooper and Lulu Graves cofounded the AND in 1917, in response to dietary needs of soldiers in World War I. Cooper had worked as a governess for nutritionist/physician John Harvey Kellogg, who sponsored her to get her BS in nursing at his Battle Creek Sanitarium (of which he was CEO and chief physician). She picked up dietetics on the fly by working as his apprentice, espousing his principles along the way. In other words, she had no dietetic training beyond what she learned from Kellogg. Like him, Cooper was a proponent of a low-protein, high-carbohydrate diet, believing "The proportions in the menu should be 10 percent protein, 30 fats and 60 per cent carbohydrates. It is impossible to emphasize too strongly that our health and energies depend on our foods." In 1913, she authored *The New Cookery,* a low-protein vegetarian cookbook. She's also responsible for this little ditty: "In many ways, the breakfast is the most important meal of the day, because it is the meal that gets the day started," quoted in *Good Health* magazine, edited by none other than Dr. John Harvey Kellogg. After all, Frosted Flakes, they're GRRRREEEEEAAAATTTT!

Conversely, Graves was a home economist who was trained and certified as a hospital dietitian. She had plenty of experience dealing with hospitalized diabetic patients and knew that high-protein and high-fat diets were the only effective therapies against hyperglycemia at the time. She even sponsored a 1921 treatise in *Modern Hospital* called "A high-fat diet for diabetic patients." Indeed, up to that point, a high-fat diet was the only rational treatment for diabetics; Dr. Frederick Allen, the successor to Dr. Elliott Joslin at the Joslin Diabetes Center at Harvard, argued in 1919 that a 70 percent fat, 8 percent carbohydrate diet was optimal for diabetics. But 1921 was a watershed year for diabetes with the discovery of insulin. And insulin meant that carbohydrate was back on the menu for diabetics, and treatment was now easier to institute than prevention. The high-fat paradigm for treatment of diabetes was destined for the trash heap (at least until ninety years later). Cooper and Kellogg won out, and the low-protein, high-carb diet became codified into dietetic lore.

Nutrition and Religion

Dr. Kellogg is quite a story unto himself, brought to life in T. Cora-ghessan Boyle's 1993 novel *The Road to Wellville,* which was turned into a 1994 major motion picture with Anthony Hopkins playing Kellogg. His Battle Creek Sanitarium was part spa, part hotel, part church—it catered to the rich and famous, who would flock to Battle Creek for various manifestations of twentieth-century burnout. Kellogg's paradigm of health was peculiar to say the least, and his methods were equally grotesque. Kellogg espoused a philosophy he called *biologic living* with two primary nemeses: constipation and masturbation, both of which he claimed stemmed from poor nutrition. The Battle Creek Sanitarium was committed to stamping out these two biologic vices. In *Plain Facts for Old and Young: Embracing the Natural History and Hygiene of Organic Life* (1887), he wrote, "If illicit commerce of the sexes is a heinous sin, self-pollution is a crime doubly abominable." Kellogg cataloged thirty-nine different symptoms of a person plagued by masturbation, including general infirmity, defective development, mood swings, fickleness, bashfulness, boldness, bad posture, stiff joints, fondness for spicy foods, acne, palpitations, poor digestion, memory loss, impaired vision, heart disease, epilepsy, and of course insanity.

The sanitarium employed several questionable methods to dispel patrons of these two scourges. Chewing thirty-two times before swallowing (known as *fletcherizing*), sinusoidal current (yup, electrocuting people), forty-six different kinds of baths, fifteen-gallon enemas, and vibrating chairs were among the more conventional. But some were a bit more Gothic. To break young boys of the habit, Kellogg suggested procedures such as tying their hands, bandaging the offending organ, or putting a cage over it. If that didn't work, he recommended circumcision without anesthetic—"As the brief pain attending the operation will have a salutary effect upon the mind," he wrote in *Plain Facts for Old and Young.* Kellogg had an even more gruesome set of treatments for girls, including the application of pure carbolic acid to the clitoris or, in more extreme cases, surgical removal.

The good news is that Kellogg's medical practices are long gone. The bad news is that Kellogg's dietary practices are still with us, and in greater force than ever. Kellogg's primary nutritional nemesis was meat, which was the devil incarnate—he said it caused constipation (well, there's no fiber, so maybe he was onto something there), and he was absolutely convinced that meat-eating was the cause of masturbation. Kellogg was a devout vegetarian, saying, "When we eat vegetarian foods, we needn't worry about what kind of disease our food died from; this makes a joyful meal!" Now, in Kellogg's defense, he is quoted as saying this long before Upton Sinclair wrote his famous exposé of the meat-packing industry, *The Jungle* (1906), so there may have been a modicum of truth in Kellogg's view based on the shoddy and inconsistent food preparation of the time. Early on at the Battle Creek Sanitarium, Kellogg created a "health treat" for patients that consisted of oatmeal and cornmeal baked into biscuits and then ground into tiny pieces. He called it *granula*. This became the prototype for the various breakfast cereals that would come to bear his name—and they were a hit, so much so that at least one of Kellogg's patients in the early 1890s, C. W. Post, thought enough of the idea to appropriate it for himself and set up a rival enterprise, the Postum Cereal Company, now called Post Consumer Brands.

Where did Dr. Kellogg come by his nutritional knowledge and practices? Apparently not from medical school. Proteins, discovered in 1838, were in high fashion when he graduated from NYU Medical College at Bellevue Hospital in 1875 (well before 1910 and the *Flexner Report*) (see Chapter 6). At that time, Darwin's natural selection hypothesis and evolutionary biology had superseded the Abrahamic God hypothesis for the origin of life in the medical curricula. Kellogg must have missed that lecture. Rather, Kellogg came to medicine with his views about food already ingrained (pun intended). They were formed during childhood, as he was a devout member of the Seventh-day Adventist (SDA) Church. In particular, he abided by all twenty-eight SDA fundamental beliefs. SDA #22 describes diet and drugs: "Along with adequate exercise and rest, we are to adopt the most healthful diet possible and abstain from the unclean foods identified in the Scriptures. Since alcoholic beverages, tobacco, and the irresponsible use of drugs and narcotics are harmful to our bodies, we are to abstain from them as well." Indeed, as a twelve-year-old he was employed in typesetting the book of quotes attributed to the church's cofounder and chief PR spokesperson, Ellen G. White. *A Solemn Appeal* (1870) warned of the dangers of meat-eating, which stirred baser passions, leading children to the heinous act of self-vice. White was so impressed with young Kellogg that she paid for his medical schooling.

There are many rational and defensible reasons to consider eating less meat, including: environment (see Chapter 25); animal welfare; cost; and religious objection, such as those of the SDA. But constipation and masturbation are not among them. And neither is metabolic health, at least for the type of flesh-meat that White and Kellogg were talking about (however, several things have happened to our current US processed meat supply that do render it suspect, such as the addition of nitrates, branched-chain amino acids, and antibiotics, as I will explore in Chapters 18 and 20). Despite the codification of meat (when slaughtered and prepared correctly) by both kashruth and halal traditions, the demonization of meat by religion is uniquely American (and Indian, where the Hindu population traditionally worships cows).

Like the origins of the dietetic movement, one can trace the current path of plant-based theology directly from Ms. White's SDA teachings. The SDA promotes self-denial for moral, physical, and spiritual health. She stated, "The people who lived before the flood ate animal food and gratified their lusts until their cup of iniquity was full, and God cleansed the earth of its moral pollution by a flood." She claimed God told her fleshmeat was a toxic stimulant; as harmful if not more so than alcohol or tobacco, stirring even baser passions and animal tendencies that would lead men, women, and children to the heinous act of "self-vice" (masturbation). "Those who indulge in meat eating, tea drinking, and gluttony are sowing seeds for a harvest of pain and death. . . . A diet of fleshmeat tends to develop animalism. A development of animalism lessens spirituality, rendering the mind incapable of understanding the truth."

Nature abhors a vacuum. As there was no formal national medical education in nutrition (see Chapter 3), the space was rife for squatters to set up shop and pretend they'd been there all along. The Seventh-day Adventist credo against meat continues in several guises, not just dietetics.

But the one thing I can categorically say—without hesitation—is that despite the abject decompensation of American health in this fifty-year period, the AND hasn't altered its message in one hundred years. Rather, they (and the entire healthcare establishment) blame the patient, claiming they're noncompliant with medical and dietary advice. If Einstein was correct about the definition of insanity (doing the same thing over and over again and expecting a different result), then the AND has truly lost its mind.

Plant-Based and Public Legitimacy

Fast forward to the 1970s when Dr. Nathan Pritikin, an adjunct professor at Loma Linda University (the Seventh-day Adventist University; indeed they advertise it, and known until 1961 as the College of Medical Evangelists), codified the first plant-based diet in his book *The Pritikin Diet* (1979). At the same time, South Dakota Senator George McGovern's aide Nick Mottern (who is said to be a member of the SDA Church himself) was put in charge of cobbling together the original 1977 Dietary Guidelines, which eschewed saturated fat. Mottern hijacked the recently elaborated but fatally flawed synthesis of saturated fat, via LDL-C (see Chapter 2), as the primary driver of heart disease. Thus, these two lines of overlapping doctrine—the religious and the scientific—came together in 1977 to alter Modern Medicine and subsequent public health directives for decades to come.

At the same time, the seeds were planted for yet another combined organization of the scientific and the religious—the Christian Association of Lifestyle Medicine (CALM), which was incorporated in 2003 at Loma Linda and changed its name to the American College of Lifestyle Medicine (ACLM). The "15 Physicians Core Competencies in Lifestyle Medicine" was coauthored, corroborated, and codified by a group of Adventist physicians currently embedded in the AMA. Except for one thing—there is no science. And the reason is because "God is the author of science." Therefore, how could there be science, because that would put the "created" over the "Creator." In fact, a sizable portion of the medical establishment pushing vegan diets are Adventists.

One such "educational" directive of the ACLM is the Lifestyle Medicine Education Collaborative, whose goal is to develop a global medical curriculum to ensure every health professional will write energy balance prescriptions advising people to "move more, eat less . . . meat." They specifically call attention to the plant-based *Garden of Eden Longevity Diet.* The plant-based diet craze leverages our concern for our health with our concern for the planet. But how did this come about? And is it based on science?

More recently, a third thread of climate change has entered and given new impetus to the anti-meat and plant-based factions. While climate change would appear to be a compelling common sense argument to reduce or eliminate meat from the diet, in fact the science doesn't support this view—I will postpone this argument until later, where I will devote an entire chapter to its debunking (see Chapter 25).

The vehemence and dogma of the plant-based movement was on full display on a recent episode of *The Doctors,* in which I debated bariatric surgeon and vegan proponent Garth Davis, author of *Proteinaholic: How Our Obsession with Meat Is Killing Us and What We Can Do about It* (2017), about the thirty-seven false claims in the movie *What the Health,* one of which says "One egg is as bad as five cigarettes."

There's just as much medical evidence for the benefits of the low-carb high-fat (LCHF) or ketogenic diet as there is for the vegan diet. The reasons both work, when they work, is because they: *1) protect the liver, 2) feed the gut* (see Chapter 11). Either diet is a choice, not a mandate. Either diet can be easily co-opted by charlatans and bad influencers. The two factions could learn a lot from each other, because there's valid science on both sides. But one faction doesn't talk to the other, in part out of religious fervor.

In my opinion, the science of nutrition has been co-opted by the religion of nutrition. The information contained in this book is my attempt to end this usurpation of the science by the "hunters" and the "gatherers."

CHAPTER 5

Dentists Lost Their Way

Have you ever experienced excruciating tooth pain? An ever-present dull ache in your mouth? You can't chew, can't sleep, and can't think about anything else. Maybe you accidentally cracked your tooth, but more likely you have a cavity, known in the business as dental caries, which affects 92 percent of adults. You thought that the xylitol chewing gum would help, but it didn't make a damn bit of difference, so you finally get yourself a crown—and not the sparkly kind—or worse a root canal, setting you back over $3,000, likely paid out-of-pocket even if you have dental insurance. There goes that Mexico vacation.

Since then you've been brushing your teeth as instructed by your dentist, but you still need payment plans for unscheduled dental procedures. Why? Dentists knew how to protect teeth; they used to learn nutrition in dental school until 1947. But then they left it behind. They never really forgot it; rather, nutrition became the "inconvenient truth" that got in the way of Modern Dentistry.

Dentists Were the Original Anti-Sugar Advocates, So Why Do They Give Out Lollipops?

In the beginning, there was the barber surgeon, who yanked out the offending tooth right after giving you a haircut and a close shave. It wasn't until the early twentieth century that Ohio dentist Weston Price (1870–1948) made oral health the purview of dentistry. In fact, dentists knew the true cause of dental caries (the disease that causes cavities) because of Weston Price. Price was arguably the most important and influential dentist in the history of dentistry, but today he's a (mostly) forgotten man—and not because he was proved wrong. Because he was proved right.

The disease is called *Mountain Dew mouth*. It's the scourge of Appalachia, all the way through Nashville, Tennessee, where Mountain Dew was invented, and beyond. Dental caries is the number one cause of chronic pain worldwide, as well as tooth loss, a chronic condition experienced by children, cause of outpatient anesthesia, and source of income for practicing dentists in the US. And it's getting worse, not better. It's the bane (or boon, depending on the dental professional's point of view, as cavities are good for business) of dentists' existence.

I recently had the opportunity to poll 340 Santa Clara, California, dentists at their annual meeting—would their practice benefit or suffer if somehow dental caries magically disappeared? All but one said their practices would suffer, yet all but one said they wished they would never see another cavity again.

Dental caries is a modern phenomenon. Our ancestors didn't brush their teeth, and they also didn't have *appreciable* dental caries. Analysis of fossils dating back to the Paleolithic era demonstrates bad tooth mineralization and only occasionally poor dental alignment, but little in the way of dental caries. Even starting with recorded history (3000 BCE and forward), the prevalence of dental caries among European populations was at a relatively low 1 to 5 percent, and it stayed that way, until the early to mid–Industrial Revolution. Then there was a huge jump in prevalence to 25 percent in a very short period of time. How come?

Nowhere was this epidemic more noticeable than in England. The Brits are frequently the butt of jokes about their bad teeth—witness *Austin Powers* (1997)—although that's not the case anymore; in fact British teeth currently outclass American teeth, at least in regard to dental caries. But Great Britain of the 1800s was the test kitchen for processed food; white flour and sugar were mixed with everything. Working long hours in the mills and mines, British workers didn't get time for a proper meal, but were afforded a biscuit (often laced with sugar). They also drank tea imported from India with at least one lump of sugar, if not two. As a result, the prevalence of dental caries increased markedly.

But now the Brits are back on top (or bottom, depending on your metric), at least in the cavity competition. Why? It's not because they're brushing more frequently. It's because, as a country, they consume less sugar than we Yanks do.

The Beginnings of Nutritional Dentistry

Weston Price watched the rise in prevalence of dental caries in his Cleveland practice. His assessment that the reason was the "displacing foods of modern commerce" was accurate. The culprits were and are white flour and rice, packaged pastries and baked goods, refined sugar and jams, canned and chemically preserved goods, and processed vegetable oils. Price abandoned his lucrative practice to travel the world—he spent the decade 1925 to 1935 visiting primitive cultures and industrializing countries, in order to understand the anthropology of tooth decay, heart disease, and cancer. Irrespective of the race of the isolated groups that he studied—be they Inuit, Swiss or Peruvian Indian mountaineers, Australian Aborigines, Kenyan Watusi or Maasai—Price found that they universally maintained near-perfectly aligned teeth and jaws, as well as no dental caries, as long as they followed their traditional diets. Conversely, every country that migrated to the processed food diet saw an exorbitant rise in dental disrepair. He labeled this process *modern degeneration*, and authored his now classic volume, *Nutrition and Physical Degeneration* (1939). By examining isolated populations south of the US, Price came to this simple conclusion—it's all about the diet. His teachings were seminal to the foundations of the burgeoning field of nutritional anthropology.

On March 27, 1934, perhaps the most consequential debate in the history of dentistry took place at the Hotel Pennsylvania across from Penn Station in New York. In front of an audience of 1,500 health professionals, the dentists duked it out over what causes dental caries. In one corner was Team Bacterial: Dr. Thaddeus P. Hyatt of Metropolitan Life and New York University; Dr. Alfred Walker of New York University; and Dr. Maurice William of the Oral Hygiene Committee of Greater New York. They came armed with the evidence that clean teeth don't decay. Brush them often enough and everything will be fine. In the other corner were the members of Team Nutritional: Dr. Elmer V. McCollum of Johns Hopkins University; Dr. Arthur H. Merritt of the American Academy of Periodontology; and, of course, Weston Price. They were armed with the evidence that other countries brushed less than we did and still didn't experience decay.

On the bacterial front, we know that the flora of the mouth and gut have changed considerably over human evolution. Our ancestors' native oral bacterial flora are no longer native, at least not in the oral cavity; there's been a mass migration of bacteria to different ends of the gut. When an environment becomes inhospitable, it's time for those denizens to up and move somewhere else or die in the process. For example, by examining the DNA in ancient calculus deposits of the teeth, we know that one particular bacteria type, *Proteobacteria*, was rare in the mouth among our hunter-gatherer ancestors, but as biological and cultural evolution changed over time, they came to dominate it. Conversely, another type of bacteria, *Firmicutes*, was prevalent in the mouth of our ancestors, but has since migrated and taken up residence in our lower gut, where it's now causing all sorts of ruckus (see Chapter

19). In fact, there used to be numerous types of bacterial species in the mouth contributing to bacterial diversity, but with the advent of the Industrial Revolution, that diversity has dwindled, and new previously "alien" bacteria have colonized the oral neighborhood. In its place we have this new squatter in the mouth, a particularly onerous species of bacteria called *Streptococcus mutans*, which have been shown to be a major producer of lactic acid and demineralize (burn holes in) teeth. While this bacterium isn't the sole perpetrator of dental caries and subsequent tooth rot, it is the prime suspect.

What could account for this wholesale microbial cleansing and bacterial migration? In the early 1910s, the dental biofilm was discovered and shown to harbor various bacteria. Despite evidence at the time to the contrary, the biofilm was considered by many dentists to be the source of caries, and therefore frequent brushing was espoused as the method to rid the teeth of unwanted bacteria.

Some believe that the toothpaste industry was responsible for this stance, as Pepsodent advocated this policy as early as 1919, before there was any data in either direction (Big Business strikes again). But even though debunked, it's one of the reasons that dentists promote the concept of frequent brushing as a preventative for dental caries, a notion that remains with us today. Maybe there is something to it—for instance, frequent brushing was recently shown to be associated with reduced risks for heart failure, just not for dental caries. You would have to brush within ten minutes of eating saltwater taffy in order to remove the lactic acid fast enough to prevent caries just from brushing; this is untenable as a strategy.

On the nutritional front, it's generally assumed, even by dentists, that carbohydrates are a primary driver of dental caries (cavities). This is technically true but misleading, and actually misses the point. After all, as stated earlier, our foraging/gatherer ancestors ate tons of carbohydrates and didn't develop caries.

There are three different forms of digestible carbohydrate: 1) monosaccharides (one sugar molecule—glucose or fructose or galactose; high-fructose corn syrup is an example of two monosaccharides at once); 2) disaccharides (two sugar molecules bound together; maltose (e.g., beer) is glucose-glucose, sucrose (e.g., fruit) is glucose-fructose, and lactose (e.g., milk) is glucose-galactose); and 3) starch, which is a string of glucose molecules polymerized together. But only the first two, monosaccharides and disaccharides, can cause dental caries. The reason is that the oral bacteria can only metabolize carbohydrates that are "fermentable"; that is, single free molecules. This is particularly true in sugared beverages, since the glucose and fructose are not bound, and they aren't trapped within a food matrix, giving the bacteria immediate access. Starch, because it's polymerized, isn't immediately fermentable by bacteria; rather, it is actually protective against dental caries because it contributes to the biofilm surrounding the tooth. However, *Streptococcus mutans*, the most cariogenic bacterium in the mouth, has a neat trick; it possesses an enzyme called *fructanase* that can cleave the glucose-fructose bond of sucrose in about a nanosecond, making *Streptococcus mutans* a champion cavity-maker.

The relationship between the sucrose molecule and dental caries goes back to 1954, with the seminal Vipeholm study—436 individuals observed for five years showed that increased frequency of sugar consumption between meals resulted in a marked increase in caries, while withdrawal of sugar halted their progression. Shortly thereafter, caries incidence was directly tied to sugar consumption in children and adults. Even getting rid of the sugar in the school cafeteria reduced caries rates in New Zealand children.

The Dentists Got It . . .

Price's admonitions seemed to carry weight back in the 1930s. His colleague McCollum wrote, "It seems that were we to turn to a low sugar, high fat type of diet, such as is prescribed for diabetic patients, we might expect a prompt and marked reduction in caries susceptibility. This type of diet is practicable in many countries, but fats are in many regions considerably more expensive to produce than are starches and sugars." Another colleague, William Davis, summed up the conundrum quite nicely: "Most people would prefer some decay rather than to eliminate the sweets . . . let us hope our research workers discover a more practical means of controlling or preventing dental decay."

Listen, I get it. I like ice cream, and I brush twice a day. Like most people, I hate going to the dentist. But, what if in eliminating most of your dietary sugar, you could avoid the dentist entirely?

. . . But Then They Lost It—Because of Fluoride

Davis's prayers were answered in 1945, as a third hypothesis of dental caries entered the fray. Team Tooth took over, and forever changed dentistry. It was discovered that a simple compound, sodium fluoride, at a low concentration of 0.1 parts per million, could inhibit dental caries formation. It did this in two ways: it reduced the amount of time that the pH of the saliva was low, thus reducing the time of burning a hole in the tooth; and it bound to the calcium hydroxyapatite crystals in the enamel itself, rendering them harder to dissolve in response to a low pH. Fluoride was on its way to overtaking modern dentistry. Dental researcher Frank McClure said, "In 1945, Grand Rapids became the first city in the world to fluoridate its drinking water. . . . During the 15-year project, researchers monitored the rate of tooth decay among Grand Rapids' almost 30,000 schoolchildren. After just 11 years, [Dr. H. Trendley] Dean—who was now director of the NIDR (National Institute of Dental Research)—announced an amazing finding. The caries rate among Grand Rapids children born after fluoride was added to the water supply dropped more than 60 percent." Consequently, the government got involved; fluoride started to be added to drinking water around the world, and the prevalence rate of dental caries was cut in half. It was a major public health win.

But, similar to Kellogg's thumb on the scale of nutrition research, the ostensibly positive triumph of fluoride has a darker side, and likely shields an industrial conspiracy driven by politics and profit. The story of fluoride's transition from industrial contaminant to public health panacea has been the fodder of countless treatises on environmental health over the decades. The original discovery of the "magic" of fluoride was quite serendipitous, first pointed out by dentist Frederick McKay, who noted in 1909 that despite the fact that seven out of eight children residing in Colorado Springs manifested brown indelible stains on their teeth, they nonetheless appeared to be protected from dental caries. McKay isolated the reason to the fluoride in the water supply.

In 1927, McKay implored the U.S. Public Health Service (at that time a division of the U.S. Department of the Treasury) to assist. Simultaneously, the same brown dental stains became manifest in the residents of Bauxite, Arkansas (named for its high aluminum content), following the drilling of three water wells by the Aluminum Company of America (ALCOA) corporation. These two isolated dental oddities independently rose to the notice of none other than Andrew W. Mellon (of Carnegie Mellon), who just happened to be both the U.S. Secretary of the Treasury (1921–1932) and the cofounder of ALCOA.

Up to that point, fluoride was considered to be a toxic waste product of the aluminum and phosphate mining industries, and a chief contributor to environmental pollution. Clearly, aluminum needed a shiny new façade. Mellon made three quick calculations. First, in 1930 he assigned dentist Gerald Cox at the newly founded Mellon Institute at the University of Pittsburgh to investigate the effects of fluoride in dental caries prevention; his work paved the way for community water fluoridation. Second, in 1930 he assigned ALCOA chemist Henry Churchill to work with the Kettering Laboratory at the University of Cincinnati to find the "sweet spot" where fluoride could prevent dental caries without producing brown dental stains like those seen in Colorado Springs and Bauxite. They arrived at a dose of one part per million. Last, in 1931 Mellon reassigned dentist H. Trendley Dean from a U.S. Marine Corps hospital to the NIH—specifically to carry the positive message of fluoride back to the dental community. Dean had no formal research training, but it didn't matter for the purpose. In 1932 Dean reported to the U.S. Surgeon General that the brown stain, termed *dental fluorosis*, was really the entrée to combatting dental caries. Dean spent the rest of his career advancing fluoride as a dental panacea. Dean got his reward—he was appointed the first director of the National Institute of Dental Research in 1948.

Fluoride in the public drinking water and toothpaste appeared to be a magic bullet, touted as the "end of dental caries." Or was it? Between 1971 and 1988, caries rates in the US dropped from 25 percent to 19 percent in toddlers, and from 55 percent to 24 percent in six-to-nine-year-old children. Definitely an improvement—but despite dentistry's best efforts, they never got lower than that. They tried everything: standard fluoride toothpaste (1,500 ppm), which led to a 30 percent reduction in adult caries prevalence; yet increasing the fluoride to 5,000 ppm only led to a 40 percent reduction. They never even broke 50 percent. Hardly a miracle.

Moreover, the dentists started to lament—"If we somehow got rid of dental caries, who will fill our chairs?" Caries prevention may be a public health issue for countries, but caries promotion is an economic issue for dentists and Big Business, pushing a myriad of toothpastes, mouthwashes, dental x-rays, and sealants. Slowly but surely, rank-and-file dentists backed away from Weston Price and their original anti-sugar stance, and more and more dentists started handing out lollipops to children after their exam (after all, dentists are scary; they come at your mouth with needles and drills). And in response, the last seventy years has seen an increase in Mountain Dew mouth, which has continued to flourish in this country, with variable changes in health patterns to boot.

The Failures of Fluoride

The dental profession bet a lot on fluoride, and they're not going to give that up easily. But there's been a recent wave of public dissent and distrust around the country about fluoride. In fact, Portland, Oregon, has banned public fluoridation since 1956. If you've seen *Portlandia*, you might chuckle to yourself about their residents' granola personae. But now seventy-four cities around the country have followed Portland's lead and also banned fluoride. Do they know something you don't?

There are a lot of pseudo-reasons for getting rid of fluoride. Some think it boosts the sugar lobby by enabling people to eat more sweets without getting cavities, and some believe that health officials are just plain afraid to stop fluoridation after having supported it for decades. And, of course, there were the conspiracy theorists who were convinced it was a Soviet plot for mind control (in *Dr. Strangelove* [1964], General Jack D. Ripper says, "Fluoridation is the most monstrously conceived and dangerous communist plot we have ever had to face!"). New data also shows a small but statistically significant negative correlation between fluoride exposure and childhood IQ, which appears to be exacerbated when fluoridated water is used to mix infant formula.

Now, to be honest, the effect is small, and correlation is not causation. I'm not a fluoride expert by any means; I'm agnostic on the issue. Here's what I do know: fluoride is a tried and true *adjunct* to prevention, but it's not a primary prevention in and of itself. If it were, the dental profession would have done better than a 50 percent reduction in caries. My take on this is very simple. Do that which works. What does the science say?

Sugar restriction is the most effective way of reducing and preventing the modern scourge of dental caries. Based on UK dental epidemiologist Aubrey Sheiham's estimates, a reduction of dietary sugar to less than 5 percent of calories would reduce the prevalence of caries significantly; this method is nontoxic, and it wouldn't cost anything. Then, maybe we wouldn't even need fluoride.

Can't Fight Tonight Honey, I've Got a Toothache

Mountain Dew mouth may sound innocuous enough, but this is serious stuff. Especially for the U.S. Armed Forces. In 1994, 30 percent of Army recruits couldn't be deployed into the field because of stage 3 dental caries (when the dental pulp gets infected), which can go on to abscess. By 2008, the U.S. Department of Defense documented stage 3 caries at 42 percent of recruits—this means that almost half of the Army can't be deployed because of their teeth, because of Mountain Dew mouth.

This isn't rocket science. It's barely even dental science. Without sugar, caries would be negligible. The profession knows the score, but the professional doesn't seem to. The American Dental Association issued its guidelines for caries, and sugar restriction isn't even mentioned as an option. They list eight nonsurgical therapies to *treat* dental caries. Nutrition is not even mentioned as a prevention.

Conversely, the World Dental Federation (FDI)—composed of two hundred member organizations—has no choice but to *prevent* dental caries, especially in the most impoverished countries of South America and Asia. There just aren't enough dentists to drill all the fillings, and there certainly isn't enough money to pay them. In the FDI's White Paper, sugar restriction is the #1 strategy to deal with dental caries. This should be a slam dunk worldwide, but it's not. Because of the money.

The good news is that dentists are starting to get back on the anti-sugar bandwagon, as they feel they now have cover from the medical profession, because of the burgeoning science demonstrating metabolic and cardiovascular detriments due to sugar toxicity. When physicians, dentists, dietitians, and patients are all on board together, when we medical/dental/dietary professionals can speak with one loud and clear voice, that's when the food industry and Washington will listen. Until then, it's business as usual.

CHAPTER 6

=

Because Big Pharma
Was Their Teacher

For six years during my postdoctoral fellowship, I was a minion of the academic bastion the Rockefeller University in New York City, bridging the Laboratory of Biochemical Endocrinology and the Laboratory of Neurobiology and Behavior. When the weather was inclement, in order to get between the two labs indoors, I had to wander through Flexner Hall. All those years, I attributed the name to the wrong Flexner. I thought the building was a monument to Abraham Flexner, the author of the seminal *Flexner Report*, which by all accounts heralded the birth of Modern Medicine. As it turns out, the hall is actually named for his brother, Simon Flexner, the first president of the Rockefeller Institute for Medical Research, founded in 1901 (in 1959, they started handing out degrees, and it evolved into a university).

But I might be forgiven for my ignorance, because the Flexner brothers were joined at the hip, and both beholden directly to none other than John D. Rockefeller himself. It was this bizarre patron-client triangle that set Modern Medicine on its current path, for both good and bad, on its quest for Drug Money, kowtowing to Big Pharma all along the way.

The Flexner Posse

Most medical pundits consider the *Flexner Report* a watershed in the evolution of evidence-based medicine. Throughout the nineteenth century, US medicine was akin to the Wild West. Anything went, snake oil was a big seller, cocaine and heroin were available without prescription, and there was a panoply of medical colleges across the country with fluid curricula and no standardization. In addition, the end of the nineteenth century saw the creation of two alternative branches to challenge traditional medicine—osteopathy, which believed in a holistic approach to the patient; and chiropractic, which believed that many diseases came from disorders of the spine. At the same time, Johns Hopkins School of Medicine in Baltimore was trying to reform itself with rigor into a beacon of evidence-based medicine and science, by adopting the German hierarchical learning pedagogy. At the top of each lab there was Herr Professor, and everyone else was an underling and therefore expendable (Rockefeller University adopted the same organizational structure).

It was against this backdrop that the nine Flexner children of Louisville, Kentucky (seven boys and two girls), came to the fore. In Jewish families of the time, you were either educated, or religious, or in some cases both. There were no slouches in the Flexner household, but this story focuses on the brothers Simon and Abraham. Abraham got his undergraduate degree after two years at Johns Hopkins, where he was exposed to this German academic paradigm. He readily adopted it and put this organizational structure into practice when he opened his own college preparatory school back in Louisville. Abraham did quite well both administratively and financially, and used his knowledge of education and running a school to write a seminal work denoting the flaws in American higher education, entitled *The American College: A Criticism* (1908).

Abraham made enough money as an educator to send his pharmacist brother, Simon, back to medical school, and afterward urged him to move on to postgraduate work at Johns Hopkins. And so Simon was also indoctrinated into the German system and received training to become a pathologist, bacteriologist, and researcher. His mentor was the iconic Canadian physician and chairman of medicine Sir William Osler, the creator of the residency program system for young physician trainees (note the German hierarchical paradigm here as well). Simon was a favored son, and Osler eventually secured him a faculty appointment in pathology at the University of Pennsylvania.

That might have been as far as it went for the Flexners, but for a dash of serendipity combined with a splash of avarice. In the late 1800s Baptist minister Frederick Gates befriended Baptist philanthropist John D. Rockefeller, and in 1892 they founded the Baptist University of Chicago (which has since become nonsectarian). Gates became Rockefeller's business advisor, who continued to help rehabilitate his cutthroat business reputation through strategic philanthropy, similar to Andrew Carnegie, and not much different from what is seen by people like Bill Gates (no relation) and Mark Zuckerberg today.

The O.G. Drug Kingpin Johnny D.

In the summer of 1897, Frederick Gates, a voracious reader, read Osler's *The Principles and Practice of Medicine* (1892). Seeing the disarray in the US medical profession, he believed that American medicine needed some of the same discipline Rockefeller brought to Standard Oil, and prodded Rockefeller to provide the funds to start his eponymous medical institute. Rockefeller was hardly a progressive, and believed in folk medicine as cure. But he also believed in money.

Standard Oil had an untapped asset/liability—coal tar, a by-product of coal mining and oil refining. Medical practitioners of the day used various preparations of coal tar to treat numerous proliferative skin diseases such as eczema and seborrhea (short-term treatment with coal tar is still occasionally used for this purpose). Rockefeller had product to push, and he needed to create a mass market—so he founded the Rockefeller Institute to engage in medical research so long as it researched the benefits of coal tar. It was up to Gates to find its first director. He contacted Osler directly, who recommended Simon Flexner. The institute opened for business in 1901, and Simon, namesake of Flexner Hall, assumed the helm in 1903.

But Rockefeller was just getting started—in the drug business, that is. Aside from the Rockefellers, the next biggest shareholder in Standard Oil was German chemical conglomerate IG Farben, best known for creating Zyklon B, the nerve gas used in Auschwitz. By the early 1900s, Farben had developed a successful pharmaceutical industry, with drugs such as aspirin, salvarsan (an arsenic compound used for syphilis), and novocaine. Rockefeller saw yet a new drug opportunity and untapped market—but he also saw that American physicians didn't know about these new pharmaceuticals, in part because they didn't learn about them in medical school. Rockefeller needed distributors to sling this product, and so green-lighted a project to completely evaluate the American medical school system in order to dismantle it and reformulate it to focus on medical research and drug therapy.

Who should spearhead such an evaluation? How about an educator who believed in the German system? Simon nominated his brother Abraham. An easy sell, as Henry Pritchett, chairman of the Carnegie Foundation, had read *The American College*. The last vote came from the American Medical Association, who stood to rid themselves of pesky alternative therapy schools and would become the regulatory body for medical education going forward. These American oligarchs "embraced scientific medicine as an ideological weapon in their struggle to formulate a new culture appropriate to and supportive of industrial capitalism."

The *Flexner Report* and Its Aftermath

Never mind that Abraham himself knew nothing about medicine—after all, physicians were the problem, right? To bone up, he spent two years evaluating the organizational structure of several European medical schools, including those in England, France, and Germany. In 1910, Flexner published his *Flexner Report*, which decried the state of American medical education for lack of evidence-based medicine (the same cry we hear today, by the way), and advocated for far-reaching reform in the training of doctors.

Flexner doubted the scientific validity of all forms of medicine other than those based on research; everything else was quackery and charlatanism. To be fair, much of it was. Medical schools had to drop electromagnetic field therapy, phototherapy, physiomedicalism, naturopathy, homeopathy, and several other questionable practices. And, most important, nutrition went AWOL. Neither Flexner brother ever embraced the concept of diet or nutrition as part of the new medical curriculum because there was no money to be made in it (to its credit, by the 1970s Rockefeller University did eventually agree that nutrition was important; two of my personal heroes were full professors there—Edward "Pete" Ahrens studied lipids, and Jules Hirsch studied obesity).

The *Flexner Report* of 1910 pissed a lot of people off. It led to the closure of most rural medical schools and complementary and alternative therapy schools. In particular, his report helped close all but two African American medical colleges, because in his view, "The practice of the Negro doctor will be limited to his own race, which in its turn will be cared for better by good Negro physicians than by poor white ones. . . . The Negro must be educated not only for his sake, but for ours. He is, as far as the human eye can see, a permanent factor in the nation." Perhaps this was because the AMA was segregated, and had no plans on integrating? Hmmm . . .

African Americans weren't the only ones who were unhappy with the *Flexner Report*. Eighty percent of medical colleges nationally were forced to shutter for either not meeting standards or not overhauling their curricula. The osteopathic and chiropractic schools were directly in the crosshairs, and while they protested, there wasn't much that could be done. The fix was in.

Although almost all the alternative medical schools listed in Flexner's report were closed, the International Association of Chiropractic Schools and Colleges (IACSC) was formed, with nineteen member colleges. The American Osteopathic Association (AOA) also brought a number of osteopathic medical schools into compliance with Flexner's recommendations to produce an evidence-based practice. The curricula of DO- and MD-granting medical schools are now nearly identical, except that osteopathic schools still teach osteopathic manipulative medicine (OMM).

If osteopathy was flawed and dangerous to patients, why are osteopathic schools still thriving? From 2010 to 2016, the number of actively licensed DOs in the US increased by nearly 40 percent, from over fifty-eight thousand to over eighty-one thousand (in my clinical retirement, I teach weekly at Touro University California, a Jewish osteopathic medical college. I can state from experience, DO students are as research-focused as their MD student brethren—the big difference is that DO students are devoted to studying the whole patient, not just the diseased organ. Oh, and they *get* "Food as Medicine").

Rockefeller, Pritchett, and the AMA presented the *Flexner Report* to Congress in 1911, which adopted it without change. Since then, it's never been updated. The report aligned well with Flexner's strategy, the AMA's strategy, Johns Hopkins's striving for preeminence among major American medical schools, and the quest for new drugs that could advance the nascent pharmaceutical industry's (and Rockefeller's) objectives.

Science is a tool; it's neither good nor bad. Such value judgments depend on the user. Science should and must be promoted, as it's a primary driver of societal advancement. However, it's also clear that the overtly political nature of the *Flexner Report*, and the effort of Big Business, Big Pharma, and now Big Medicine to capitalize on it, has left a big hole in the profession, which keeps expanding and threatens to engulf us all.

Big Pharma on the Rampage

Big Pharma has exacted some major victories, like antibiotics (although even that claim is now tenuous, see Chapter 2). But one thing you can't argue with is their profit. Big Pharma's top eleven corporations have generated net profits on the order of $75 billion per year; for instance, the net profit for 2012 among those top eleven amounted to $85 billion in just that one year (and that's *net*, not *gross*). That's a lot of pills—and more each year. The majority of these largest pharmaceuticals are headquartered in the US—including the top four: Johnson & Johnson (#39 on the Fortune 500 list), Pfizer (#51), Merck (#65), and Eli Lilly (#129), along with Abbott (#152) and Bristol Myers Squibb (#176). American sales of prescription drugs were $457 billion in 2015, and worldwide sales topped $1.2 trillion in 2018. With that kind of obscene money to throw around, what Big Pharma wants, Big Pharma nearly always gets.

And they aim to keep it that way. Experts say the industry contributes about two-thirds of the FDA's budget, so the government has little impetus to impugn them. Big Pharma also employs a small army of 1,378 lobbyists to spread its influence on Capitol Hill. And they're great peddlers. Every single drug company spends more on marketing than on research and development. Some, like Johnson & Johnson, spend double their R&D budget on marketing. The rest of the top ten (Novartis, Pfizer, Roche, Sanofi, Merck, GlaxoSmithKline, AstraZeneca, Eli Lilly, and AbbVie), in the years between 1997 and 2016, doubled their annual marketing budget as well, from $17.7 billion to $30 billion. Schmoozing doctors went from $15 to $20 billion, while direct business-to-consumer advertising increased fourfold (from $2.1 to $9.6 billion). For every $1 spent on "basic research," Big Pharma spends $19 on promotions and advertising.

The hidden business model of Big Pharma is to turn one drug into many—by turning out minor variations that extend patent life; and through clinical trial administration, research publication, regulatory lobbying, physician and patient education, drug pricing, advertising, and point-of-use promotion to create distinct marketing profiles and brand loyalty for otherwise similar products. Why? Because generic drugs are cheaper; by slightly tweaking their ingredient list, they get more time on patent protection. Hey, if it didn't work, you know they wouldn't be doing it.

Big Pharma on the Ropes

Big Pharma also had some major screwups along the way. Between 1997 and 2016, civil fines totaling $11 billion were levied for illegal marketing of drugs and hiding data on health harms. But that's chicken feed compared to what we saw in 2019 with Purdue Pharma ($12 billion and counting) having to file for Chapter 11 bankruptcy, and Johnson & Johnson with fines of $572 million due to its fomenting of the American opioid crisis.

Despite all of its successes, only 28 percent of Americans have a good opinion of Big Pharma. In fact, Big Pharma is the third most hated industry in America, after tobacco and petrochemicals. Perhaps the reason they're both so successful and hated is because they're treating the symptoms of disease, not the disease itself (see Chapter 1). There are more and more people with more symptoms to treat. They've altered their portfolios to invest money and effort into chronic therapies (that you'll be on for twenty to thirty years) that are palliative, rather than acute therapies that are curative (like one week).

Nowhere is this exemplified better than in Big Pharma's response to the coronavirus, because vaccines don't generate enough profit. The US government initially entertained eighty-nine separate proposals to develop a vaccine. A total of seventy-seven came from universities. Of the hundreds of US pharmaceutical firms, only twelve submitted proposals. Does Big Pharma not do virology?

Polypharmacy Kills People

As the world's life span has been expanding consistently over the last one hundred years due to public health improvements and antibiotics, so has the number of older people, both in absolute figures and as a percentage of the population. In the US, people older than sixty-five now account for 16 percent of the population and consume one-third of all prescription medications. In fact, 20 percent of people over the age of sixty-five are taking at least five different medications. In the UK, the same age group accounts for 18 percent of the population and consumes close to 45 percent of all prescription drugs.

There have been several prospective studies on this topic, although none with a global or multicountry scope. Yet the conclusion is damning: polypharmacy—taking more than five prescription pills a day—is associated with increased mortality risk; and it's not just because people are old. In fact, the third most common cause of death today is prescription medication. Perhaps as a result of the overmedication of America, with drugs vying to occupy a share of the medicine cabinet over the past ten years, hospital admissions of the elderly due to medication side effects have tripled.

Too many pills might kill you, but that's only one part of the problem. Pills, no matter how many and how good, don't cure chronic diseases— they just treat the symptoms (see Chapter 2). To be sure, single-pill fixed-dose combination therapy shows improved compliance with some diseases, like hypertension and HIV. But at what cost? An example is Zegerid, a combination of over-the-counter omeprazole (Prilosec) and bicarbonate of soda. Great for raising the pH of the stomach if you have an ulcer. But we now know that raising the pH of the stomach can lead to vitamin B_{12} malabsorption, altering the gut microbiome to increase the risk of gastrointestinal bacterial diseases like *Clostridioides difficile*. Is this such a good idea? And for these fixed-dose combinations, the drug company socks it to you on the price; a recent study argues that Medicaid spends an extra $1 billion per year on the combo version.

And now there's new data that even some of the inactive fillers or excipients in most pills (e.g., dyes like tartrazine [yellow], lactose, fructose) that make up 75 percent of the mass of the pill may in and of themselves be harmful in some patients, causing allergies, irritable bowel syndrome, and other inflammatory conditions. Mo' pills, mo' problems.

Big Pharma, Little NIH

How about public health? Big Pharma made great contributions to public health efforts, until twenty to thirty years ago, with antibiotics (though their efficacy is dwindling) and vaccines. But since then there's been very little progress. Between 2000 and 2008, a total of 667 drugs were approved by the FDA, yet only 11 percent of them were deemed truly innovative; the rest were knockoff analogs in an attempt to bully their way onto the market.

Doctors know how to prescribe medicines—because that's what they're taught in medical school; and because doctors are the primary prescribers, they're also the target of Big Pharma's educational push. Currently, 70 percent of the US population is taking at least one prescribed medication. Is that because 70 percent of the population is sick? Well, actually yes. In fact, 88 percent of the population is thought to be metabolically ill. But does that mean that medicine is the treatment?

If you ask Big Pharma, the answer is an unequivocal yes. Ever since government got out of medical research, it has left the playing field wide open. Starting with Ronald Reagan, there's been a steady push from successive US administrations away from research, and by the time George W. Bush assumed office in 2001, the transformation was complete.

Under George W. Bush, NIH Director Elias Zerhouni announced a new plan, known as the NIH Roadmap for Medical Research. Euphemistically, the NIH Roadmap initiatives "are designed to speed the movement of research discoveries from the bench into practice for the benefit of the public." In reality, this plan shuttered clinical research centers nationwide; as Zerhouni said, patient research should be done by Big Pharma. I've witnessed this paradigm shift firsthand. Most clinical research has been cut back at the government and university level, leaving it open for Big Pharma to invest in whatever will turn the biggest profit.

Except that Big Pharma's reports of their own research are highly suspect. A meta-analysis by the Cochrane institute demonstrates that when the same drug is evaluated in two studies—one sponsored by Big Pharma and one independently—though the results are similar, the conclusions drawn are completely different. The industry reports were less transparent, had few reservations about methodological limitations, and had more favorable conclusions than the independent studies.

Spin is everything. Can doctors trust what Big Pharma says about its own drugs? The answer is unfortunately no, we can't; industry studies harbor a 37 percent bias toward their own drug.

In the new millennium, Big Pharma has primarily contributed to increasing morbidity, in other words, keeping sick people with chronic diseases (cancer, diabetes, etc.) alive—so they can cost more money. And with no governmental regulation, medicines that have been around for a century have tripled in price in just one decade (e.g., insulin). For diabetics, insulin is indispensable; and it's what the market will bear. For another egregious example, just look at what happened to the price of the EpiPen; kids with anaphylactic allergic reactions were forced to pay four times the original cost, because they had no choice—it's literally a matter of life or death.

But what if life feels like death? Staying alive in poor health is not a big winner. Between 2000 and 2008 the odds of surviving for at least five years after diagnosis increased 10.2 percent, and one additional drug approval increased the odds of surviving five years by 2.4 percent. Most of this life-span gain went to increasing time spent with morbidity. Adding extra time to morbidity is not a big winner either. In addition to cancer, a million people with diabetes are on dialysis; that's an extra five years of life, but it's all morbidity and costs $88,000 per patient per year.

An Uneasy Symbiosis

Big Pharma needs doctors to power the machine that generates their profit. Only one-third ($26 billion) of their annual $85 billion profit comes from over-the-counter drugs that patients can buy without a prescription—and so Pharma *has to* keep doctors prescribing. The best way to do that? Control the medical school curriculum. And how to do that? Pay for stuff.

Individual datapoints for American medical schools are harder to come by, but we know what's going on with our Canadian friends north of the border. Canadian pharmaceutical company Apotex gave the University of Toronto CAN$2,875,077 over one decade for research projects, GlaxoSmithKline contributed CAN$4,566,930 over two decades, Janssen donated CAN$1,642,998 over five years, Allergan gave CAN$272,696 over two years, and Bristol Myers Squibb sponsored the salaries of two physician-scientists. We can only assume that American medical schools are reading from the same script.

And it's in the university's best interest to maintain these industry relationships, for two reasons: 1) direct drug money as above; and also 2) potential drug money for in-house discoveries. Congressional passage of the Bayh-Dole Act of 1980 gave universities the right to patent any discoveries stemming from federally funded research, to own that IP, and then to license those discoveries to Big Pharma in return for institutional royalties.

Before Bayh-Dole, universities were the wallflower. But after, universities joined Big Pharma on the dance floor for the Grand Waltz.

Junkets and Junk Food

Another way for Big Pharma to maintain the green gusher in the drug pipeline is to bypass the institutions altogether and co-opt the prescribers directly. In the past, to get their drug out into the world, drug companies would sponsor their own medical symposia—in places like Cancun or Hollywood or Maui—and would invite medical school faculty members to both talk and be talked to. Oh, and their wives' expenses were paid as well.

The mornings would be all science, and the afternoon would be all scuba diving. I myself had joined the faculty at the University of Wisconsin in July 1990, and by February 1991 I found myself in a lagoon spearfishing in Fort Lauderdale. All because I could prescribe human growth hormone. Of course, these symposia got expensive, and by the 2000s, the American Medical Association was beginning to scrutinize this practice—so it began to fall on the Big Pharma detail reps in the field to do the massaging. They would show up to clinic every week without fail, lunch in tow, ostensibly to provide clerical assistance in filling out the paperwork to start a new patient on growth hormone. I can't tell you how many burritos I didn't have to pay for. Sometimes we had reps from two different drug companies vying for our stomachs at the same time.

In 2013, in an attempt to limit their influence, academic medical centers banned pharma reps from their campuses, and subsequent prescriptions for brand-name medications fell while generics increased. Yet only 36 percent of private hospitals have followed their lead—Big Pharma reps continue to lobby doctors in hospitals nationwide. And the Empire is striking back. A 2017 U.S. Supreme Court case, *Sorrell v. IMS Health Inc.*, argues that Big Pharma can data mine information from patients, leaving open the possibility that drug companies can access patient records.

Recently, a group of AstraZeneca-affiliated clinicians argued that by reducing access to reps, doctors weren't up-to-date on medical breakthroughs. So now medical schools are blaming the doctors instead of the pharma companies, by tightening regulations on professors who exhibit conflicts of interest. Point being, Modern Medicine and Big Pharma remain caught in a vicious cycle: doctors need Big Pharma because they're taught to treat rather than cure or prevent; but the reason they don't know any better is because medical education has been co-opted by Big Pharma itself. And so the cycle repeats.

Disease A Plus Treatment B Still Equals Death

All medicines are selective toxins, poisoning one specific pathway in the body. Pharma grew in the 1950s because of the success of antibiotics that poison the cellular pathways of bacteria (which are like plant cells) without poisoning other necessary animal cell pathways. This is why they've been effective in eradicating most acute infectious diseases.

But when we're dealing with chronic conditions, the dysfunctional pathway is the human's energy metabolic pathways (not the bacteria's), primarily our mitochondria (see Chapter 9). But there's no medicine that can get to and fix the mitochondria. In fact, treating with antibiotics for acute infectious diseases may have altered the bacteria in our gut so severely that new and resistant bacteria have moved in to take their place. The bacteria battling in our intestines can cause leaky gut and systemic inflammation, furthering chronic disease. Further, our gut microbiomes have been altered by the antibiotics added to our food supply (see Chapter 18), which also drives systemic inflammation, making us even sicker.

All of our medicines are treating the symptoms that come from these various mitochondrial perturbations: for instance, blood pressure medicines fix the blood pressure, but not the mitochondria. Yet by treating solely these symptoms, the pharma industry has lulled people into a false sense of security that their disease has been ameliorated. Wrong. The symptoms of their disease have been ameliorated. Until the actual cause of the condition is addressed, there's no quick fix. *And there's no pill for this.*

So, what's the solution? Some in the profession think they're just doing their job, while others know that they're taking money under false pretenses. How do we hold the medical profession accountable for spinning its wheels addressing the symptoms of the problem rather than the problem itself, and making money off the victims? Big Pharma is the **first of the three *immoral hazards*** delineated in this book, creating the problem, and making money off the misfortunes of others. More to come, stay tuned.

Part II

Debunking "Chronic Disease"

===

CHAPTER 7

The "Diseases" That Aren't Diseases

Diseases tend to have difficult medical-technical names that no mere mortal can pronounce, so they're often assigned more manageable monikers, based on the name of the doctor who first described it (e.g., Alzheimer's disease), or its most famous patient (e.g., Lou Gehrig's disease). Sometimes it's even based on the country of origin (e.g., Jamaican vomiting sickness), on the tissue of interest (e.g., foot-and-mouth disease, polycystic ovarian syndrome), or on the symptoms expressed (e.g., fibromyalgia). However, sometimes naming the disease after the symptom can be quite cryptic. For instance, "diabetes" is a Greek word that means *siphon*, because you're in the bathroom peeing your brains out, but it doesn't say anything about glucose, insulin, or the subcellular dysfunction that causes it. Cardiovascular disease localizes the problem to the heart and blood vessels, but doesn't really say what's happening there or how it got that way. Hypertension tells the patient there's high blood pressure, but unless they have such high blood pressure that they get a headache or stroke, they don't feel it, don't know what it means, don't know what to do about it, or whether they should even care. Many of them will make contractions of disease processes to take the onus off—for instance, "I got the high blood," "I got the low blood," "I got the sugar." They might be tempted to think that the process is just a part of normal aging, or that since their parent had it as well that it might be genetic.

In any case, the prevailing wisdom is that these diseases are inevitable. And doctors don't do anything to alter that illusion. I can't tell you how many patients I've seen who said, "Well my mother had diabetes, so I'm not surprised I got it." These lay formulations couldn't be further from the truth. But do you know of any doctors who disabuse their patients of these mythologies? That's because they don't understand them either.

The US population, and indeed the populations of most developed and developing countries, is verifiably sick. While this metabolic dysfunction is exacerbated by body weight, it's not even remotely dependent on it (remember "thin-sick" from Chapter 2). Yes, the adult American population is 67 percent overweight, but the data argues that 88 percent of the population exhibits some level of metabolic dysfunction. Is obesity the problem, or the symptom (see Chapter 2)? And what do the doctors tell the other 21 percent who aren't obese but still metabolically ill? What disease do they have? After all, if doctors don't know how to diagnose, treat, or prevent an unknown disease, why would they even bring it up?

Sadly, *you're* going to have to bring it up. And that means being facile with the science. I offer Part II so that you have the option of understanding the science, to take ownership over it. Unavoidably, I'm going to have to introduce some new concepts and biochemistry that address food, cancer, and aging. If the science is daunting, then just skip to Chapter 9, which will provide you with the do-it-yourself approach to your own personal health and well-being.

Metabolic dysfunction is the "disease without a name." The cells of the body, and often of the brain, are sick, due to eight—count 'em, eight—intracellular processes that have gone awry. These eight processes are not mutually exclusive—often if you have one going on, you likely have more than one. Also note that these eight processes, when working right, contribute to longevity; but when not working right underlie the various chronic diseases that result in mortality. They're not considered diseases per se—as they don't have an easy lab test or biomarker. They don't have an ICD-11 code, so they aren't reimbursable. They don't have a drug target (see Chapter 10), so doctors don't talk about any of them with their patients—because why would you want to bring up something you can't solve? It recalls a saying I learned while I was a visiting professor in Paris, "If there is no solution, there is no problem."

But scientists who work in the field of chronic disease do know about them. Each of these eight processes can work *for* you, in which case you'll live to be one hundred playing tennis—or *against* you, in which case you'll be disabled, depressed, on dialysis, or dead before your time. Further, they're not mutually exclusive—each interacts with the others, and so they tend to cluster together. They are the processes belying most, if not all, of the chronic diseases that are killing people and costing billions of dollars. And they are all exacerbated by processed food.

Cell Bio 101

To explain these eight subcellular pathologies, I first have to explain a cell and its contents. That means an ultra-short course in cell biology. For this exercise, I'll limit the syllabus to energy metabolism only, which is the root of all eight subcellular pathways.

The cell is nature's basic building block of life. Each of us is composed of ten trillion cells, most of them specialized and residing in different organs. In order to stay alive, a cell has to burn energy. Any cell can (and normally does) burn glucose, a simple sugar and the building block of starch. The liver and adipose (fat) tissue need the hormone insulin (released from the pancreas) to open the metabolic door within the *membrane*, the bag that holds the cell together, to let the glucose enter the cell; however, other organs don't need insulin for glucose entry. But if glucose is in short supply and insulin levels are low, then adipose tissue will give up some of its stored fatty acids to enter the bloodstream, and the liver will turn those fatty acids into ketones, which then seep back into the bloodstream, so that any cell can burn those ketones instead, even without insulin.

Cells are magicians. They either make glucose disappear, or if there's too much, then presto-change-o, they turn glucose into fat, which wreaks havoc on metabolism. But how and when is the key. Once inside the cell (**Fig. 7-1**), glucose undergoes breakdown through a series of metabolic steps called *glycolysis* to the intermediate pyruvic acid,

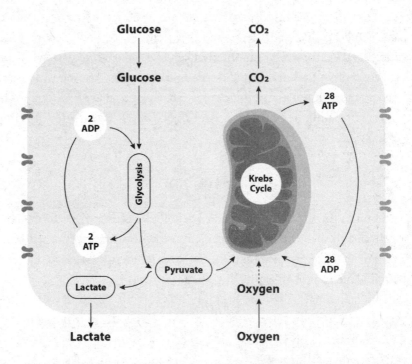

Figure 7–1: Energy metabolism 101. The cell imports glucose and converts it into pyruvic acid (glycolysis, left side), yielding two ATPs. If the mitochondria are functioning, the pyruvic acid is metabolized by the Krebs cycle (right side), yielding twenty-eight ATPs and carbon dioxide.

releasing only a small amount of energy, which is captured within a molecule called adenosine triphosphate (ATP). From there, the pyruvic acid has one of two choices: 1) either enter the *mitochondria* (the energy-burning factories inside the cell), where the metabolic breakdown continues, a process called the *Krebs cycle*, to yield a lot more ATP (and making the waste product carbon dioxide, which you breathe out from the lungs); or 2) if the mitochondria are busy or dysfunctional, the pyruvic acid diverts to a process called *de novo lipogenesis* (new fat-making) to turn into a fatty acid called *palmitic acid*, which is then bound to a glycerol molecule and exported out of the liver cell as a triglyceride particle.

These two pathways of energy metabolism, especially within the mitochondria, consistently release toxic by-products inside the cell called oxygen radicals (kind of like what hydrogen peroxide does on a wound). If not detoxified, these can damage the cell, and even cause it to die. Therefore, the cell has another structure called a *peroxisome*, which is where various antioxidants are stored to neutralize the oxygen radicals.

1. Glycation

Why do we get cataracts and wrinkles as we get older? Each of these is an example of an undeniable and inevitable fact of life—the *Maillard* or *glycation* or *browning* or *caramelization* reaction. All four terms describe the same process, which is the primary process of aging. First described by Professor Louis Camille Maillard in 1912, this process occurs in all living cells. It doesn't need any energy or enzymes or cofactors or other nutrients, it just happens. It's a by-product of living, yet it's the primary reason for dying. We're all browning, all the time, and the only way to stop it is by dying. The faster the Maillard reaction occurs, the faster you age—you get wrinkles, your arteries become sclerotic, and you eventually reach the pearly gates. But you can slow this process down—and if you're successful, you'll be a lot healthier for a lot longer.

The Maillard reaction only needs two molecules to occur: a carbohydrate (fructose or glucose), plus an amino acid (e.g., proteins). Put them together and the protein starts to "brown" and become less flexible. Ideally, these damaged proteins will be cleared away by cellular waste processing systems, but if the reaction occurs faster than the waste can be cleared, eventually the buildup of *advanced glycation end products*, or AGEs, will lead to cell, organ, and human dysfunction. The question is not *if* the Maillard reaction will occur, but rather *how fast*.

And this is where the metabolic differences between glucose and fructose becomes important (see Chapters 2 and 12). One might think that glucose and fructose, both being molecules found in dietary sugar (sucrose, high-fructose corn syrup, honey, maple syrup, agave—they're all metabolically the same; take your pick), would drive this reaction at the same rate. You would be very wrong. Yes, they're both carbohydrates, and yes, they both bind to proteins, but that's where their similarities end. Because glucose has a six-member-ring structure (see **Fig. 7-2**), it's more stable and engages in the Maillard reaction relatively slowly. Conversely, fructose's five-member ring is more easily broken apart, and engages in the Maillard reaction seven times faster than glucose. It also generates one hundred times the number of oxygen radicals (see *Oxidative Stress* below). Furthermore, our research group has shown that a specific breakdown product of fructose, called *methylglyoxal*, drives the Maillard reaction 250 times faster than glucose.

All in all, when it comes to aging, fructose is worse than glucose, and therefore sugar is worse than starch. That doesn't make glucose "good"—it raises insulin and drives obesity—but compared to fructose, it's a walk in the park.

2. Oxidative Stress

Oxygen (O_2) is a peculiar molecule. Our brain is completely dependent on it; in fact, the brain dies in four minutes flat without oxygen, while the rest of your body can keep on living. However, many types of cells

a.

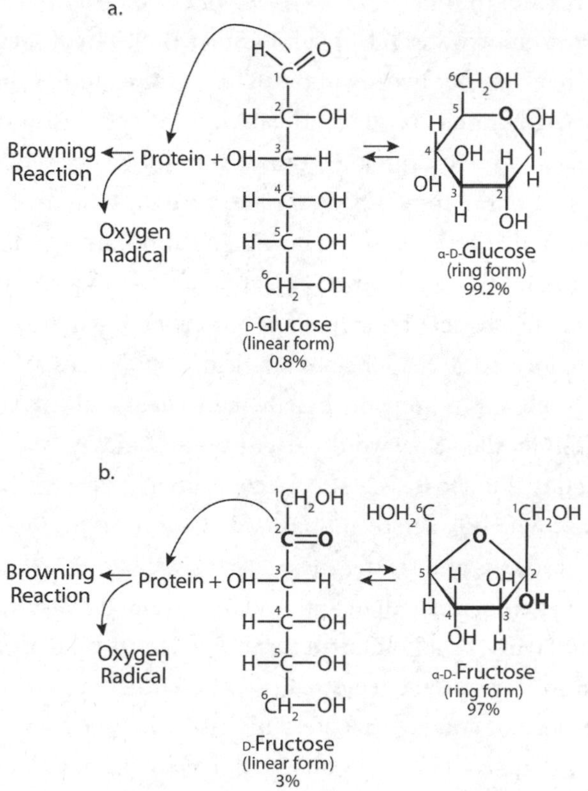

b.

Figure 7–2: Structures of a) glucose and b) fructose, in the linear form and the ring form. This figure demonstrates that a sugar is not a sugar. Glucose is a six-membered ring and is more stable than the five-membered ring of fructose, which breaks down more easily to the linear form. Only the linear form can engage in the Maillard reaction. Therefore, fructose drives the Maillard reaction seven times faster than glucose, causing seven times the damage.

grow specifically when they're deprived of oxygen; this is particularly true of cancer cells (see Chapter 8). Oxygen also has the unique capacity to create an inhospitable environment for foreign invaders (like bacteria), but also for our own cells.

Inside our white blood cells, oxygen undergoes a reaction catalyzed by an enzyme called *superoxide dismutase* (SOD), which turns O_2 (the stuff we breathe) into O_2—, an *oxygen radical* or *reactive oxygen species*, similar to how water (H_2O) can be turned into hydrogen peroxide (H_2O_2). When you put hydrogen peroxide on a wound, it bubbles and fizzes as the liberated oxygen radicals kill everything in sight. And that's great if you're cleaning a wound. But this process occurs in all of our cells all of the time. Oxygen radicals are a standard by-product of three normal reactions in the body: glycation; energy metabolism in our mitochondria; and iron metabolism (equivalent to rusting, which is constantly occurring in all of our cells). Furthermore, oxygen radicals are formed in response to anything that causes inflammation. Thus, each cell in our body ordinarily has to deal with an oxygen radical pool; if unleashed they would kill us pretty quickly.

Each of our cells possesses specialized subcellular organelles called *peroxisomes*, which is where antioxidants lie in wait to quench incoming oxygen radicals and render them inert (see Chapter 19). But if there are more oxygen radicals than antioxidants (termed *oxidative stress*), it causes cellular dysfunction, structural damage to lipids, proteins, or DNA, and in the extreme, cell death. When this happens in the liver and the pancreas, you get diabetes. It's also why we need to consume Real Food that has color, because color is an indication that these plants contain the antioxidants we can't make on our own.

3. Mitochondrial Dysfunction

Imagine an old-style factory with a coal-burning furnace. The coal is transported on railroad cars, and there are able-bodied furnace stokers working in shifts to feed the furnace. As long as the rate of arrival of the coal and the offload by the stokers are matched, the factory runs at full capacity. Now imagine that many of the furnace stokers are old and infirm, or perhaps stricken ill at once. There just aren't enough stokers for continual twenty-four-hour work. As a result, they're not going to generate enough energy for the furnace to burn at full capacity, and the factory will not put out the best product. There's also the scenario where the railroad cars filled with coal start arriving inside the factory walls faster than the furnace stokers can unload it—the cars build up, taking over the factory floor, and eventually the factory will be overwhelmed, will choke off, and shut down.

Now imagine both of these issues happening at the same time. That's *mitochondrial dysfunction*. Chronic disease *is* mitochondrial dysfunction, and mitochondrial dysfunction *is* chronic disease. They are one and the same.

Mitochondria are really bacteria that decided eons ago that they were happier living inside of animal-based cells than facing the cold, cruel world on their own. Bacteria were great at burning energy, while animal cells were great at fending off invaders—so they made a symbiotic decision to stick together. To this day, mitochondria have their own DNA and their own genetic program apart from the human DNA found in the nucleus of the cell. But like the shift workers, mitochondria tend to go defective with time and are prone to oxidative stress and damage. Mitochondria are finicky, lose capacity easily, and constantly need to be renewed and replenished. They need to divide, and the cell needs to clear the old ones out. The single best stimulus to make more and fresh mitochondria is exercise—but even your mitochondria can't outrun a bad diet (see Chapter 10). Not surprisingly, the pharma industry has identified increasing mitochondria as a primary drug target for metabolic disease—yes, they believe you can market "exercise in a pill"—but *there is no magic pill*.

When glucose and oxygen availability, as well as mitochondrial capacity, are all matched, everything goes smoothly. Using the coal factory analogy, when the glucose comes in faster than the mitochondria (stokers) process it, the excess chokes off the factory. The mitochondria have no choice but to divert the excess pyruvic acid into fat, a process called *de novo lipogenesis* (new fat-making). When this happens in the liver, you get fatty liver, which leads to liver insulin resistance (see *Insulin Resistance* below). If instead this happens in the pancreas, you get fatty pancreas and insulin deficiency. And fructose (in processed food) makes twice as much liver fat as does glucose.

The sicker your mitochondria, the earlier you die. The organs that need mitochondria and energy production the most are the brain and hormone-secreting organs—because neurotransmission and hormone secretion are energetically expensive. If the mitochondrial DNA is defective, you end up with a class of nasty diseases known as *mitochondrial encephalomyopathies*. I took care of one girl with a mitochondrial disease called Kearns-Sayre syndrome who came to my practice at age nine with seizures and droopy eyelids (keeping your eyes open is a high energy task!). Over the next ten years, she slowly developed diabetes, a heart rhythm disturbance, inability to walk, and finally went comatose at age twenty. She died at twenty-three, and there was nothing we could do for her. Mitochondria can be defective because of genetics, or because of the pathologies discussed in this chapter. Either way, the results are disastrous.

4. Insulin Resistance

As we've explored, most people think of insulin as the "anti-diabetes" hormone; it lowers the blood glucose, which prevents diabetic microvascular complications (eye, kidney, nerve disease) from occurring. This is only half of the story. Insulin's main job is actually to store energy for a rainy day.

Just two organs in your body need insulin to function: the liver and adipose tissue. Too much insulin can get in the way, forcing glucose clearance from the bloodstream into tissues. It can also lead to hypoglycemia (low blood glucose) and inadequate glucose delivery to the brain, which can make you dizzy or unconscious or seize or die, depending on its severity. The pancreas senses the drop in the blood glucose, and stops releasing insulin before you lose consciousness.

But nowadays, more often than not, the opposite problem occurs; different types of cells are not responding to the insulin in the bloodstream. This is called *insulin resistance*. When glucose can't get into certain cells, those cells starve, which leads to organ dysfunction. When the liver or muscles are resistant, glucose builds up in the blood, leading to diabetes. The fact of the matter is that insulin resistance isn't due to low insulin levels, but rather high ones—because the cell isn't responding to the insulin signal. Of course, genetics can play a role—but then again, genetics haven't changed in fifty years, but the environment sure has.

Various problems that can lead to defective insulin signaling are: obesity; chronic stress; environmental chemicals that drive weight gain (obesogens like estrogen, bisphenol A [BPA], phthalates, PBDE flame retardants); and, our favorite, processed food (see Chapters 18, 19, and 20). High insulin levels cause cellular dysfunction, which ultimately leads to chronic disease, morbidity, and early death. Insulin resistance is the central problem in metabolic syndrome, and different people can have different reasons for insulin resistance—but processed food is by far the biggest player. Even those who are overweight and those who are under stress don't exhibit metabolic syndrome if their diet is unprocessed.

5. Membrane Integrity

Every cell has an outer membrane to protect and contain its contents. When membranes get damaged, cells spill their contents and all hell breaks loose, usually leading to cell dysfunction and death. Then the mop-up crew follows behind and does even more damage during the cleanup (see *Inflammation* below).

Membranes are composed of a lipid bilayer, like a sandwich; lipids on the inside facing the cellular contents, lipids on the outside of the cell facing the bloodstream, and proteins forming the filling of the sandwich. Membranes can be damaged through two mechanisms: the lipids themselves are damaged either from toxins or from oxidative stress (see *Oxidative Stress* above); or the lipids are inflexible, like rubber tubing where cracks appear due to plastic that has gotten old and dried out. Membranes should be flexible and malleable like a balloon, called *membrane fluidity*—they should give somewhat when poked from one direction. When they don't, they can burst.

There are seven different types of fats in your diet, and all can impact

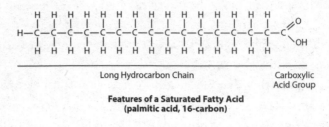

Long Hydrocarbon Chain   Carboxylic Acid Group

**Features of a Saturated Fatty Acid
(palmitic acid, 16-carbon)**

HO *trans*-palmitoleic acid

HO *cis*-palmitoleic acid

H₂C—O   fatty acid 1, palmitic acid

HC—O   fatty acid 2, oleic acid

H₂C—O   fatty acid 3, linolenic acid

glycerol backbone

Features of a Triglyceride

Figure 7–3: a-c) Structures of free fatty acids. a) palmitic acid (16-carbon saturated), b) *trans*-palmitoleic acid (16-carbon *trans*-unsaturated), and c) *cis*-palmitoleic acid (16-carbon *cis*-unsaturated). Note that the COOH carboxyl group (which is inflammatory) is free. d: Structure of a triglyceride, which is composed of three different free fatty acids (at least one of which must be unsaturated), linked to a glycerol backbone, so that the inflammatory COOH carboxyl groups are not free and available to do damage.

your cell membranes in different ways. But for this exercise, we only need to consider three of them, as shown in **Fig. 7–3**.

Problems with lipids can damage outer membranes in one of two ways. First, saturated fatty acids (which are different from saturated fats; see Chapter 12) are completely flexible because they don't have any double bonds, which normally apply a degree of inflexibility to a fat's structure. This means that saturated fatty acids can conform in any shape, which normally is good for membrane integrity. However, new research suggests that because they're so fluid, they can sometimes layer on top of each other and form a clump of lipid within a membrane, the subcellular version of cellulite, which reduces the cells' overall fluidity.

Unsaturated fats are almost always better for you than saturated ones, which themselves are none too problematic in regard to metabolic syndrome. Because of their *cis*-double bonds, unsaturated fatty acids have fixed angles built into them, which prevents them from layering. But there are two problems with unsaturated fats. First, those *cis*-double bonds are exactly where toxins and oxidative stress like to do their damage, by oxidizing that double bond. And when they do, they release an oxygen radical (see *Oxidative Stress*). Second, when an unsaturated fat is heated beyond its smoking point, the *cis*-double bond can "flip"—and now you've got a *trans*-fat, which is deadly to the cell (see Chapter 20). Even though the FDA finally got around to banning *trans*-fats in commercial foods, you can still accidentally make them on your own (see Chapter 18).

6. Inflammation

Foreign invaders (e.g., viruses and bacteria) can damage cells directly. Our body has developed an inflammatory response, which recruits various white blood cells to release toxins like oxygen radicals and cytokines (peptides with killing activity) to destroy the invaders. While we need an inflammatory response (or we would be eaten by the maggots), unfortunately there are four downsides.

1) The process kills normal tissues, too, which can lead to longstanding damage after the invader is cleared (e.g., kidney disease after *E. coli*, coronary aneurysms after Kawasaki disease, and now we are learning about long-term damage with COVID-19).

2) The inflammatory process can sometimes be triggered against a body tissue because a body tissue molecularly resembles a foreign invader, a phenomenon called *molecular mimicry*. This is why, for instance, some people develop rheumatic fever, kidney disease, and even psychiatric disease after a strep infection.

3) Bad bacteria can proliferate in the gut in response to an aberrant environment (either the food itself or the antibiotics in the food; see Chapter 20), which can cause pathogenic bacteria to predominate, such as *Streptococcus mutans* in the mouth and dental caries. The inflammatory reaction will cause breaks in the intestinal barrier, allowing toxins and bacteria to pass across the intestinal wall into the bloodstream; they then head to the liver and cause insulin resistance, a process known as *leaky gut*. Leaky gut is one reason for the dramatic increase in food allergies and autoimmune disease in people (see Chapter 14).

4) Body fat (subcutaneous or visceral fat) can release palmitate, an inflammatory lipid, which in turn drives up the inflammatory response. Palmitate can also be formed in the liver in response to excessive sugar intake, resulting in liver inflammation, which makes chronic disease even worse. In fact, palmitate is the real bad actor in the story of metabolic syndrome (see Chapter 12).

There are connections between metabolism and inflammation in both directions. For instance, when fat cells get so large that they spill their grease, macrophages come into the fat depots to mop it up, and then release a set of cytokines that directly interfere with liver insulin signaling, driving chronic disease.

There are also connections between specific foods and inflammation. For instance, increased dietary fructose reaching the liver spurs on an enzyme called *c-Jun* N-terminal kinase-1 (JNK1 for short), which inactivates the insulin signaling pathway as well.

The key to the chronic disease kingdom is that there are not four separate problems (nutrition, metabolism, inflammation, immunity); there's only one, and they are all related. Screw up one and you screw up the other three.

7. Epigenetics

Lots of effort has been placed on looking for genetic reasons behind metabolic syndrome, but the studies say only 15 percent is genetic—the rest is environmental. But environment can change genes as well, through a phenomenon called epigenetics. *Epigenetics* refers to changes in the areas around our genes that can cause them to be turned on or off, usually inappropriatcly, altering responses to these pathologies, and which over time can result in the development of various diseases.

Think of it this way: epigenetics is the on-off switch attached to the dimmer on your living room chandelier. The gene is the lightbulb, the epigene is the light switch. If the lightbulb is defunct or the switch is frozen in the "off" position, the dimmer function is useless. Likewise, epigenes control the effect to which the gene turns on. Epigenetic modifications acting on various tissues typically only influence the physiology of the exposed individual, changing the risk of disease development later in life. This might partly explain the developmental origins of health and disease.

In some cases, environmental factors alter the epigenetic programming of germ cells in the sperm or egg, and alterations in disease can appear in future generations without further direct exposure. This is known as *transgenerational epigenetic inheritance.* So far, it's been shown to affect as many as four generations going into the future. So it's not just what you ate; it's what your mother ate. In fact, it's what your great-great-grandmother ate. And as you can imagine, if each person has two offspring, these epigenetic changes can multiply across the population pretty fast. These changes might be a plausible partial explanation for the pandemic of obesity and related diseases that cannot be fully accounted for by genetic variations and lifestyle factors.

Altered nutrition also appears to be a primary driver of altered epigenetics. For instance, take the vitamin folic acid, a necessary and limiting cofactor for the nuclear enzymes called *DNA methyltransferases* (DNMTs), which adds a methyl group to DNA to alter whether genes are being activated. Folic acid is so important to normal fetal development in order to prevent the occurrence of spina bifida that the FDA has remanded the baked goods industry to add it to grocery store–bought bread. In addition, folic acid is necessary to catalyze the breakdown of a metabolite called homocysteine (Hcy; see Chapter 9), which has been linked to one form of early heart disease, although its role in general heart disease remains controversial. Some people carry a mutation in the gene that activates folic acid; these people have higher Hcy levels and greater risk for heart disease, but supplementing their diet with extra folate can reduce some of their risk.

Other nutrients such as vitamin B_{12} (cyanocobalamin), vitamin B_6 (pyridoxine), vitamin B_2 (riboflavin), methionine, choline, and betaine are also involved in epigenetics. And nutrients such as retinoic acid, resveratrol, curcumin, sulforaphane, and polyphenols can also modulate it (see Chapter 14 for more on supplements).

Last, epigenetics has also been shown to be at work in the long-lasting effects of some endocrine-disrupting chemicals (EDCs), which mimic hormonal actions and alter long-term metabolism. Examples include elements that come in contact with our processed food supply, such as BPA and phthalates found in processed food cans and plastic bottles (see Chapter 20), both of which can lead to insulin resistance and obesity.

8. Autophagy

For years, we've dumped garbage into landfills and then built on them. In the San Francisco Bay Area, we owe our airport and several lower income housing areas, such as Treasure Island and Foster City, to reclaiming land by adding garbage to it. But what happens when you run out of places to put the garbage? Or worse, what happens when there's nobody to pick up the trash? And the garbage starts to settle and the whole Bay Area starts to stink, and to sink? As you might expect, it's much better to clear the garbage than to build on it. And that goes for the human body as well.

Clearing biological waste products is a process known as *autoph-agy*, and it plays a key role in healthy aging, especially in the brain. The brain uses more energy than any other organ, and so there are lots of mitochondria, oxygen radicals, and therefore lots of damage in it. Omega-3 fatty acids (see Chapter 19), which we need for healthy brain functioning, are particularly susceptible to damage—which equals lots of cleanup.

And as you might imagine, there's not a lot of extra room in the brain for this waste, so the brain has to be particularly adept and rapid at removing debris. That's what sleep is for—our intracerebral pressure goes down during sleep, which opens small pores within the brain called *glymphatics*. An ebb tide fluid shifts slowly during sleep to remove damaged cellular components into the bloodstream for disposal. In other words, in the brain, every night is garbage night. And if you don't get enough sleep, it's like having your brain's garbagemen on strike.

But this isn't just good for the brain—all organs do better with autophagy, which is an essential process that maintains healthy cells by removing damaged proteins and malfunctioning organelles, especially mitochondria. Old mitochondria make a lot of oxygen radicals. Therefore, to improve metabolism and slow aging, it's essential to get rid of the old mitochondria by autophagy. In fact, people who clear their mitochondria more efficiently live longer.

There's also evidence to support that autophagy is under various nutritional controls. For instance, vitamin D deficiency is associated with cellular aging; and vitamin D appears to play an important role in promoting autophagy, by increasing calcium influx into old cells, which induces a cellular program to purposefully kill it. Paradoxically, vitamin B_1 deficiency accelerates neurodegeneration, while supplementation appears to promote autophagy and slow neurodegeneration, by reducing oxygen radical formation. The biggest effect of nutrition on autophagy has to do with the metabolic improvements that can be seen with the now-popular maneuver of intermittent fasting, which lowers insulin and raises ketones, both of which promote autophagy (we'll get into more detail in Chapter 14).

The "Hateful Eight"? or the "Grateful Eight"?

As you can see, none of these eight processes evoke disease outright. In fact, when they are working right, they contribute to longevity and good health. But, screw up a few, and you have the makings of a very short and miserable life. More important, all eight processes are related to chronic disease, and also related to each other and to food. See a pattern here? These are the true diseases of processed food; they're just not called diseases or taught in medical school. But they should be taught before any mention of any drug, so that medical students can triangulate, "How does this drug impact these eight processes?" Only in this way can we unlearn doctors to focus on what's important and patients to understand the limits of disease therapy. Otherwise, both Big Food and Big Pharma win again and again and again.

CHAPTER 8

Checkpoints Alpha, Bravo, Charlie: Nutrient-Sensing and Chronic Disease

Food drives both illness and wellness; it's the poison and the antidote. Metabolic syndrome could colloquially be redefined as *cells eating badly*, as every one of the eight subcellular pathologies is made worse by providing the wrong food in the wrong place at the wrong time. In fact, there are really only two processes that handle energy properly—growing or burning. And there are two proper outcomes—living or dying. Every cell has to grow at one time in its life versus burn at another time—but never both at the same time. Similarly, every cell has to live and die, but clearly not both at the same time.

What determines when a cell grows or burns, and what determines when a cell lives or dies? What if a cell is burning when it should be growing, and living when it should be dying, or vice versa? Any perturbation of the growing/burning or living/dying pattern will lead to disease. It's through this lens where we find the clues to the real reasons for metabolic syndrome (spoiler alert: it's processed food!), and also for both treatment and prevention. It's complex science, so feel free to skip to Chapter 9, but it's very cool; it's Nobel Prize–winning work—twice.

Oxygen Is So Overrated

Does life need oxygen? Plant life clearly doesn't. In fact, green plants need carbon dioxide for photosynthesis, making oxygen as the by-product. But does animal life need oxygen? The first clue to this puzzle came in 1924. German biochemist Otto Warburg made an astounding observation—cancer cells didn't need oxygen to grow. While Warburg never figured out why this was the case, his observation was important enough that he won the 1931 Nobel Prize in Physiology or Medicine.

So regular cells need oxygen, but cancerous ones don't? Aren't cancer cells just regular cells sped up? They divide way faster than normal, which is why some chemotherapies work—they poison the dividing process (called *mitosis*). But how can growing cells not need oxygen? Doesn't every cell need oxygen?

The answer is a resounding no. In fact, there's very little oxygen in the gut. The intestinal microbiome has adapted to it; 99 percent of the bacteria in our intestine, called *obligate anaerobes*, don't need oxygen. In fact, many bacteria grow just fine without it and don't have mitochondria.

But that's all the bacteria in your gut do—they grow. They don't burn. They generate a lot of lactic acid, because that's the waste product of glucose metabolism without oxygen, but those bacteria stay (or, at least, are supposed to stay) in the gut. Your muscles can also produce lactic acid, which causes pain when you've run a marathon (so I've heard, but running a marathon is still on my bucket list). The bacteria in your gut don't make or release stuff. They divide and increase in mass, just like cancer cells. Cancers double every fifty to two hundred days. And they make boatloads of lactic acid in the process.

Any idea about what cells grow even faster than cancer cells? Fetal cells. A sperm and an egg meet, called *fertilization*, to make one cell called a *zygote*. That zygote doubles (divides in two) over and over to achieve 36 doublings (2^{36} cells) over 270 days of pregnancy for a total of 68 billion cells at birth; that averages doubling about every 7.5 days. This growth happens in the lowest oxygen environment imaginable (the placenta delivers to the fetus a partial oxygen pressure of 30 millimeters of mercury (30 mm Hg), compared to the 100 mm Hg that the lungs deliver to adult cells). So how do fetal cells grow so fast with so little oxygen?

The discovery of the metabolic signal for this effect that drives cancer and fetal cells to grow without oxygen is so important the Nobel Prize was awarded to its discoverers (Gregg Semenza, William Kaelin Jr., and Peter Ratcliffe) in 2019.

If you're a cell in growth phase without oxygen—making structural components and the by-product lactic acid—do you even *need* mitochondria? Do you even *want* mitochondria? There are only four states of increased lactic acid production in humans: post-exercise, cancer, mitochondrial diseases like Kearns-Sayre syndrome (see Chapter 7), and metabolic syndrome—because that's mitochondrial dysfunction as well. As cells divide, mitochondria have to divide, too (remember they have their own DNA); and they can't divide fast enough to keep up with the cell's growth, especially in cells that are growing rapidly—meaning mitochondria become an unwanted luxury for a rapidly growing and dividing cancer cell or fetal cell. However, these cells still need to generate ATP (the fuel of your cell) to power them.

How do they do that without mitochondria or oxygen? This conundrum perplexed scientists until recently.

Blood Flow Restriction for Muscle Growth

This phenomenon of growth without oxygen has recently been exploited to treat a common disease of aging, called *sarcopenia*, or loss of muscle mass. As people advance into their seventies, they can lose half their muscle mass, which renders them frail and susceptible to falling and fracture. To treat this, exercise physiologists have started putting tight bands around the patient's arms and legs with low-intensity resistance and endurance training. Lo and behold, muscles increase in mass and strength—because depriving muscle cells of oxygen switched them from burning to growing.

Two Metabolic Programs—One for Growth, One for Burning

Growing cells need all sorts of structural components in order to divide and make new cells. They need lipids for membranes, ribose (a 5-membered monosaccharide) as the backbone for DNA and RNA, and amino acids for proteins. Where do all of these building blocks come from?

They're not imported in the blood, but instead are created on-site from available materials. Imagine a piece of wood in your house. That wood could be used to make furniture, or it could instead be used for firewood, but not at the same time. It's the same for glucose inside the cell. Will it be used for growth and structural components, or will it be burned? There are two linked metabolic pathways inside the cell; when the cell is burning, they run in tandem, but when the cell is growing, they can dissociate from each other (see **Fig. 7-1**).

The first pathway is called *glycolysis* (see Chapter 7), which prepares glucose to be used for structural components, and *pyruvic acid* is the end product. If the pyruvic acid is not used for burning in the next stage, it can leave the cell as lactic acid. Glycolysis provides the added bonus of generating a grand total of two ATPs, all without needing oxygen.

The second pathway is called the *Krebs cycle* (see Chapter 7). The pyruvic acid enters the mitochondria, where it burns all the way to completion, at the end of which you have twenty-eight ATPs and carbon dioxide. If the goal is burning (e.g., aerobic exercise), you need both glycolysis *and* the Krebs cycle working in tandem. If the goal is structural components for growth (e.g., blood flow restriction, or body-builders using high-intensity interval training to build muscle mass), then you only need glycolysis, and the pyruvic acid will be diverted for building muscle.

Nutrient-Sensing, Kinases, and the Setup for Chronic Disease

Both of these pathways, *glycolysis* for growth and the *Krebs cycle* for burning, are *adaptive*. Basically, they're the superhighways of your cell. If they get blocked, then the detours can be highly excruciating, even killing you. Essentially, when energy metabolism goes awry, those eight subcellular pathologies of Chapter 7 become *maladaptive*. And this is where processed food becomes maladaptive.

There are three protein checkpoints (like traffic lights) inside the cell called *kinases* that determine what happens to each molecule of glucose or fructose; these are turned on and off within seconds by the addition of a phosphate molecule generated from the food we eat.

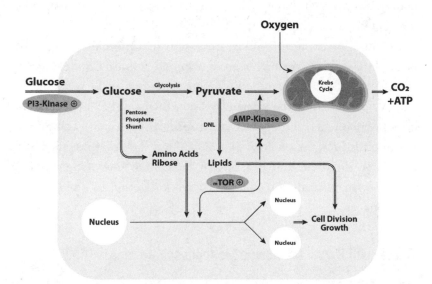

Figure 8–1: The three enzymes that determine cell fate. PI3-kinase lets glucose into the cell; AMP-kinase directs that energy either to produce structural components for the cell or to enter the mitochondria to burn all the way to carbon dioxide; and mTOR determines whether the cell lives or dies.

When the three checkpoints (which we'll call Alpha, Bravo, Charlie) are coordinated in one direction, you get growth. When they are coordinated in the opposite direction, you get burning. But when they are uncoordinated, that's when you get a traffic jam and chronic metabolic disease happens.

Checkpoint Alpha: Phosphatidylinositol-3-kinase (PI3-kinase)

Glycolysis generates a total of two ATPs from a glucose molecule, hardly enough to power a cancer cell. But who said anything about just one glucose molecule? Cancer cells import two hundred times the amount of glucose than normal ones do—meaning they're not making two ATPs, they're making four hundred. Lewis Cantley of Weill Cornell Medical College in New York City showed that this first enzyme, called *PI3-kinase*, opens the glucose floodgates of the cell. Lots of glucose entry means that cell has lots of fuel to power itself, all without mitochondria or oxygen. No wonder cancer cells and fetal cells have high levels of PI3-kinase.

So could blocking PI3-kinase stop cancer? Originally, drug trials of PI3-kinase inhibitors had been disappointing, until Cantley's group showed that if you first cut down on insulin signaling by reducing the amount of dietary refined carbohydrate, then the PI3-kinase inhibitors became much more effective. Insulin drives cancer cell growth because it's how the glucose gets into the cell in the first place; it's the key to the door, and PI3-kinase determines how wide the door swings open. Insulin and PI3-kinase work together to flood the cell with glucose.

Checkpoint Bravo: Adenosine Monophosphate-kinase (AMP-kinase)

OK, the glucose is now inside—then where does it go? If the cell is low on energy, it needs to burn. The second checkpoint, *AMP-kinase*, is the cell's fuel gauge. It knows the difference between *full* and *empty*.

When a cell has used up its ATPs, the mitochondria need to burn pyruvic acid completely, to generate twenty-eight new ATPs to replete the cell's energy stores (with the waste product of carbon dioxide). AMP-kinase has the added bonus of signaling the cell to make more mitochondria in order to burn more glucose to make even more ATP. Anything that gooses AMP-kinase, like exercise or the anti-diabetes drug metformin, will keep mitochondria functioning optimally and improve insulin sensitivity.

But on the other hand, when a cell has too much ATP, AMP-kinase gets turned off. Mitochondria aren't burning, and the cell will divert the pyruvic acid to make structural components. Anything that impairs AMP-kinase will drive fat synthesis and worsen insulin resistance. And what food impairs AMP-kinase the most? *Sugar*, of course.

Checkpoint Charlie: Mammalian Target of Rapamycin (mTOR)

If a cell has plenty of energy but limited oxygen or mitochondria, it may decide to divide; while if a cell has adequate oxygen and glucose, it may just hang out. Finally, if a cell has limited energy and is getting old, it may decide to die to make room for new ones (*autophagy*). What signals this three-path Rubicon of fate? That's the job of the third checkpoint, *mTOR*, which determines a cell's commitment to growth, quiescence, or death.

The discovery of mTOR highlights its central role in cell fate. In the late 1970s, a soil sample from Rapa Nui (the native name for Easter Island) yielded a compound called *rapamycin* that had bizarre effects. Rapamycin turned out to be not just an immunosuppressant, or an anticancer drug, or a fungicide—but all three at once because it alters the growth phase of the cell. mTOR determines whether a cell lives or dies, so autophagy can clear out the debris. It's the major regulator of growth in animals and the key link between what's in the cell versus what happens to the cell. mTOR is the holy grail of cell fate, and the target of most current longevity drugs. However, because it's so multifaceted, the medical establishment hasn't yet figured out how to harness its power.

As you might expect, mTOR is highly sensitive to diet. A high protein composition of your diet activates mTOR, thereby promoting cell division, development of lean body mass, insulin sensitivity, and bone and cardiovascular health. Conversely, caloric deprivation (see Chapter 14) leads to lowering of ATP levels, which reduces mTOR, making growth an impossibility. Also, activating AMP-kinase can shut down mTOR in its tracks because now you're burning, not growing. So while mTOR is its own checkpoint for cell survival, it's also dependent on the cell's AMP-kinase status. This will become important when we see how dyssynchrony of these three checkpoints can cause chronic disease.

Growth Versus Burning, and Everything in Between—the Eight Combinations

These three enzyme checkpoints together explain how the cell metabolizes energy: PI3-kinase imports glucose into the cell; AMP-kinase directs the energy to mitochondria for burning; and mTOR determines whether a cell lives or dies. While cell metabolism has *everything* to do with *energy*, it has *nothing* to do with *calories*. It's not calories that drive growth or burning, it's what the chemicals that reach the cell, and especially the mitochondria, do to these three enzymes. And it is these three enzymes that show why *everything* we thought we knew about nutrition is wrong.

Here's why. Each of these three enzymes can exist in one of two states—on or off. Therefore any cell's metabolic status can be described by one of a total of 2 x 2 x 2, or 8 different combinations of these three enzymes. I want to state that this is a hypothesis, not proven—but this is a new way to think about the role of diet and nutrition, and it fits the available scientific data of nutrients and their effects on growth, burning, and disease. One biochemical constraint on this hypothesis is that when AMP-kinase is turned on, it preempts mTOR, which turns off. These three enzymes explain health and longevity when they are working in harmony, but when dyssynchronous they explain the eight subcellular pathologies, metabolic syndrome, and even cancer.

Table 8-1 numerically lists each of these eight combinations. The combinations of the three enzymes for normal growth are listed in column 1, and for normal burning in column 2; both of which are needed for the cell to survive, and programmed to occur at different times in your life. But when the combinations of those enzymes are dyssynchronous, which means energy is not being handled in a normal way, it sets you up long-term to develop a disease. The scenario for each combination and its metabolic result follows. For instance, neurons are supposed to burn, not grow—but if the combination is defective, they can turn into a neuroblastoma, a devastating pediatric tumor. Any of the other combinations (columns 3 to 8) occur due to an energy fork-in-the-road, and can lead to one or more chronic pathologies, which if unchecked could foment different types of NCDs. We don't know that the last two combinations actually occur (because when AMP-kinase is turned on, it preempts mTOR), but they make sense to include for completeness. Each of these permutations are subject to dietary manipulation, either for good or for bad.

1. PI3K +, AMPK−, mTOR +

    This combination leads to **growth** and occurs in the absence of oxygen. When PI3-kinase and mTOR are turned on and AMP-kinase is turned off, cells will import lots of glucose, and use it to make lipids for membranes, amino acids for proteins, and ribose for DNA. It can also increase the risk for cancer; every time a cell divides there's a chance that a mistake will be made in the DNA copying, which could lead to cancerous mutations.

2. PI3K−, AMPK +, mTOR−

    This combination leads to **burning** in the presence of oxygen. Because PI3-kinase is turned off, glucose will be in low supply, thus glycation and oxygen radical formation will be low. More AMP-kinase means healthier mitochondria. Since mTOR is turned off, old cells can be cleared. Risks for metabolic syndrome and cancer development are low.

3. PI3K +, AMPK–, mTOR–

    This combination leads to classic **metabolic syndrome**. Glucose enters the cell but mitochondria aren't activated, so it has nowhere to go. Glycation, oxidative stress, and inflammation will increase. Even though mTOR is turned off, the high glucose supply will mean that the cell will likely not die of autophagy. Insulin will be high, driving production of lipids/fat, and eventually type 2 diabetes.

4. PI3K–, AMPK–, mTOR +

    This combination is likely to lead to **early aging**. Without glucose flooding the cell, glycation and oxidative stress is low and cell damage will be slow. Lack of AMP-kinase means mitochondria won't be generating oxygen radicals. But because mTOR is turned on, there is no autophagy, and damage will accumulate slowly.

5. PI3K–, AMPK–, mTOR–

    This combination is likely to lead to early **cell death**. Less glucose is imported, but it's not being burned; and there is also increased autophagy. The cell is likely to die more easily, allowing for quicker turnover, and very little risk for cancer; but excessive early death could lead to organ dysfunction.

6. PI3K +, AMPK +, mTOR–

    This combination is likely to lead to low-level **inflammation**. It is similar to (5), but with more autophagy, so there would be less long-term damage.

7. PI3K +, AMPK +, mTOR + becomes–

    This is similar to (6). This combination is likely to lead to high-level **vascular injury** and heart disease. Increased glucose entering the cell means glycation and oxidative stress. The glucose will be burned by mitochondria; as AMP-kinase partially inhibits mTOR, there will be some but not complete autophagy, and some clearing of dead cells. This could result in heart disease.

8. PI3K–, AMPK +, mTOR + becomes–
    This is similar to (2) and should lead to **burning,** occurring only in the presence of oxygen. Not much glucose, and the burning is aerobic, so not much oxidative stress, and mTOR reduced.

As you can see, these eight combinations of three enzymes (on or off) will cause cells to grow, burn, or create disease. Does this hypothesis stack up with the data in the literature? One way to assess its veracity is to look at the effects of specific drugs utilizing these enzymes on the cell and the organism. We have data on PI3-kinase inhibitors, AMP-kinase stimulators, and mTOR inhibitors at our disposal, and they demonstrate reduced cancer growth and increased longevity, therefore supporting this hypothesis.

Again, the scourges of chronic disease are all about how energy is handled at these three checkpoints. And each checkpoint is modulated

Kinase	1	2	3	4	5	6	7	8
PI3K	+	—	+	—	—	+	+	—
AMPK	—	+	—	—	—	+	+	+
mTOR	+	—	—	+	—	—	+ —> —	+ —> —
	Normal Growth	Normal Burning	Metabolic Syndrome	Early Aging	Early Cell Death	Low-level Inflammation	Becomes #6	Becomes #2

Table 8–1: The activity of three enzymes (PI3-kinase, AMP-kinase, and mTOR), in two different states (on [+] or off [–]), leads to eight separate permutations. In any given cell at any given time, each enzyme can either be (+) or (–), although AMP-kinase (+) activation automatically results in mTOR (–) inactivation; thus combinations 7 and 8 are theoretical.

by your diet. However, there's currently no blood test to measure any of these checkpoints. So what can you or your doctor do to assess your health? Chapter 9 will show you how to use the information your doctor gleans from standard tests in order to diagnose yourself. It's time to take charge of your own health, because no one else will.

Assembling the Clues to Diagnose Yourself

Y ou make an appointment to see your doctor for a routine clinic visit. They're booked solid (because the only way they make more money is by seeing more patients) and are an hour and a half late in seeing you. They've got you slotted in for a ten-minute visit, and their hand is already on the doorknob before they say hello, because that ninety minutes has got to be made up somehow, and it's likely at your expense.

Sound familiar? Look, I'm a doctor, and I know how I feel when I'm running late. But you, the patient, shouldn't be the victim of my frustration—so it's up to you to become an educated patient. **Rule #1: Don't take "busy" for an answer.**

The medical assistant checks your weight and blood pressure, the doctor does a cursory physical exam (just to be able to say they did, to justify a higher CPT code and a greater reimbursement), and then looks at the report listing your lab tests. The first column is the name of the test, the second is the normal range, and the third column, some-times color-coded, lists next to each test a designation of high, low, or normal.

That third column is the biggest scam in medicine. Each of those designations is an "interpretation," and $10 is charged against your in-surance. Whatever interpretation your doctor offers is worthless. You must *never* use or accept the word *normal* from your doctor, yourself, or anyone else. I mean, what does normal actually mean? Normal for who? At what age? And in what circumstance? This term must disap-pear from your lexicon. And it should disappear from the entire medi-cal lexicon. **Rule #2: Don't take "normal" for an answer.**

As an example, let's take (body mass index) BMI. A "normal" adult BMI is 19 to 25. Between 25 and 30 is overweight; between 30 and 35 is Class 1 or mild obesity; between 35 and 40 is Class 2 or moderate obesity; and over 40 is Class 3 or morbid obesity.

But as discussed in Chapter 2, there are MHO (metabolically healthy obese) people and TOFI (thin on the outside, fat on the inside) peo-ple (again, both are established terms in the medical literature). BMI doesn't tell you any of these things, because obesity and metabolic health aren't the same thing. BMI is a good measurement for popula-tions (because populations regress to the mean), but not for people (be-cause each of us is an "n of 1"). The real issue is insulin. If you look at the degree of insulin sensitivity at any given BMI, there's a huge spread, meaning at any given weight, some will be healthy, and some won't. What determines this isn't the subcutaneous fat, but the liver (and sec-ondarily, muscle) fat. You can't determine these factors by looking at a patient's BMI.

Let's explore another example of why "normal" means nothing. While not specific for liver fat accumulation, the liver enzyme alanine ami-notransferase (ALT) is cheap and easy to assess on a standard blood draw, and is sensitive (although not that specific) for measuring the de-gree of liver fat. The question is where to draw the line between nor-mal versus high, especially when the range is a moving target and has shifted to the right (for instance, a size 10 dress twenty years ago is now a size 6, even though it's the same amount of fabric). When I entered medical school in 1976, the upper limit of normal (two standard deviations from the mean) for ALT was 25. Now the cutoff on the lab slip says 40. How come? Did the *ALT assay change*? The name changed (back then it used to be called *serum glutamate-pyruvate transaminase*, or SGPT), but the assay is the same. So why is the cutoff 15 points higher—maybe because *humans changed*? Yes, because 45 percent of the general population now has some modicum of fatty liver disease, and the entire "normal" distribution has shifted to the right.

However, these people don't know they have fatty liver disease because they have no overt symptoms. And neither do their physicians (because they just read off the designation in the third column). So these people are thought to be normal, thus the widening of the normal range. But just because you haven't been diagnosed as "sick" doesn't mean you aren't.

Further, the threshold for concern is dependent on a host of other factors. This includes whether you're Caucasian (above 25), African American (above 20), or Latino (above 30); whether you're Asian (ALT will start to rise at a lower BMI); and whether you have a genetic predisposition to liver fat (19 percent of Latinos have one of two genetic alterations that predispose to liver fat accumulation, which may in part account for the very high incidence of metabolic syndrome in this population). Your ALT is also influenced if you're an alcohol drinker. Do you think your doctor has factored all that in?

The medical literature argues that 88 percent of Americans have some level of metabolic dysfunction that's likely gone unrecognized, whether it's fatty liver, high blood pressure, high blood uric acid (the cause of gout), high blood lipids, or high blood glucose. All of these are due in some measure to insulin resistance, which is due to metabolic dysfunction. Do those 88 percent of people know that they're metabolically ill? Or is it that 88 percent of doctors don't know what to look for? Do you really think your doctor is telling seven out of eight patients that their health is suboptimal? What would they advise if they did? If 88 percent of people have a problem, maybe it would be smart to assume you do, until such time as your doctor proves you don't? **Rule #3: Don't take paternalism for an answer.**

Assembling the Clues

Sadly, figuring out your true metabolic status will likely be up to you, because your doctor never learned how to synthesize the patterns of demographics, physical measures, or all of the lab results that attend chronic disease. In fact, your doctor has likely never heard of MHO or TOFI, because these aren't taught in medical school (and I know, because I'm the one who has to teach it even though I'm a pediatrician— how ridiculous is that?). So, how can you use the information your doctor skimmed, validated, or discarded, in order to determine your own biochemical profile, so that you can take control of your health?

In order to become an educated patient, you must also become a pattern recognizer, which is hard, because the only pattern you know is yours, and only if you get all the information. Luckily I know the patterns, so I'm giving them to you here. However, you also have to understand the subcellular processes that are going on in your membranes, mitochondria, and nuclei, and in your liver, muscles, and brain. These are all clues pointing to potential problem pathways possibly fixed by controlling your environment, and especially your diet.

All in all, there are four pieces of data you have to diagnose yourself: family history, vital signs, waist circumference, and the standard fasting lab panel done at your doctor's office. **Rule #4: Get the numbers.**

• *Family history.* The good news is you know your family history better than your doctor does. That being said, it's important to write down and give your doctor a list of the diseases your parents, grandparents, aunts, and uncles had and how they died. At the same time, just because you have a family history of a certain disease doesn't mean it's genetic. Virtually every chronic disease is *polygenic*, which means that multiple genes are involved in risk; and by most scientists' estimations, genetics accounts for a maximum of 50 percent of the risk, and usually less. No one gene is going to answer all questions (now with 23andMe, your genetic risk profile can be assessed, but for chronic diseases it's pretty useless).

For instance, let's say you're tall, but both of your parents are medium height. How could this happen? When I went to medical school in 1976, the joke was it was the 3M hypothesis—a "mistake," "mutation," or the "milkman." We've learned a lot in forty-five years; now we know there are forty-four genes that determine your height. Probability is like playing craps in Las Vegas—on any given role of the dice, a 7 is most likely to come up because there are more combinations of that than any other number.

Well, on any given roll of the genetic dice, what's the most likely result? You would get equal numbers of tall (twenty-two) and short (twenty-two) genes from both parents, so you'd be an average of the two. But on any given roll of the sperm-egg combinations, maybe you got all the tall genes and none of the short genes. Or you could just as easily have lost the genetic lottery, getting all the short genes instead.

Now, let's talk obesity. There are thirty-nine genes that determine risk here. Only two—called MC_4R and FTO—have any real clinical import, and are only found in about 16 percent of the obese population, never mind the general population. If you had every other obesity risk gene, it would only explain ten kilograms or twenty-two pounds of weight, hardly enough to explain the population rise in obesity. Genetics are important, but not the biggest reason for obesity.

Similarly, for Alzheimer's disease, even if you have a double dose of the high-risk ApoE4 gene, your risk is nine times higher than the general population—that's high, but still not remotely a fait accompli. Nonetheless, knowing your family history can help you determine relative risk.

The good news is that for chronic disease, genetics only explains about 15 percent of the variance in risk. The other 85 percent is environmental, which means there's plenty you can do to mitigate your risk for diabetes, cancer, heart disease, dementia, and virtually every other chronic disease. Just because your mother developed diabetes doesn't mean you're going to get it. She probably got it through her 85 percent environmental risk, and her risk is likely the same as yours—because you eat the same processed food that she introduced you to. The bad news is that what your mom ate while you were gestating inside her womb likely had its own effects. It changed the expression of your DNA—called *epigenetics* (see Chapter 7). So, if she was obese during her pregnancy, your epigenetics were changed, putting you at greater risk for disease. However, if she had bariatric surgery between the birth of you and your sibling, then your sibling didn't suffer those same epigenetic changes. This is why family history is even more important than genetics—it takes both genetics *and* epigenetics into account. But in no way is any of this information a death sentence. You can't alter the *propensity* for chronic disease, but you can alter the *outcome* once you know what to do.

• *Vital signs.* In general, your vital signs are always normal or you wouldn't be walking around or reading this book. If they were abnormal, you would likely be in an ICU hooked up to a dopamine drip or an EKG monitor, with a balloon catheter in your aorta, sucking on some oxygen through an endotracheal tube. However, there are nuances of normal. Your pulse rate and blood pressure are very much dependent on your psychological state. If you're at the doctor's office, you're likely already anxious. Your pulse rate may be 5 to 10 beats per minute higher, and your systolic blood pressure 5 points higher than your baseline, just from fear and activation of the sympathetic nervous system, which is your body's fight-or-flight mechanism.

However, if your blood pressure rises at the doctor's office above 130/90 on the first measurement and then goes down on the second, this is often referred to as *white-coat hypertension*, and is usually passed off by your doctor as benign. It's not. Having white-coat hypertension is a sign that you have an overly active sympathetic nervous system (which would have served you well in ancient times when you needed to flee lions), putting you at increased risk for permanent hypertension later in life. The question is whether you can obtain your baseline vital signs at home and away from the doctor's office—and, most important, while you're sleeping. You can buy a finger blood pressure cuff at your local pharmacy to check your blood pressure at home, both before you go to sleep and immediately upon waking but *before* you get out of bed. This is when psychological forces and your sympathetic nervous system are minimized. If you do have hypertension, your doctor might send you home with an ambulatory blood pressure monitor (ABPM) to wear overnight to see if your vital signs reduce while sleeping. If they come down, you're likely in the clear. But if they remain elevated, then you perhaps might actually need a medicine for high blood pressure.

Doctors' assessments of blood pressure have continued to change as well. When I was in medical school in the 1970s, a blood pressure of 140/90 was considered the upper limit of normal. Then, due to the high incidence of stroke in the population in the 1990s (or was it the appearance of anti-hypertensive drugs on the market?), this threshold was ratcheted down to 130/85. Then, we learned that every extra 2 mm of mercury to the blood pressure reading increases the risk for stroke by 10 percent. So in 2019, the upper limits were reduced again, this time to 125/80.

So is your blood pressure really normal? Refer to the American Heart Association guidance for whether you should worry about it; your doctor doesn't always keep up with the newest data.

Pulse rate and blood pressure are both highly variable, and much of the variability depends on age, sex, race, BMI, pregnancy, exercise capacity, and, most important, diet—especially processed food. Most people talk about the dietary salt in processed food as being the most important factor in hypertension, because when it was reduced in the UK, the prevalence of stroke declined. And for about 20 percent of the public, that's absolutely true—they're exquisitely salt-sensitive and consistently need their dietary salt restricted. But most people with functioning kidneys should be able get rid of their excess salt just fine. So why aren't they? Because we're dealing with a population-level epidemic of insulin resistance.

One downstream manifestation of insulin resistance and hyper-insulinemia is being unable to excrete excess salt, which drives up blood pressure. Furthermore, sugar directly increases blood pressure by increasing uric acid (see Chapter 2). Therefore, cutting salt consumption to reduce hypertension works, but only in the face of underlying insulin resistance—the result of our processed food pandemic. If your nighttime blood pressure is higher than normal and doesn't come down during sleep, you might consider reducing your sugar intake for a week, and repeating the exercise to see if it helps.

Waist circumference. Waist circumference is a sign of either visceral (belly) fat, liver fat, or both. All the diseases of metabolic syndrome are associated with increased waist circumference—even in normal weight people—and so waist circumference is much more sensitive for disease risk than is BMI; in fact, waist circumference is increasing faster than BMI in the population, because it's the visceral fat that's going up more than the subcutaneous fat. An increased waist circumference suggests inflammation (leaky gut), mitochondrial dysfunction, and insulin resistance (three of the eight subcellular pathways; see Chapter 7), as well as oxidative stress. All in all, waist circumference is the biggest clue of all, and it's free. Adult males should have a waist circumference of less than 40 inches, and adult females less than 35 inches. Don't have a tape measure? Just use your belt size.

Fasting lab tests. There's a boatload of information to be gleaned from fasting lab tests, but it often takes an experienced clinician who's up-to-date in their medical knowledge and expertise to know how to order and interpret them properly. Here's the list of the tests you need to make sure your doctor orders: lipid profile (LDL-C, HDL-C, TG), homocysteine (Hcy) level, alanine aminotransferase and aspartate aminotransferase (ALT and AST), uric acid, fasting insulin, fasting glucose, and hemoglobin A_{1c}.

First, since you want to assess diet and risk for heart disease, let's start with the lipid profile. Virtually everyone in America (children, too) now gets a fasting lipid profile (aka cholesterol test). It's actually a better assessment of insulin resistance than it is heart disease—but there's a lot more to the lipid profile than meets the eye. The absolute numbers themselves mean very little, and total cholesterol means less than nothing. In fact, it's actually detrimental—and the FDA knows it, which is why they've removed dietary cholesterol from the Nutrition Facts label (see Chapter 24). Rather, it's the pattern and ratio of the various lipid fractions that are important (see Chapter 2). Remember, the LDL particle number (LDL-P), rather than the LDL cholesterol level (LDL-C), is what we care about, because it factors out the dilution of the large buoyant LDLs that aren't important. But LDL-P is still considered a research test and done in only a few specialized labs around the country. It's also not usually covered by health insurance. So then, how do you determine if you have large buoyant or small dense LDL?

The serum triglyceride (TG), when unloaded of its fat at the adipose tissue, becomes the small dense LDL. Therefore, the TG:HDL (high-density lipoprotein) ratio—the real ratio of bad to good cholesterol—is the best biomarker of small dense LDL, the best biomarker of cardiovascular disease, and the best surrogate marker of insulin resistance and metabolic syndrome. The reason TGs were ignored until now is that we had statins as treatment for high LDL-C, but until about fifteen years ago, we didn't have treatment for high TG levels other than diet, which doctors didn't employ.

The second thing to look at is the HDL. If it's over 60, it almost doesn't matter what the other fractions are, as this is a sign of good cardiovascular health. If the HDL is under 40 (men) or under 50 (women), then your predisposition for heart disease is much higher.

The third thing to look at is the LDL-cholesterol. If it's below 100, the small dense fraction can't be high enough to be harmful. If it's over 300, you might have the rare genetic disease familial hypercholesterolemia (FH) and you can't clear your LDL, in which case a low-fat diet, and likely a statin added, will be essential to prevent a future heart attack. If it's between 100 and 300, then you need to look at the TG level. If the TG level is above 150, that's metabolic syndrome until proven otherwise. Finally, tell your doctor to look at your TG:HDL ratio. For reasons that are completely unclear, race matters with TG levels. If it's over 2.5 in Caucasians or over 1.5 in African Americans, that's a

correlate of metabolic syndrome. Your doctor needs all this information to prognosticate on your behalf, and she has to understand what
she is looking for, and why.

But there is yet another dietary pathway to heart disease, and it has
nothing to do with LDL or triglycerides. If you have a family history of
heart disease, tell your doctor to look at your diet and epigenetics by
drawing a serum homocysteine (Hcy) level. This is a lab test that is not
routinely ordered because it's not correlated with genetics and heart
disease, only with diet and heart disease. Hcy is an amino acid associated with heart disease, but it does not come from eating protein. Hcy
should be completely cleared from the bloodstream and eradicated or it
will build up in the blood vessel and cause inflammation. The enzyme
that clears Hcy is responsive to the vitamin folic acid. But if you have
low folic acid in your diet, or you're on chemotherapy, such as metho-
trexate, or you have a genetic problem with this enzyme, then your Hcy
levels go up and your risk for heart disease goes up as well.

Fourth, you need to assess diet and liver function. As stated before,
while not specific for liver fat accumulation, the liver enzyme alanine
aminotransferase (ALT) is easy to assess and reasonably sensitive and
specific for measuring the degree of liver fat. If it's over 25, you definitely should investigate further. You also want to look at the aspartate
aminotransferase (AST) level, which is a measure of mitochondrial
function. AST levels rise acutely with alcohol or acetaminophen consumption, but also with hepatitis from any cause. If the AST is elevated,
you can assume your liver is either under acute (infectious, alcohol-, or
toxin-related) assault, and if your ALT is elevated, then it's likely under chronic metabolic assault (e.g., liver fat). If both are elevated, you
then want to know whether there's been any liver damage. For that your
doctor will need to order a nonstandard but inexpensive test called a
gamma-glutamyl transpeptidase, or GGT. If this is over 35, you've got
a problem, and likely need a liver ultrasound to assess your liver fat.
You're also going to need to do something different about your sugar
and alcohol consumption or both.

Fifth, you can also assess diet and mitochondrial function by measuring uric acid, which rises with sugar consumption. High uric acid levels lead to gout and hypertension, and also generate liver fat. Uric acid is a by-product of liver carbohydrate metabolism, especially when it metabolizes sugar. This prevents the mitochondria from metabolizing pyruvic acid to carbon dioxide, which forces the liver to turn excess energy into liver fat. Levels above 5.5 indicate mitochondrial dysfunction and insulin resistance.

Sixth, you want to investigate glucose control parameters. Every practitioner gets a fasting glucose on all their adult patients, looking for type 2 diabetes. Yet this is the single worst parameter to measure, because it's the last thing to change. Once the fasting glucose rises over 100 mg/dl (signifying glucose intolerance; 126 means diabetes), metabolic syndrome is in full force, and there are no options for prevention anymore; now you're in full-fledged treatment mode. But in fact, a fasting blood glucose of 90 is already questionable. The same is true for hemoglobin A_{1c} (HbA_{1c}), the blood test that assesses glucose control over the preceding three months. By everyone's estimation, under 5.5 percent is normal, while over 6.5 percent is frank type 2 diabetes. It's what goes on in between that's up for grabs, and it's in this gray zone where most adults live. The higher it is, the greater the glycemic excursions, and the more risk for metabolic disease. The body will do everything it can to maintain a fasting serum glucose below 100, including increasing the insulin (that's insulin resistance!). So, irrespective of the fasting glucose, you want to have a simultaneous fasting insulin level, which tells you how hard the pancreas is working. A fasting insulin of greater than 15 microunits/ml usually means significant insulin resistance, and risk for metabolic disease. From the glucose and insulin levels together, you can calculate an index called the *homeostatic model assessment of insulin resistance* (HOMA-IR = glucose x insulin ÷ 405), which assesses your risk for diabetes. A HOMA-IR of less than 2.8 is excellent, 4.3 is average, and anything higher means trouble.

However, many academic societies (including the American Diabetes Association) don't advocate getting a fasting insulin level. They have several arguments against it such as cost (about $15), reproducibility, and the fact that fasting insulin doesn't correlate with BMI—which is exactly the point. It's *not* about obesity; it's about metabolic health. If you don't measure fasting insulin, you're missing all the TOFIs—the normal-weight metabolically ill people (see Chapter 2).

Further, there are two insulin disorders associated with obesity. A fasting insulin will only tell you about insulin resistance, but won't tell you about insulin hypersecretion, which drives weight gain but not metabolic syndrome. In order to make the diagnosis, you have to stimulate the beta-cell with an oral glucose tolerance test (OGTT) with insulin levels. Most doctors don't know about insulin hypersecretion, because they've never looked for it—but you wouldn't know you need to look for it if you hadn't gotten a normal fasting insulin first.

Ultimately, if you're obese, you've got a 75 percent chance that you're insulin resistant, a 10 percent chance you're an insulin hyper-secretor, or a 5 percent chance you're both at the same time. And since rational treatment is dependent on the pathology, at UCSF we were very quick to perform a three-hour oral glucose tolerance test (OGTT) with insulin levels (see Chapter 14). From these data we can compute indices of insulin secretion and resistance, which will help determine what diet pattern might work best for each patient. **Table 9-1** lists the disease processes and the lab tests that will alert you to them.

	Laboratory
Fatty liver disease	ALT >25 in Caucasians, >20 in African Americans, >30 in Latinos
	GGT >35
	Uric acid > 5.5
Glucose intolerance	Fasting glucose > 100 or 2-hour glucose > 140; HbA_{1c} > 6.0 percent
Type 2 diabetes mellitus	Fasting glucose > 125 or 2-hour glucose > 200; HbA_{1c} > 6.5 percent
Dyslipidemia and heart disease	Lipid profile: TG > 150, HDL < 40, TG:HDL > 2.5, LDL-C >300, LDL-P >1000
	Homocysteine > 15
Insulin resistance	Fasting insulin > 15
Insulin hypersecretion	3-hour OGTT with insulin levels; measure insulin secretion and resistance indices

Table 9–1: Lab tests for chronic metabolic disease and normal ranges

Mitochondria under the Microscope

Why go through this painful exercise? Chronic disease has many definitions—but perhaps the best one is: how well your mitochondria perform at baseline and in response to the stress of living and eating. If your mitochondria are fresh, fit, and functional, it doesn't matter how much you weigh. If your mitochondria are dull, dilapidated, and under duress, it also doesn't matter how much you weigh. But there's no simple blood test for mitochondria, which is why doctors don't know how to assess them. But you will, because now you have all the clues assembled. And then you will know what types of food and food pattern might be best for you.

Your waist circumference is a key. If it's high, expect that there is some metabolic problem, and that you will have to change your diet to improve your insulin resistance.

If your waist circumference is high and your blood pressure is also high, assume the problem is sugar, not salt. If your blood pressure is high and your waist circumference is low, the problem might be salt or stress.

Fresh, fit, and functional mitochondria burn glucose and ketones to completion (see Chapter 8), and generate few oxygen radicals. They don't need insulin to work, so insulin stays low. Mitochondria are inhibited by uric acid, low folate, and fructose, which both cause mitochondria to be overwhelmed in order to divert energy to fatty acid and triglyceride production. Signs of poor mitochondrial function are high uric acid and high homocysteine. Signs of liver fat are high ALT and high fasting insulin. Signs of poor peripheral clearance of fat are a high triglyceride and a low HDL. This pattern would argue for reducing your refined carbohydrate and sugar consumption. Conversely, signs of poor liver clearance of fat include a high LDL without a concomitant high triglyceride, as well as a normal fasting insulin level. This pattern would argue for a very low-fat diet. Last, if none of these are true, but your weight is still a problem, then you might be an MHO and insulin hypersecretor, in which case your doctor could be persuaded to perform the three-hour OGTT; or if not, you might try a very low-carb diet to suppress insulin release.

Once you know your family history, anthropometric, and metabolic status, it's much easier to figure out what kind of diet intervention you need (e.g., low-carb, low-fat, paleo, keto, vegan, Mediterranean, low salt). From there, match it with your cultural and religious preferences, and see it go to work. Be forewarned: there's no processed food on any menu.

CHAPTER 10

Foodable, Not Druggable

Chronic diseases have been known to medicine for at least a millennium, but they've come to dominate medicine in the span of just fifty years. Currently, 88 percent of Americans are metabolically ill, irrespective of weight. As stated in Chapter 2, obesity is a red herring. It's a symptom of the disease, not the cause. The Endocrine Society has finally acknowledged this fact by issuing guidelines that implore physicians to check for metabolic health apart from obesity.

There are three commonalities to all the diseases that we call metabolic syndrome: 1) despite all efforts, these diseases are all increasing in incidence, prevalence, and severity at a faster rate than obesity; 2) they're all exacerbated by obesity, although not specifically caused by it; and 3) while there are drugs to treat the *symptoms* of each one (including obesity), there are no drugs to either treat, cure, or prevent the diseases themselves. Further, as explained in Chapter 2, physicians treat the symptoms of each of these diseases with drugs, in order to prevent other disastrous sequelae like stroke, heart attack, amputation, or dialysis. And that's because each of these diseases is due to problems inside the cell—and we don't have medicines to treat them. Therefore, none of these diseases will remit, no matter the drug. The patient will continue their inexorable slide to oblivion, whether it be diabetes or cirrhosis or dementia—and if they don't die of one of those diseases, then they'll most assuredly develop another because the subcellular pathologies are still there. The three enzyme checkpoints (Chapter 8) are still dyssynchronized.

A Bitter Pill to Swallow

However, every single one of these pathologies can be prevented, mitigated, and in many cases reversed, by changes in diet. And none of these changes in diet have anything to do with calorie restriction. In most cases, reversal can be accomplished just by removing processed food and substituting Real Food (see **Part IV** for a full definition of each component and its disease potential).

Let's take mitochondria as an example. While lots of research on treating mitochondrial disease is underway, no drug has yet made it to market. People will try to sell you stuff that purports to be a mitochondrial tonic, a wonder drug—just check out Amazon. There's a lot of charlatanism in this space. For instance, coenzyme Q10 has been shown to be ineffective against the diseases of metabolic syndrome, with the exception of heart failure (which isn't a disease of metabolic syndrome). These supplements don't get where they need to go in the cell to be effective, but because they are *nutraceuticals* (a food with purported health properties), the FDA can't regulate them (see Chapter 24).

There's a reason that drugs and nutraceuticals don't work for metabolic syndrome. If you look at those eight subcellular pathologies at the biochemical level and 1) examine their transcription factors (the proteins that turn them on); 2) their co-activators and co-repressors (the proteins that bind to the DNA to amplify or inhibit them); and 3) their second messengers (proteins that mediate the effects within the cell), our drugs don't touch them. None of the underlying causes are responsive to medicines in our current drug armamentarium (see Chapter 14). Treating the symptom doesn't treat the problem.

However, all of them are driven by, and therefore responsive to, specific components of food, because Real Food gets where it needs to inside the cell. People think processed food is food, because it's calories and macronutrients, but in fact processed food gets in and poisons those pathways instead.

People think supplements are the antidote for bad food. They're not. Rather, Real Food is the treatment, while bad food is the poison. In particular, we've learned that sugar, the main component of processed food, is the primary driver of four chronic diseases. It's also a likely candidate for another five, listed in order below. These nine diseases together total about 75 percent of the healthcare burden in the US, and 60 percent globally. Processed food is behind them all, sugar makes them worse, and there's no drug that prevents or reverses any of them. Below is a comparison of how well drugs versus food work to ameliorate these nine different chronic diseases.

Diabetes—the Modern Scourge

To this day, the American Diabetes Association continues to tout drug therapy to reduce blood glucose levels as the prime directive of diabetes therapy. They also promote weight loss as the primary strategy for prevention. While it's true that a 10 percent weight loss over one year can reverse type 2 diabetes, only 30 percent of the subjects were able to achieve it, leaving most people out in the cold. The ADA doesn't own up to the fact that diabetes can be reversed by dietary changes apart from weight loss, and their own dietary recommendations fall short on many counts.

Changes in food composition instead of quantity accomplishes the same result, which is exactly what Virta Health attempted to do. Using a ketogenic diet (see Chapter 14) for two years without caloric restriction, they reversed diabetes in 80 percent of their patients, were able to discontinue insulin in 94 percent of their patients who were injecting, and induced a twenty-nine-pound weight loss as well.

It's the consumption of refined carbohydrate that's associated with type 2 diabetes. In particular, dietary sugar, even more than starch, drives the metabolic reactions that lead to type 2 diabetes, especially because of effects in the mitochondria. The glucose in the dietary sugar drives the insulin release, which drives the weight gain, while the fructose drives the liver fat accumulation that drives the insulin resistance. Processed food is the primary vehicle.

While drugs can lower the plasma glucose, they can't reverse the insulin secretion driving the weight gain, or the insulin resistance at the core of the disease. Furthermore, mitochondria generate more oxygen radicals with processed food than with Real Food. New studies from the UK and Europe demonstrate that it's the degree of food processing that predicts diabetes (see Chapter 17). Food can either prevent, cause, or reverse diabetes. Drugs may lower the blood glucose, but they can't fix the diabetes.

Heart Disease—Don't Have a Coronary . . .

In Chapter 2, we saw that statins lower LDL-C, but don't reduce risk of heart attack (except in those who've already had one). One scientific study argued that triglyceride-lowering agents, such as fenofibrate, could prevent deaths from coronary events. But then the authors of that report issued a correction that amended the finding to total nonfatal events, so it's not as clear what fibrates really do. On the other hand, fish oil, a dietary supplement, reduced incidence of heart attack by 8 percent—as well if not better than statins—because most of us are omega-3 deficient to start with (see Chapter 19).

It's processed food that foments heart disease risk. The relationship between food and heart disease is somewhat more complex than that of diabetes. The first issue is the role of omega-3 fatty acids (see Chapter 19), which act in two ways: by reducing general levels of inflammation, risks for heart disease are lower; and by reducing serum triglyceride levels, there's less chance of plaque buildup. The second issue is insulin, because insulin increases coronary artery smooth muscle proliferation, making it more likely to get a clot. And the third issue is sugar—the percent of calories in the diet as added sugar predicts risk for dying of a heart attack, exclusive of calories or obesity. Conversely, removing added sugar from the diet removes the atherogenic particles (the small dense LDL), lowers triglycerides, and raises HDL—all protective against heart disease.

Nonalcoholic Fatty Liver Disease (NAFLD)—Human Foie Gras

NAFLD is now the leading cause of liver transplant in the US. It was unheard of prior to 1980, and now affects 25 percent of the world's population, and 40 percent of the adult US population. Every pharmaceutical company is looking for the magic bullet to treat or reverse it. Scientists have tried novel drugs with funny-sounding names (obeticholic acid, selonsertib, elafibranor, cenicriviroc), but the best of them demonstrated only a 10 to 30 percent success rate. Noticing a common theme here? Drugs don't do it. But diet does.

While many things in the environment can damage the liver, there are two stages of fatty liver disease both driven at least in part by processed food and drinks. And guess what? Alcohol and soda have the same detrimental effects. The first stage is the deposition of liver fat, and the second is inflammation. If you eat a processed food diet, you're vulnerable at both stages. The high fructose content in sugar-sweetened beverages and the high *trans*-fat content in highly processed and fried food (even though *trans*-fats have been removed by the FDA from processed food, the heat of frying can create them anyway; see Chapter 18) are damaging at both stages. In fact, sugar-sweetened beverage consumption has been shown to be an independent predictor of NAFLD.

Tooth Decay and Periodontitis—Oral Hazard

The primary role of sugar in dental caries is and has been quite clear for at least a century (see Chapter 5). But what hasn't been discussed is the relationship between caries and other metabolic syndrome diseases.

Doctors don't think about the mouth, because we're not trained to. Dentists don't think about the heart or liver, because they're not trained to. But the same processes are going on everywhere, and there's a strong association between the rotting of your teeth and your liver. Dental caries are associated with NAFLD, whether separately or linked is undetermined, but the instigator of both is sugar.

There's an even more pernicious disease process going on in the mouth—periodontitis, which affects half of all Americans. There's no question that periodontitis is associated with heart disease; there are defined mechanisms linking the two. But that's not even the big kahuna. How about oral disease and dementia? Another oral bacterium, *Porphyromonas gingivalis*, has been associated with the development of Alzheimer's, and researchers have found DNA for *P. gingivalis* in the brains of people who died from it. How did it get from the mouth to the brain? And what is it doing there? We don't know yet, but we know it's concerning.

Cancer—the Emperor of All Maladies

Like diabetes and heart disease, the degree of food processing has been shown to increase risk for cancer, regardless of calories or obesity. Chapter 8 explained why; if you stimulate PI3-kinase, block AMP-kinase, and disinhibit mTOR, you're going to drive cell growth and risk for cancer. Sugar does the same thing. In fact, sugar consumption has been implicated in many cancers of endodermal (the inner lining of the embryo) origin, including breast, lung, bladder, ovarian, and pancreatic cancer. It also increases risk for cancer recurrence. But sugar is just one reason as to why processed food drives cancer.

Refined carbohydrate is its own driver, by increasing insulin release. Processed meats are laden with nitrates, known to cause colon cancer and breast cancer. And fiber has been known to prevent colon cancer for decades, but did you know that fiber can also prevent breast cancer? Processed food is dangerous because of the lack of fiber—thus flooding the liver and starving the gut (see Chapter 11). This is why cancer centers like Memorial Sloan Kettering in New York and MD Anderson in Houston are experimenting with fiber-rich and low-carb diets in many cancer treatment plans.

Dementia—Brain Drain

Given the $290 billion annual cost of dementia in the US and that there've been 146 failed trials, it's almost laughable that we keep trying to develop a drug. The fact of the matter is, diabetics are four times more likely to develop dementia than the general population. Furthermore, both forms (Alzheimer's disease and vascular dementia) are increased in people with diabetes—because insulin resistance affects the brain.

New research shows that sugar consumption is associated with the development of Alzheimer's disease. It appears that fructose alters mitochondrial function in the brain, reducing energy generation, which puts the identified neuronal proteins amyloid and tau at risk for clumping, forming the classic *neurofibrillary tangles* of Alzheimer's. A processed food eating pattern has been shown to be predictive of future Alzheimer's disease, although no one has yet demonstrated that switching to Real Food lessens one's risk.

Obstructive Sleep Apnea (OSA)—Not a Snoozer

OSA has many causes, many unrelated to body weight (see Chapter 16). But obesity of the neck can reduce the diameter of the airway, cutting down on oxygen delivery to the lungs, which causes fitful and restless sleep. The sympathetic nervous system and stress hormones get kicked up when you don't sleep, and the cortisol spikes drive insulin resistance. Lack of sleep also increases the hormone ghrelin, which makes you eat more, driving weight gain. But there's a reciprocal relationship between OSA and metabolic disease—the lack of oxygen to the liver likely inhibits AMP-kinase, causing the liver to turn more sugar into fat, thus increasing the amount of triglyceride and fomenting more obesity, inflammation, and heart disease.

Although OSA is clearly linked to obesity, which increases the risk of diabetes, there's also evidence that OSA can cause diabetes independent of obesity. Indeed, OSA, processed food, and metabolic syndrome travel together. One may lead to another and they often coexist.

Autoimmune Disease—the "Leak" in Your Gut

Autoimmune diseases are a disaster and there are no good medicines available (steroids work, but the treatment is worse than the disease). They've been around for centuries, but there's been a clear uptick in the last fifty years. Why? Two hypotheses have been proffered to explain it: the *barrier hypothesis* (our skin or lungs are letting in antigens) and the *hygiene hypothesis* (we don't eat dirt and are *too* hygienic). But in fact, in the gut, they're the same thing; because the gut is the dirtiest place in the world—one hundred trillion bacteria to have to fend off at all times—you don't need an intestine, you need a fortress. We've known for a while that leaky gut is akin to chinks in the walls of that fortress. Antigens, like enemy soldiers, escape through those chinks into the bloodstream, where T cells and antibodies react against them. But in a case of mistaken identity, these immune cells then accidentally identify parts of your body as foreign invaders and generate an immune response to kill them off, a process termed *molecular mimicry*.

Then there are two new twists. First, it appears that one autoimmune disease, called *ankylosing spondylitis*, produces antibodies to a gut bacterium called *Klebsiella pneumoniae*. Conversely, a different autoimmune disease called *rheumatoid arthritis* produces antibodies to a second gut bacterium called *Proteus mirabilis*. Now, this might not seem that earth-shattering, but recent work has shown that the refined carbohydrates in processed food feed those two bacteria in particular, and that carbohydrate restriction improves both of these diseases.

Indeed, a low-sugar, high-fiber Mediterranean diet has been shown to be efficacious at prevention and treatment of rheumatoid arthritis. Furthermore, introduction of fiber to the diet appears to improve asthma (frequently an autoimmune disease), likely by improving gut function and reducing inflammation.

Depression—the Moody Blues

Insulin resistance has been shown to be a primary cause of clinical depression in humans. Sugar is a specific driver of insulin resistance, and one cause of depression in both rats and humans. So it should be no surprise to anyone that two studies, one in Europe and one in China, showed that ultra-processed food consumption is associated with depression in people.

The foods that drive metabolic syndrome are those that are most clearly associated with the foods that people binge on—refined carbs and sugar. The question is, does the depression drive the food choices, which then drive the metabolic syndrome; or do the food choices drive the metabolic syndrome, which then drives the depression? Which is cause and which is effect? We still don't know. But what we do know is that many people can eat their way both out of their metabolic disease *and* out of the depression by switching to a Mediterranean diet. The fact that your food choices can lift your mood certainly argues that the food is one driver, though many changes in our society are associated with depression and other mood disorders.

You Can't Outrun a Bad Diet

Inquiring minds want to know: can't I just exercise past my bad diet? Won't an extra ten minutes on the elliptical trainer solve everything? Amateur Finnish triathlete Sami Inkinen tried and failed. Sami was one of the original founders of Nokia, sold his share early, and moved to the US to attend Stanford Business School. There he started the real estate website Trulia, which was bought by Zillow for $2.5 billion. In other words, Sami had more money than God—and he exercised five hours per day.

Nevertheless, by age thirty-eight, his performance was down. His glucose tolerance test revealed that he was a prediabetic. He didn't get it—how can a triathlete be a prediabetic? He consulted UC Davis professor and low-carb physician Dr. Stephen Phinney, who had the answer: it was the sports drinks. Caffeine has its own effect on insulin resistance separate from fructose, and together they can cause their own brand of insulin resistance and glucose intolerance, ratcheting down some of the beneficial effects of exercise.

Point being, exercise without dietary change can help to affect five of the eight subcellular pathologies (see Chapter 7): mitochondrial dysfunction by generating newer and fresher mitochondria; insulin resistance by reducing skeletal muscle and liver fat; improvement of propensities toward autophagy and reduce inflammatory markers; and maybe even epigenetics, although this effect appears to be mediated through exercise's suppression of inflammation. However, exercise alone won't improve glycation, oxidative stress (exercise actually makes this worse), or membrane integrity and fluidity. In other words, you can stop some of the aftermath of bad food by engaging in exercise, but exercise can't undo it all.

Recognizing the limitations of exercise on health improvement, Sami, Steve, and low-carb physiologist Jeff Volek went on to found Virta Health, a ketogenic diet start-up that proves diet matters more than exercise in reversing type 2 diabetes. The results have been impressive, so much so that the former chief medical officer of the American Diabetes Association, Dr. Robert Ratner, signed on to be their chief executive officer after having previously eschewed the low-carb diet.

The bottom line of this complete scientific analysis is that processed food results in acceleration of the eight subcellular pathologies that lead to metabolic dysfunction, inappropriate cell proliferation, and cell death. Nutrition, on the other hand, is the overarching paradigm to live a long and healthy life free from disease. There's no pill for this. Exercise alone can help mitigate some of the damage, but not all. *It's about the food.*

As you will see in **Part III**, nutrition is easy to do right, as we did it for ten thousand years. But sadly, it's even easier to do wrong, and that's what we've stupidly done for the last fifty.

Part III

Notes from the
Nutritional Battlefield

CHAPTER 11

What Does "Healthy"
Really Mean?

Which is worse: no food or bad food? The answer might seem obvious, but it's not. In fact, when I asked José Graziano da Silva, the former director general of the UN Food and Agriculture Organization (FAO; part of the WHO, located in Rome), he didn't have an answer—and for good reason.

The pains of hunger are real and acute, but the pains associated with limb amputation and burning in your toes (peripheral neuropathy) from type 2 diabetes can be likewise incapacitating. No food is usually the *result* of upheavals such as drought, floods, war, or pandemics. The FAO estimates 140 million people were starving worldwide in 2019, and this is increasing to 270 million in 2020 because of COVID-19. This social upheaval is heart-wrenching, but it's a statistic that might move people to action and donation, as there's a resulting imperative to improve. On the other end of the spectrum, bad food isn't the result of upheavals, as it's been engineered to be insidious. It's very bad *chronically*, as it is the *cause* of NCDs, social disparities, healthcare collapse, mental health crises, societal devolution, and in time, an even greater risk for social upheaval. Ultimately, even more people die—just slower, and it's under the wire, as the cause isn't as clear, so no one does anything about it, and it only gets worse. In addition, bad food puts you at increased risk of getting seriously ill or dying from COVID-19 (see Chapter 13). You don't know you're dying until it's too late, you don't know why, and you and society have racked up untoward medical, productivity, societal, and environmental costs in the process.

Nutrition vs. Nutritionism

Nutrition is the most important and malleable factor influencing people's life span (how long we live) and health span (how well we live). Studies on fraternal vs. identical twins show that genetics account for 25 to 30 percent of a person's longevity. The other 70 to 75 percent proves that while favorable genetics clearly play a role, the environment, including a bad diet, can easily overcome those gifts, hence why the US has seen reduced life expectancy four years in a row. It's impossible to specifically calculate what percentage of someone's life span is attributable to nutrition, but given what's happened to chronic disease incidence, prevalence, and severity statistics over the last fifty years, food plays a huge role. It always has.

But what is it about the food? Everyone has a theory, but very few facts—and those facts are being ignored by various stakeholders in order to tout their own ideas and advance their own agendas. That includes the public (see Chapter 12), because everyone's a nutrition "expert"; after all, each and every human is their own "n of 1"; that is, they have their own experience as to what worked (or didn't work) for them, but they have no idea of what works for you.

Since the publication of *The Omnivore's Dilemma* (2006), food journalist Michael Pollan has made the point that *nutrition is religion*—because it requires believing without seeing. After all, nutrition must be all about *what's in the food*. With the discovery of the first vitamin

(B$_1$, or thiamine) in 1912, scientists became convinced that there were chemicals in food that conferred health, so there must also be chemicals in food that conferred illness. This in turn has led to the concept of *nutrients* as being the lowest common denominator for any eating paradigm, giving rise to the religion of *nutritionism*. This is the procedure that the dietitians and the food industry have been promulgating for decades—just add up the good stuff and the bad stuff, and call it science! It's how we got the FDA food label (see Chapter 24), which empowered the plethora of nutritional pundits on YouTube and Reddit and Medium. You don't have to have an advanced degree to be a nutritionist. Which means that *everyone* is a nutritionist. And this has given rise to faith over science—because nutritionism is about zealotry.

The Knights of the Dinner Table

Every nutritional pundit has a drug to sell if they have money to invest in it to bring it to market. Otherwise, they have a supplement to sell, or at worst case, a diet. On their late night televised infomercials or on YouTube, they offer "n = 1" testimonials as to the power of their diet in reversing disease. All anecdote, no data.

Sometimes these infomercials are disguised as documentaries, in order to make them look fair and balanced. Look, if a moviemaker is making a documentary about diet and health, the opposite viewpoint must at least make an appearance at some point. Check out the latest fodder on vegan diets—for instance, *Forks Over Knives* (2011) or *The Game Changers* (2018), and find any mention of alternatives. I've had my own public run-in with Kip Andersen and protein-phobic Dr. Garth Davis, the director and talking head, over their scaremongering movie *What the Health* (2017) (an egg is the same as five cigarettes?); and all I can say is there wasn't any science offered in explanation, either in the movie or in the debate. But it's true on the other side of the street as well. Check out *The C Word* (2016), a story with an "n of 1" that extols the benefits of a ketogenic diet for cancer, and *The Magic Pill* (2017), which lauds dietary fat—no mention of any alternatives.

Nutritional mythology has never been more fervent than it is now, in part because life span and health span are declining—everyone wants to blame someone, or something, including me. But it has to be done with science. Otherwise nutrition is no better than hydroxychloroquine, just hearsay. It's time to adjust the current paradigm.

"Developed World" Kwashiorkor

In order to understand how diet affects our eight pathologies and three enzymes, you need to understand the difference between nutrient deficiency and excess. If we feed a healthy individual with the "right" amount of calories per day—say 2,500 to 3,000—but provide only sugar as the food source (say 700 grams/day), that person will exhibit *weight loss* and not survive more than two to three weeks. In contrast, as we saw in the documentary *Super Size Me* (2004) by Morgan Spurlock, the same number of calories supplied as processed food rapidly devolves into massive *weight gain* with miserable and adverse health outcomes.

It's more than enough calories in both cases; one caused weight loss, and the other weight gain—but both put health at risk. As Mr. Spurlock developed nutrient excess (energy), he also became nutrient deficient (micronutrients). Nutrient deficiency diseases can bear striking resemblances to nutrient excess diseases.

Recall two different diseases made known to the public in the 1960s as the US attempted to solve the malnutrition epidemic in Africa; marasmus and kwashiorkor. Marasmus babies are "skin and bones"; they don't get enough to eat, and suffer from protein *and* calorie deficiency. This is what happens if you consume straight sugar for three weeks; sugar alone without any nutrients can't even be absorbed from the intestine. Kwashiorkor is a different disease, resulting from protein deficiency *without* calorie deficiency. These babies have huge bellies because their livers are filled with fat—they've got nonalcoholic fatty liver disease (NAFLD). What caused the fatty liver? Cassava flour—a high-carbohydrate, low-fiber food, resulting in glycation, oxidative stress, mitochondrial dysfunction, insulin resistance, poor membrane integrity, and inflammation (see Chapter 7). In other words, they have "developing world" metabolic syndrome. Well, guess what? We have instead "developed world" kwashiorkor.

People with metabolic syndrome are frequently both overnourished and undernourished. They consume plenty of calories, but they are also deficient in rare amino acids like tryptophan (needed to make serotonin) and methionine (needed to make glutathione, the liver antioxidant). They're deficient in micronutrients once the grains have been stripped of their germ (location of the vitamins, polyphenols, and minerals).

Another disease explains the dissociation of overnutrition and obesity with metabolic syndrome. This disease, called *lipodystrophy*, is a disorder of subcutaneous fat production. Because people with lipodystrophy don't make fat cells, they are not obese; rather, any extra energy ends up as ectopic fat in the liver and muscle, which leads to all the diseases of metabolic syndrome.

Whether people get lipodystrophy has nothing to do with calories. No surprise, whether people get metabolic syndrome has nothing to do with calories. In each case, it has to do with whether the liver mitochondria is working right to process the energy to keep itself healthy. And in kwashiorkor, lipodystrophy, and metabolic syndrome, those mitochondria are not working right, leading to those eight subcellular pathologies (see Chapter 7). That's what chronic disease is really all about.

Nutritional Naysayers

There are several reasons why these truths took a back seat to mythology and why the science of nutrition took a wrong turn in favor of zealotry. First of all, most pundits in the field aren't bench scientists or clinicians; they tend to be nutritional epidemiologists, and nutritional epidemiology has significant limitations.

Epidemiology means *correlation*, not *causation*. Like John Snow's cholera/Broad Street pump exercise (see Chapter 2), nutritional epi-demiology studies are discovery, and discovery can be very important in posing the questions that truly need answering. However, it almost never answers the questions by itself; you need to design a proper study to answer them (see below). Just because A is associated with B, does that mean that A causes B? Or could it be reverse causality (B causes A)? Or could it be intermediate causality (C causes A or B)? Could it be irrelevant (C is associated with B and D, and D causes A)? As an example, ice cream consumption correlates with frequency of drownings. Does that mean eating ice cream causes you to drown? Or do survivors of the drowned victim bury their sorrows in a baked Alaska? More likely we eat ice cream when it's hot, we swim when it's hot, and some unfortunate people drown when they swim. Correlation does not automatically imply a cause-and-effect relationship. But the media, in its effort to sell newspapers or snatch eyeballs, treats almost all epidemiological studies as causation. Therefore, the public doesn't understand the difference either.

Some investigators and news sources tout *meta-analyses*, an attempt to conglomerate multiple studies. It's the gold standard to prove your point. And meta-analyses *can* do this well, when the individual studies are independent of industry and are also scientifically sound. But many such analyses are GIGO—"Garbage in garbage out"—as they are only as good as the data they are based on. And when the food industry is in charge, the results are suspect.

Another reason why nutrition remains an academic backwater is because we don't have good biomarkers (e.g., blood tests) that measure what people are actually eating. Most of the data in nutritional studies are obtained through memory recall to food questionnaires. You can see for yourself—try asking someone what they've eaten for the last three days. Most people can't tell you what they've eaten in the last three hours. Which doesn't even factor in that sometimes people lie, not always intentionally, but perhaps they put on rose-colored glasses when it comes to memory recall.

For example, Leann Birch at Penn State University asked a group of eleven-year-old girls what they ate, and videotaped them while they ate it. She then divided up the group into weight tertiles—thin, normal weight, overweight—and showed that the thin and normal weight kids reported correctly, while the overweight kids underestimated the candy, soda, and desserts that they ate—except for one item. They reported their juice intake correctly because they thought juice was healthy (we'll deal with juice more fully in Chapter 19).

Dr. John Ioannidis, an internist and accomplished statistician from Stanford University, has proposed that we do away with nutritional epidemiology entirely, as the studies are impossible to control, the data is perennially abused, and the results are virtually guaranteed to be wrong. I disagree. There's no doubt that people read too much into these studies, but they also need to be educated. No single nutrition epidemiology study is ever the final word, because they don't rise to the level of causation. There are only two types of studies that can approach the rarified air of causation. One, called *econometric analysis*, looks at the natural history of both consumption and disease prevalence, but also accounts both for confounders and for time (time is essential to causation). Developed by iconic UK statistician-epidemiologist Austin Bradford Hill, this level of evidence provides what we call *causal medical inference*; the level of proof we have today for tobacco and lung cancer. The second is called *randomized controlled trials* (RCTs), where the investigator varies only the one nutrient under study. However, such studies must have a placebo control group to be able to rise to the level of proof.

But, aside from study design, there's yet another and more prescient reason why these epidemiologic studies, even those that purportedly assess causation, are suspect. They measure what goes in the mouth and assume it's what's absorbed in the intestine and ends up in our bloodstream—which isn't true. Think of what really happens as analogous to eating for two. When pregnant, the mother's intake is wildly increased over baseline. She gains weight, but we don't care because we know about 30 percent of the energy is going to the growing fetus. Well, even without being pregnant, each of us is always eating for two, because we also have to feed our own intestinal microbiome, which receives and metabolizes about 30 percent of our ingested nutrients. If the nutrients didn't enter our bloodstream, did we really get them?

The discovery of our symbiotic relationship with our intestinal microbiome changed everything. We now know that we have to feed it to stay healthy. When we don't feed it right (e.g., depriving it of dietary protein), those bacteria send blood-borne and neural signals that tell our brains to alter our behavior so that they can get the nutrition that they do need. Whether you like it or not, you're eating for two—you're in a symbiotic relationship with your gut, and if you hurt your gut, your gut will hurt you back.

The argument I'll make throughout the rest of this book is that it's not *what's in the food*, it's *what's been done to the food* that matters. Because the real nutritional question is: who and what are you feeding? Are you feeding the human? Or are you feeding the intestinal microbiome? And is your liver working right based on the share that you get? Based on our current eating paradigm and Nutrition Facts label, you can't figure either of those two questions out.

Who Decides What's Healthy, and for Whom?

In a population where 88 percent have some level of metabolic dysfunction, the entire concept of healthy has been obfuscated. And who obfuscated it? All the usual suspects, plus some. The American Heart Association demonized saturated fat; we took the fat out of milk and got cheese and chocolate milk instead—but they're healthy, or so we're told. The American Diabetes Association pushed whole grains, so we foisted whole-grain bread on the public, except that as soon as it's milled, it's not whole grain anymore (see Chapter 19). The Academy of Nutrition and Dietetics told people that eggs had cholesterol, so Americans opted for refined carbs like breakfast cereal. But my personal all-time favorite is the U.S. Institute of Medicine, which in 2004 codified an upper limit for added sugar at 25 percent of total calories. In what universe is 25 percent of calories as added sugar justifiable? This gave the food industry carte blanche to add as much as they possibly could, making us sicker and sicker.

When it comes to food, the only labeling rule is for allergies like eggs, gluten, peanuts, shellfish, and the like—things that can kill people acutely. After that, anything goes (see Chapter 23). Most people trust and buy products based on the way they're promoted on the package, rather than their actual nutritional value, which still means nothing—because it's not *what's in the food*, it's *what's been done to the food* that counts. But that's nowhere to be found on the label.

My Definition of "Healthy"

The key to fending off chronic disease is to keep those eight subcellular pathways running right—and each and every one of them can be made to run right with two simple dictates:

1. **Protect the liver.** You have to protect the liver from fructose, glucose, branched-chain amino acids, omega-6 fatty acids, iron, and other oxidative stresses—all of which end up causing fat accumulation and liver damage, and generate insulin resistance. This can be done by either reducing the dose of dietary liver stressors (e.g., a low-sugar diet) or their flux (e.g., a high-fiber diet, which blocks sugar absorption, thus reducing the rate by which fructose and branched-chain amino acids reach the liver).

2. **Feed the gut.** If you don't feed your microbiome, your microbiome will feed on you; it will literally chew up the mucin layer that protects your intestinal epithelial cells, which increases the risk for leaky gut, inflammation, and more insulin resistance. The goal is to deliver more nutrients farther down the intestine (e.g., a high-fiber diet).

Fiber is an essential nutrient—not for only you, but also for your microbiome. The fiber in Real Food is of two kinds: soluble, which is globular, like what holds jelly together (e.g., psyllium, pectin, inulin);

and insoluble, like the stringy stuff in celery (e.g., cellulose, chitin, peptidoglycan). You need both, as they do different jobs; and you also need the geometry in order to make fiber work for you.

Here's a thought experiment: imagine a spaghetti colander. You run the water, it goes right through the holes. Now throw a glob of petroleum jelly into the center of the colander. You run the water, it might bounce off the jelly, but it still runs right through the holes. Finally, take your finger and rub the petroleum jelly all throughout the inside of the colander. Now run the water—you have an impenetrable barrier. When fiber (soluble and insoluble) is consumed within food, the insoluble fiber (stringy) forms a latticework on the inside of the duodenum, while the soluble fiber (globular) plugs the holes in the lattice. Together, along with this geometry, they form an impermeable barrier along the duodenal wall, which has numerous biological benefits. It's because of this geometry that dietary fiber, when occurring naturally in food and without adulteration, protects against metabolic syndrome—by protecting the liver and feeding the gut.

Cellulose is an insoluble fiber. Alone it could form the latticework, but not plug the holes. Psyllium is a soluble fiber. It can swell and absorb water, but can't lay down the scaffolding. To get the benefits on delay of absorption to protect the liver, you need both. Real Food has both. Could you put both into one pill? Perhaps. But the side effects would be highly problematic. Cellulose isn't compressible, so in order to lay down the latticework, you would have to take a high dose of cellulose. On the other hand, psyllium swells with exposure to water and doesn't release it, causing severe bloating, distress, and diarrhea. It also doesn't absorb macronutrients, just water.

On the other hand, intact fiber—found in Real Food—has many benefits, and not just short-chain fatty acids (SCFAs). In the processed food industry, the germ of the grain (the nucleic acids, flavonoids, polyphenols) is removed along with the fiber because they can go rancid (see Chapter 19). Protecting the liver means maintaining the fiber and keeping the germ intact as well.

Two simple precepts—*protect the liver, feed the gut*. Real Food (low-sugar, high-fiber) does both. Processed food (high-sugar, low-fiber) does neither. Processed food is the primary suspect in our current health and healthcare debacle, because it doesn't improve our eight subcellular pathologies, our three nutrient-sensing enzymes, and our two physiologic precepts.

CHAPTER 12

Nutrition "Unwrapped"

Politics is often spread through myths, which themselves are easily turned into propaganda, thus perpetuating the politics—a vicious cycle. These three are replete within nutrition, perhaps more so than any other medical discipline, because there are so many stakeholders with their own beliefs and agendas. That's why we need the science; it's the only way to debunk the myths. Then and only then can the propaganda be shattered, clearing the way for a new political landscape. The healthcare professionals didn't create the myths or the propaganda, but they've bought them hook, line, and sinker. Let's start with the myths surrounding terminology. Here are just three examples:

1. **The word "weight"**—when did it become a synonym for *health*? When we decided that health was the new morality. Political correctness meant you couldn't shame people for poverty or race—but fat-shaming continues to this day, because "it's your fault you're a glutton and a sloth." But the data shows that it's your liver and visceral fat that determines your health, not your weight or total body fat. Liver fat tops out at about one

pound, and visceral fat at about six pounds. You can't see that on the scale. Normal weight people have liver fat, too. It's not the fat you can see, it's the fat you *can't see* that matters.

2. **The word "fat"**—does it mean body fat or dietary fat? Or, as you will soon learn, fatty acid? Or, "do these pants make my butt look fat?" (Pro-tip: never answer this question.) Two-thirds of the US populace continue to believe and perpetuate the myth that "fat makes you fat." While it's true that dietary fat *could* become body fat, it does so only in response to insulin. And so weight isn't driven by dietary fat, which doesn't raise insulin, but rather by dietary refined carbohydrate and sugar, which do.

3. **The word "sugar"**—does it mean blood sugar (glucose) or dietary sugar (glucose-fructose)? The food industry says "you need sugar to live"—but while you do need a blood glucose level to live, you don't have to consume that glucose. In fact, your liver can make glucose from the glycerol (see **Fig. 7–3d**) released from the breakdown of triglycerides in either dietary fat or body fat, or from amino acids, a process called *gluconeo-genesis*. Conversely, you don't need fructose (the molecule that makes food sweet) to live at all. In fact, there's no biochemical reaction in any animal cell on the planet that requires dietary fructose. Which means you may *want* dietary sugar, but you don't actually *need* it.

Nutrition myths die hard, kind of like Voldemort and vampires; they seem indestructible, especially when the Dark Forces of Industry (see Chapter 23) spend a lot of money to maintain and propagate them. What follows are my best efforts to drive a stake through the heart of each of these nutritional myths, so that you can "unlearn" what you've been taught.

A Calorie Is Not a Calorie

This myth is all that is left of the legacy of Wilbur Atwater. It argues that all calories possess the same heat generation, equivalent to 4,184 joules of energy. From a physics standpoint, a calorie *is* a calorie. But so what? This has nothing to do with what happens to those calories in the human body, because weight gain is only about how those calories are stored.

The efficiency of capturing all those calories and transforming them into chemical energy in the human body is highly uneven. Understanding these various phenomena shows that in fact "a calorie is *not* a calorie," and there's an actual difference between eating a handful of almonds and a donut, even if their calorie count is the same.

The "calorie is a calorie" myth can be disproven through five examples:

1. **Fiber.** You eat 160 calories in almonds, but you only absorb 130. The other 30 are prevented from early absorption because the fiber in them prevents early absorption in the duodenum (early intestine), so the bacteria in the jejunum and ileum (middle and late intestine) will chew the 30 up for their own purposes. You ate them, so they're considered "calories in," but you didn't get them (your bacteria did).

2. **Protein.** If an amino acid is to be prepared for energy metabolism, the amino group must be removed by the liver to convert it into an organic acid (e.g., aspartate to oxaloacetate). It costs two ATPs to do this, as opposed to preparing carbohydrate, which costs one ATP. This is known as the *thermic effect of food* (TEF). *Fats generate about* 2 to 3 percent of TEF, *carbohydrate about* 6 to 8 percent, and *protein about* 25 to 30 percent—meaning it takes more energy to burn a protein than a carbohydrate. If a calorie isn't recouped because it's burned, it can't be stored.

3. **Fat.** All dietary fats would liberate 9 calories per gram if you burned them. But omega-3 fatty acids aren't burned—they're hoarded, as they're needed for cell membranes and neurons in the brain (see Chapters 7 and 19). Furthermore, *trans*-fats can't be burned, as humans don't have the enzyme to cleave the trans-double bond. They instead will clog your

arteries and kill you, unrelated to their calories. All in all, neither are burned, but one will save your life and the other will kill you.

4. **Sugar.** Added sugar is made up of equal amounts of glucose and fructose. Both provide the same number of calories, but are metabolized differently in the liver and perform different jobs in the brain. Glucose can be metabolized by all of your body's tissues and only 20 percent of a glucose load goes to your liver, and even then insulin tells the liver to turn it into glycogen (liver starch). On the other hand, fructose can only be metabolized by the liver, so the whole load goes to your liver, insulin doesn't have an effect, the mitochondria are overwhelmed, and the rest is turned into liver fat, driving insulin resistance (see **Fig. 2–1**). And on the third hand, fructose drives glycation seven times faster than glucose (see Chapter 7), doesn't shut off the hunger hormone ghrelin, and is addictive (see Chapter 21).

5. **Different fat depots.** It's not just *if* the calorie is stored, it's *where* it's stored. There are three fat depots, but they confer different risks for development of metabolic disease: 1) subcutaneous (butt) fat: you need about 22 pounds to worsen your health; 2) visceral (belly) fat: you need about 5 pounds to worsen your health; and 3) liver fat: you only need about 0.3 pounds to worsen your health. And almost all calories from added sugar are going to liver fat. If a calorie stored were a calorie stored, it wouldn't matter which fat depot was doing the storage—but it does. Protecting the liver is the prime directive.

But It's Zero Calories . . . ?

Sugar sweetened beverages (SSBs) are causative for at least three diseases of metabolic syndrome—type 2 diabetes, heart disease, and fatty liver disease—plus tooth decay. So, what about noncaloric diet sweeteners, for those with a "sweet tooth"? Stevia, sucralose, aspartame, acesulfame-K, allulose, xylitol, erythritol, and others would seem the obvious choices—no calories, so no heart disease, right? No fructose, so no liver fat or diabetes, right? Not so fast. Though the US has slowly turned to diet drinks because of the obesity epidemic—as of 2010, 42 percent of Coca-Cola sales in the US were of the no-sugar variety— 33 percent of all sugar consumption is in drinks, and 42 percent of drinks are now no-sugar, so someone somewhere should be losing weight, right?

Unfortunately, diet sweetener consumption is also correlated with metabolic syndrome. Studies of switching out sugar for diet sweeteners don't show beneficial effects on weight loss. Rather, the data show that sugar is a direct cause of metabolic syndrome—though thus far we only have correlation with diet sweeteners. So, do diet sweeteners cause metabolic syndrome, or do people with metabolic syndrome consume more diet drinks? The question really is if the substitution of diet sweeteners for sugar actually reduces caloric intake, body fat, and metabolic disease. Here are five reasons to be concerned:

1. There's a difference between pharmacokinetics (what your body does to a drug) and pharmacodynamics (what a drug does to your body). We have pharmacokinetic data on diet sweeteners to determine acute safety, which is part of the FDA's charter (see Chapter 24), but none of the pharmacodynamics. This has to do with chronic effects, which is not in the FDA's charter. The fact of the matter is, we don't know what any of these diet sweeteners do to your long-term food intake, weight, body fat, or metabolic status. The food industry doesn't do these studies because such studies are expensive and could have detrimental effects on sales. The NIH won't do them, saying it's the food industry's job. So the studies aren't done.

2. You drink a soda. The tongue sends a signal to the hypothalamus that says, "Hey, sugar is coming, get ready to metabolize it." The hypothalamus then sends a signal along the vagus nerve to the pancreas, saying, "A sugar load is coming, get ready to release the insulin." If the "sweet" signal is from a diet sweetener, the sugar never comes. What happens next? Does the pancreas say, "Oh, well . . . I'll just chill until the next

meal," or does it say, "WTF? I'm all primed for the extra sugar. Let's eat more to get it."

In one study, four groups of Danish men ate their normal diet for six months plus a liter of sugared soda per day, a liter of diet soda per day, a liter of milk per day, or a liter of water per day. No surprise, the sugared soda group gained 22 pounds. The diet soda group gained 3.5 pounds. The milk group stayed the same. The water group lost 4.5 pounds. Now, 3.5 is better than 22 pounds, but they still gained weight even without the calories. And the milk has as many calories as the sugared soda, so why didn't that group gain weight? It all has to do with insulin—meaning the diet sweetener still caused insulin release, while the lactose and fat in the milk didn't. Plus the fat was satiating, so people ate less.

A second study took diet soda drinkers and switched them to water. They lost another 6 pounds. If there are no calories in either case, why did their weight change? Insulin again. Insulin response to oral glucose tolerance testing was performed in seventeen morbidly obese adults without diabetes, both with and without a diet sweetener pretreatment. After the diet soda, the insulin response was 20 percent higher than with the seltzer control. The sweet taste alone can both stimulate appetite and insulin release, which drives energy storage.

3. Diet sweeteners might change the composition of intestinal bacteria, which could cause leaky gut, generate inflammation, increase deposition of visceral fat, and drive metabolic syndrome, unrelated to calories (see Chapter 7). The intestinal microbiome plays a role not only in what the tongue tastes, but also what the brain senses.

4. Early studies suggest that certain diet sweeteners act directly on fat cells grown in a petri dish to promote energy transport inside the cell. In other words, diet sweeteners may have insulin-like properties of their own, but this has yet to be confirmed.

5. We don't know the role that diet sweeteners may play in sugar addiction (see Chapter 21), as this field is in its infancy. However, there are animal

studies that suggest brain pathways react similarly to sucrose and diet sweeteners.

Recent studies argue that artificially sweetened beverages are associated with diabetes, cardiovascular issues, and dementia. Thus far, all of these studies have been correlative—we don't yet have causation. Nonetheless, quantitatively, the data suggests that the toxicity of two diet sodas is equivalent to one sugared soda, and that they're way worse than water in terms of obesity and diabetes development. As an example, take the case of aspartame (NutraSweet), which in animal models affects three of our eight subcellular pathologies: oxidative stress, membrane integrity, and inflammation (see Chapter 7). These health concerns are just swept under the rug—a University of Sussex report looked at the original approval of aspartame by the European Food Safety Authority (EFSA). They documented that the EFSA discounted fully 100 percent of the seventy-three studies that showed aspartame caused harm, while accepting 84 percent of the studies that showed no harm.

While none of this research closes the book on diet sweeteners in either direction, it should certainly give us pause. In the last fifteen years, American sugar consumption has dropped from 120 to 94 pounds per year, yet obesity and metabolic syndrome persist unabated. Could diet sweeteners be playing a role? The only surefire way to find out is for Americans to de-sweeten their food across the board—drinks, too. And don't start thinking juice is the answer (see Chapter 19).

Instead of worrying about calories, we should instead focus on the interaction between genetics and sugar consumption, as this determines insulin levels and where that fat will develop and deposit. Understanding the role of different foods in generating different insulin responses is paramount, and that includes diet sweeteners.

A Fiber Is Not a Fiber

As mentioned earlier, there are two types of fiber—soluble and insoluble—and you need both. The reason you hear doctors espousing a plant-based diet isn't because of the plant origin *per se*; it's because plants come with both types of fiber. Together, the two kinds of fiber form a gel on the inside of the duodenum, reducing intestinal absorption by 25 to 30 percent, thus *protecting the liver*. Reciprocally, a sizeable portion of what you eat stays in the intestine, where the bacteria can feast on it and grow, thus *feeding the gut*.

As discussed in Chapter 11, the fiber in food is perhaps the most important nutrient for health, because it singlehandedly **protects the liver** *and* **feeds the gut** in six different ways:

1. Both kinds of fiber together form a gel on the inside of the duodenum to reduce the rate of absorption of monosaccharides and disaccharides, as well as slow the breakdown of starches. Reduced absorption means reduced transport to the liver, thus preventing the liver from turning excess energy into fat—in turn preventing liver insulin resistance.

2. The reduction in the rate of absorption also reduces the glycemic excursion in the blood, keeping the insulin response down, and reducing energy deposition into fat tissue.

3. There are two flavors of bacteria that live in your gut: the *white hat* and the *black hat* bacteria—and it's a daily struggle to see which will prevail. The white hat bacteria (e.g., *Bacteroides*) need more energy to survive and grow in order to battle the black hat bacteria (e.g., *Firmicutes*). Thankfully, the good bacteria can proliferate and maintain a balanced intestinal ecosystem, but need a greater and more robust supply chain to ward off the bad guys. What's that supply chain made of? Fiber—both types.

4. The fiber transits the food through the intestine faster, generating the satiety signal (the gut hormone peptide YY_{3-36}, which is released into the bloodstream and goes to the brain) sooner, thus reducing second portions.

5. Soluble fiber is metabolized by gut bacteria into short-chain fatty acids like butyrate. They uniquely feed the microbiome of the colon (large
   intestine) and are absorbed into the bloodstream where they are anti-
   inflammatory as well as suppress insulin secretion from the pancreas.

6. Insoluble fiber acts as a mild abrasive in the lumen of the colon, which
   dislodges and sluffs old dead cells, thus reducing cancer risk.

Be forewarned: the processed food industry will tout the benefits
of "added fiber" to various products. But you can't put the toothpaste
back in the tube. Yes, they can add back some soluble fiber (e.g., the
psyllium in Fiber One bars), but they can never recapitulate the insoluble fiber lost during processing.

The same goes for *whole grain*. We've been taught that brown bread
is better for you because it has more fiber. The Whole Grains Council
says, "Whole grains or foods made from them contain all the essential parts and naturally-occurring nutrients of the entire grain seed
in their original proportions. If the grain has been processed (e.g.,
cracked, crushed, rolled, extruded, and/or cooked), the food product
should deliver the same rich balance of nutrients that are found in
the original grain seed." In other words, if it starts as whole grain, it
remains whole grain. It's not *what's in the food*, it's *what's been done
to the food*.

Fig. 12-1 is a good example of the problem. The one-pound loaf of
bread on the right is big and fluffy. If you threw it at someone's head, it
would bounce off. The slices are thick. The bread on the left is small
and dense. If you threw it at someone's head, it would knock them unconscious. The slices are thin, and they crumble easily. Which one
makes a better sandwich? Which is healthier? The bread on the right
has milled grain, and the starch and gluten are dissociated from the
bran. It generates a rapid and high glucose and insulin response, but
makes great avocado toast. The bread on the left still has its starch and
gluten within the kernel, and crumbles easily, and it's an "acquired

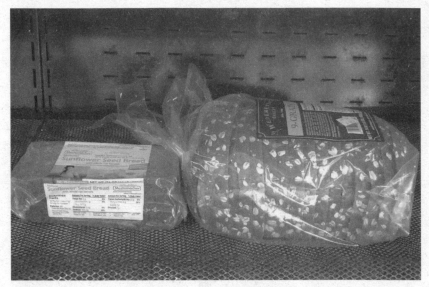

Figure 12–1: Two kinds of whole grain bread. Each weighs one pound. The one on the left is and remains whole grain, while the one on the right started as whole grain but was then milled and processed.

taste." Both have soluble fiber, but only the one on the left has structurally and functionally maintained its insoluble fiber.

A Carb Is Not a Carb

For decades, the American Heart Association, American Diabetes Association, and American Medical Association advocated a low-fat diet. By definition that means a high-carbohydrate diet. Is that a good trade? Just like "a calorie is not a calorie" and "a fiber is not a fiber," "a carb is not a carb." There are three inherent myths about carbohydrates that play a role as to whether they're causative of, or preventative against, NCDs:

1. **Sugar vs. starch.** Sugars are monosaccharides and disaccharides (one or two molecules), while starch is a complex polymer (many molecules). Sugars either have one bond or no bonds to break, so they're digested

and absorbed quickly in the duodenum, especially when they've been liberated from a food matrix, as they often are (e.g., soda, fruit juice, alcohol). Starch has more bonds to break, and is digested and absorbed slower. All of this adds up to a more rapid and higher insulin response with sugar, which drives weight gain.

2. **Type of starch (the two "Amys"):** But "a starch is not a starch." There are two kinds of starch: amylose (brown foods including beans, lentils, and legumes; carbs that are digested and absorbed slowly) and amylopectin (white foods including wheat, pasta, rice, and potatoes; carbs that are digested and absorbed rapidly). Amylose is better for you, as it's a string of glucoses with two ends; therefore, only two enzymes at a time can chew it up, resulting in slow digestion and absorption. Amylopectin is more like a tree of glucoses, with lots of branch points. Many more enzymes can chew it up at once, releasing glucose more rapidly, which is more likely to be absorbed early, flood the liver, and generate a bigger insulin response.

3. **Carbs are rarely ingested in isolation.** A slice of white bread is straight glucose. But Real Food is glucose plus protein plus fat plus fiber. Those other macronutrients, or lack thereof, influence the glucose's absorption in the intestine, the insulin response that follows, and risk for weight gain.

Carbs and Glycemic Index (GI)

Higher glucose spikes during eating are associated with more insulin, more inflammation, and higher mortality. Therefore, a primary goal of improving metabolic health is to get the insulin down. One way is to eat foods that don't make your blood glucose rise too fast. This is where amylose—the "good Amy"—comes in. Thus was born the concept of the glycemic index (GI). Tables of specific foods and their inherent GI are readily available. Some claim that a low-GI diet will keep blood glucose down and help you lose weight. But does it work to keep insulin down? Is it the glucose spikes or the insulin spikes that do the damage?

Unfortunately, GI isn't the panacea that the zealots hype. GI is defined as: how high does your serum glucose rise in response to 50 grams of carbohydrate in a given food, as compared with the glucose response in 50 grams of straight starch (e.g., white bread). However, there are four things conceptually wrong with GI:

1. **GI is an indirect proxy for insulin.** While rapid glucose spikes after re-fined starch lead to glycation and oxidative stress, it's the insulin fluc-tuation that induces the other six subcellular pathologies (see Chapter 7), drives excess energy intake, and promotes obesity.

2. **GI assumes everyone responds to the same food in the same way.** GI is computed based on responses of healthy people to certain foods, even though 88 percent of people have some form of metabolic dysfunction. Now that people are using continuous glucose monitors (CGMs; see Chap-ter 14), it's very clear that people respond differently to the same food.

3. **The important parameter is glycemic load (GL).** GL is different from GI— how much food do you have to eat to get the 50 grams of carbohydrate? GL takes into account the beneficial effect of fiber. A good example is carrots, which are high-GI (lots of carbohydrate) but low-GL (even more fiber). More fiber means a larger portion, because there's less digestible carbohydrate. You can turn any high-GI food into a low-GL food by eating it with its original fiber. Real Food is by definition low-GL.

4. **Fructose!** Fructose is the most egregious cause of liver insulin resistance and metabolic syndrome because of how the liver uniquely metabolizes it. Fructose isn't glucose—when eaten, it doesn't raise the blood glucose level (it's not measured in the glucose assay). In fact, by definition, it's low-GI, because it has no glucose. Still, this hasn't stopped the food in-dustry from trying to capitalize on the low-GI craze by adding fructose to foods. In fact, the Glycemic Index Foundation of Australia has the nerve

to label sugar as low-GI, as if somehow that was a good thing. Keep insulin low by eating lots of fiber and by avoiding added sugar. Real Food is by definition a low-GL diet.

A Fat Is Not a Fat

The epic battle between British physiologist John Yudkin and Minnesota epidemiologist Ancel Keys for control of the American Diet, detailed in my book *Fat Chance* (2012) and Nina Teicholz's *The Big Fat Surprise* (2017), is now sixty years old. Yudkin wrote *Pure, White and Deadly* (1972) targeting dietary sugar; Keys wrote *The Seven Countries Study* (1980) targeting dietary saturated fat. Both scientists had correlation but not causation; both had static data (single points in time) rather than longitudinal data (patterns over time). Both used ecologic (population) data, which is much flimsier than individual data. In other words, both had weak cases.

However, Keys had a few more things going for him than Yudkin: hubris, bombast, cherry picking, and willful denial. Keys was also the beneficiary of three scientific discoveries of the 1970s that sealed Yudkin's fate: people with familial hypercholesterolemia (FH; see Chapter 2) have high LDL and heart disease; dietary fat raises LDL levels; and LDL levels correlate with heart disease in populations. Never mind that smoking and *trans*-fats are bigger contributors, or that those countries eating the most fat had the lowest levels of heart disease. The die was cast, and the 1977 Dietary Guidelines assured that the world would go low-fat.

There are one restriction study and two substitution studies that assessed the effects of the removal of saturated fat from diet—and the latter two had to be reanalyzed to get to the truth. The restriction study was done by the Women's Health Initiative (WHI), which studied 161,000 women between 1993 and 1998 who reduced their consumption of saturated fat from 30 percent to 10 percent of calories. The verdict: no effect on either weight loss or heart disease. In the Sydney Diet Heart Study, which ran between 1966 and 1973, 458 men who had experienced a heart attack had the saturated fat removed from their diet and replaced with linoleic acid (from soybean oil), which is pro-inflammatory. All subjects experienced a decline in their LDL levels, yet their risk for heart attack increased by 62 percent, as well as their risk of dying by 70 percent. Perhaps the most egregious study was the Minnesota Coronary Study, which followed nine thousand patients over five years (1968 to 1973) at state mental hospitals and nursing homes, where meals were controlled by removing saturated fat and substituting linoleic acid (from corn oil). The study experienced the same results as Sydney—LDL went down, but heart attacks and deaths went up. The authors never published their findings, because they couldn't explain them. Instead, the data lay in wait in the basement of the lead author, only to be discovered forty years later by his Mayo Clinic cardiologist son. In 2016, he published the findings. He was astonished, but he shouldn't have been. Low-fat doesn't work, and substituting with other fats doesn't work either. It's not about the LDL; it never was (see Chapter 2).

Furthermore, the saturated fat story doesn't take into account that all saturated fats are not the same. For example, the saturated fats in red meat are *even-chain* fatty acids (16 or 18 carbons), meaning they're cardiovascularly neutral. The saturated fats found in dairy are *odd-chain* fatty acids (15 or 17 carbons), which are metabolized differently in the liver, and are associated with protection from chronic diseases like diabetes and heart disease. Therefore, the fat in dairy is likely protective—except we skim off that fat from cow's milk and turn it into processed cheese. Good for the dairy producers, as they get two products out of one, but not so good for you, as an ingredient that could be protective against chronic disease has been removed "for your own good." Even worse, sometimes we flavor the milk with chocolate or strawberry syrup for good measure (see Chapter 14).

The Difference between Saturated Fat and Saturated Free Fatty Acids

Despite all these data, and the fact that the FDA removed saturated fat from the Nutrition Facts label, people still think it's the bogeyman. Let's get the facts straight: there's a difference between innocuous *saturated fat* and pernicious *saturated free fatty acids*. Saturated fat itself isn't inflammatory, because it's packaged into triglycerides (see **Fig. 7-3d**). Rather, the unpackaged moiety called *free fatty acids* or *non-esterified saturated fatty acids* (see **Fig. 7-3a** and **c**), in particular free palmitate (see **Fig. 7-3a**), is the inflammatory component, both in the body and in the brain. In particular, free palmitate seems to be the driver of liver and hypothalamic inflammation. However, you don't eat free fatty acids. They're produced and exist in only two places in the body. When stored triglyceride is released from the adipocyte (fat cell), the glycerol backbone must be cleaved off, liberating its three free fatty acids. It also happens when the liver turns excess sugar into triglyceride through the process of *de novo* lipogenesis (DNL), as it first must produce a free fatty acid. Both of these processes are related to each other through fructose, as fructose causes both insulin resistance *and* DNL. So is the saturated fat from food the problem? Or are the free fatty acids the metabolic by-product of dietary sugar?

A Protein Is Not a Protein

Companies are touting protein as a cure-all and for weight loss/muscle gain. They're selling protein shakes, protein cookies, protein snack bars, even protein coffee. It's true that protein is neither carbohydrate nor sugar nor fat, and you need it to maintain normal growth. However, your kidneys have a limited capacity to excrete the metabolic by-products of protein metabolism, and overexcretion can cause kidney damage. Therefore, protein *quality* is as important as protein *quantity*. For example, eggs and beans both contain protein, but are very different in quality. Dietary protein is made up of twenty separate amino acids strung together in different combinations and amounts. One of those amino acids, tryptophan, is rarer and therefore more important than others, because it's the precursor of serotonin, an important brain neurotransmitter (see Chapter 19). Eggs, poultry, and fish are the best sources of this amino acid, while beans have very little. On the other hand, additional protein is needed if you're building muscle, especially branched-chain amino acids (BCAAs; leucine, isoleucine, valine), which are 20 percent of muscle (see Chapter 18). BCAAs are in high concentration in corn products, and are what's in those tubs of protein powder at the health food store. If you're a bodybuilder, you need them; if you're not a gym rat and consume excess BCAAs, your liver will take the amino groups off and turn them into organic acids, which will either be diverted into liver fat (through DNL) or into excess glucose, either of which can generate hyperinsulinemia and drive chronic disease. The goal is to get more tryptophan and less BCAAs in the protein you consume.

What about Meat?

Meat is relatively high in tryptophan, vitamins, and minerals, but it brings along several other less desirable items as well. With beef, health problems include: iron (oxygen radicals); BCAAs in corn-fed beef (DNL, liver fat, and insulin resistance); and choline, a by-product of which sticks to arteries, causes vascular disease, and leads to insulin resistance. However, red meat has a hazard risk (HR) ratio for diabetes of 1.24; in other words, high meat-eaters have a 24 percent increased risk over that of the general population. So if the general prevalence of diabetes is 9.4 percent, meat-eaters have a prevalence of 11.6 percent. While a 2.2 percent increase is not negligible, public health officials don't worry about HR ratios unless they're above 1.3. Further, when the iron and heme levels were adjusted, the HR ratio was reduced down to 1.13 (resulting in a diabetes prevalence of 10.6 percent, suggesting that other stuff in the meat isn't a big driver of diabetes). In another study, unprocessed meat had a HR ratio for diabetes of 1.12 per 100 grams, while processed meat (bacon, sausage, salami) had a HR ratio of 1.51 per 50 grams. Thus, the difference in prevalence goes from 10.5 percent to 28.4 percent. Now, that's notable. It's the processing that renders the meat dangerous.

Also, nitrates in processed meat are a known risk factor for colon cancer. Thus, it appears that processed meat is more problematic, presumably due to the additives and the iron, rather than due to the saturated fat. Some, although not all, of these concerns can be assuaged by purchasing grass-fed and nitrate-free meat instead.

Mythology Begets Propaganda; Science Begets Public Health

Old myths die hard; saturated fat still casts a long shadow. For instance, in 2016 the USDA took total and saturated fat off the Nutrition Facts label, yet the Dietary Guidelines still advise us to eat only certain amounts of saturated fat.

On the other hand, sugar doesn't cast enough of a shadow. How can the USDA say to people, eat less sugar, but then allow it in 62 percent of all foods in the grocery store and not require the manufacturers to label it as such? Science works as a change agent for public health only if the opponent is operating off the same science. The issue here is the food industry generates its own science—call it pseudoscience—and uses it to propagandize those myths that best benefit their politics.

And if we've learned one thing about propaganda in 2020, it's that if you say something long enough and loud enough, people will start to believe it.

CHAPTER 13

Food in the Time of Corona

I write this chapter during week 6 of San Francisco's shelter-in-place order to flatten the curve of COVID-19 infection. My infrequent provision trips to the supermarket in mask and gloves, along with the forty-five-minute wait to enter the store, always reveal the same story—the produce is there, the meat is there, the nuts, dairy, and eggs are all fully stocked. What isn't? Toilet paper, yeah, I got that, but what else? Pasta, bread, breakfast cereal, and candy. It's not my imagination. Kraft says, "We can't make enough mac and cheese." There are few things that render me speechless, but Kraft running out of mac and cheese has me completely gobsmacked.

To be sure, since people are eating at home, all kinds of food sales have increased, processed and otherwise. In March 2020, sales of meat and oranges were up 57 percent over the same month of 2019, while packaged soup sales were up 237 percent, and canned meat was up 282 percent. Kroger reported a 30 percent jump of sales in March. Credit Suisse projected that retail sales of packaged food companies will grow, on average, by as much as 15 percent to 30 percent in 2020.

Processed food companies have increased production by as much as 40 percent.

Now, I understand that processed food lasts a long time on the shelf. People are unsure of the resilience of the food supply, especially after the closings of the Smithfield pork plant in Sioux Falls, South Dakota, the Tyson pork plant in Waterloo, Iowa, and a meatpacking plant in Indiana. People are worried that fresh food somewhere along the food chain might have been handled by a virus carrier—not to mention everyone is stressed, driving the brain's need for comfort and pleasure, which can be found at the bottom of a package of Oreos. I also understand that parents use sugar as a reward for kids' good behavior while cooped up in the house.

But this is an incorrect, and dangerous, formulation. It's clear that anyone can be infected with COVID-19 and get pneumonia—but who dies from it? The mantra has been that those who are most at risk for serious infection and death are over sixty-five with underlying health conditions. OK, the octogenarians, that makes sense—they also die of the flu. But what are these elusive "underlying health conditions" and who has them?

Data compiled from hospital admissions during New York City's COVID-19 pandemic of the population under sixty years yield alternative hypotheses. Analysis of demographics reveal that the infection rates are indiscriminate; but hospital and ICU admission as well as death rates identify three groups at highest risk for morbidity and mortality: people of color; the obese; and those with the diseases of metabolic syndrome (heart disease, hypertension, kidney disease, and diabetes in particular). These three groups overlap. People of color bear a greater burden of obesity and metabolic syndrome in America, yet another manifestation of social disparities, which can result in increased risk of death from COVID-19. Those harboring metabolic syndrome, with or without the associated diseases, are in a state of chronic inflammation at baseline. Throw COVID-19 into the mix, and you have the makings of an inflammation tsunami.

But death is not due to the virus itself—rather it's due to the ensuing cytokine (inflammatory protein) response. When your immune system faces its biggest threats, it has to roll out its biggest guns. These proteins start the chain reaction in the immune system to kill anything in its wake. The underlying inflammation of metabolic syndrome already has the immune system on high alert, and when COVID-19 hits, it results in a disproportionate immune response.

In the lungs, COVID-19 causes acute respiratory distress syndrome (ARDS), which destroys lung tissue with abandon. But the mind-boggling fact about COVID-19 is that it affects every organ in the body. For instance, a syndrome of inflammation of the blood vessels, called Kawasaki disease, has affected young children in New York City and Italy, as well as many young adults who've died due to strokes caused by blood clots formed in the cytokine storm.

How Chronic Disease Leads to Acute Disease

Why does this domino effect happen? And what's food got to do with it? A lot, as it turns out. Scientists have been feverishly working to unlock the secrets of how COVID-19 infects cells and generates this cytokine response; and now we know three ways that processed food consumption (two direct, one indirect) could affect our susceptibility to COVID-19:

1. On the surface of each of our cells, especially those in our lungs, is a membrane receptor called *angiotensin-converting enzyme-2* (ACE2). The virus uses this receptor as its entry point into the cell. It's the genius of the coronavirus that it uses this ACE2 structure as the puncture site and a portal into our cells; the more ACE2 on the surface, the more complete the infection and the sicker one gets. Increased activity of the ACE2 is involved in increasing blood pressure and in inducing insulin resistance. But it works the other way, too, as insulin reduces the shedding of ACE2 from cells, such as the kidney, and insulin resistance increases ACE2 expression on cell membranes. More ACE2 on the cell surface means more doors for the virus to enter, and more risk for severe infection.

2. Another possible direct relationship between COVID-19 and processed
    food has to do with the lack of fiber in it. Normally, soluble fiber is me-
    tabolized by bacteria in the colon to short-chain fatty acids like butyric
    acid, which have been shown to suppress immune system activation and
    inflammation, which is what actually kills you. Processed food is notori-
    ously devoid of soluble fiber (see Chapter 19), so there's no protection
    against runaway inflammation. Also, the COVID-19 virus appears to af-
    fect gut permeability, likely exacerbating leaky gut, which puts your im-
    mune system into overdrive, while fiber could reverse it.

3. It appears that high blood glucose, as seen in type 2 diabetes, glycates
    (see Chapter 7) both the COVID-19 spike protein (which does the inject-
    ing) and the ACE2 receptor (the puncture site), making it easier for cells
    to be infected. Thus, preexisting diabetes increases the risk that an in-
    fected patient will have a bigger cytokine response and succumb to the
    infection.

Now, let's look at these three high-risk demographic groups. People of color have higher insulin levels than Caucasians at all ages and
BMI levels. As stated in Chapter 2, 80 percent of obese individuals are
insulin resistant with high insulin levels. It's well known that excess
body fat, especially visceral fat, induces immune dysregulation and
chronic inflammation, which is directly linked to the cytokine storm.
Furthermore, the obese are more likely to die from the cytokine storm.
For example, in the H1N1 influenza epidemic of 2009, 61 percent of
patients admitted to hospital were obese, compared to 30 percent of the
general population; obesity was also found to be an independent risk
factor for death.

The COVID-19 data currently available also shows that the obese
are more likely to end up hospitalized. The diseases of *metabolic
syndrome*—diabetes, heart disease, hypertension, and kidney disease—
are the diseases that are driven and made worse by insulin resistance
and high insulin levels, often resulting in obesity.

Invasion of the Body Snackers

Your ACE2, insulin, and inflammatory status are all inexorably linked—but what is it that ties them all together? Processed food, of course. There are four inherent pro-inflammatory problems with the stuff: excess omega-6 fatty acids (seed oils like soybean oil), which are pro-inflammatory (see Chapter 20); excess sugar (virtually all processed food), as the fructose (sweet) molecule in sugar poisons mitochondria, induces insulin resistance, and promotes inflammation (see Chapter 20); lack of omega-3s (oily fish), which are anti-inflammatory (see Chapter 19); and lack of fiber (all processed food), due to leaky gut (see Chapter 19).

Conversely, improving your inflammatory status is the single best way to improve your chance for survival; flavonoids, polyphenols, vitamin C, and vitamin D all have antioxidant, anti-inflammatory, and immune-strengthening capacities. That's called Real Food—the stuff that's still in the supermarket! Indeed, vitamin D was found to be effective at prevention and treatment of SARS back in 2003. It's been proposed as a maneuver for COVID-19 as well.

But what about foodborne viral transmission, you ask? While it's true that COVID-19 is very resourceful and can bind to intestinal epithelial cells, no one appears to have contracted the virus through the oral route. This is a droplet disease. The gut is not a route of infection. If you're still worried, cook the hell out of it; it's still better than eating the crap out of the box.

If there's any solace to be had within this pandemic, it's that by reducing restaurant outings and cooking at home, the world is consuming less sugar. Citigroup estimates that world consumption will be down 1.2 percent this year, the first time in forty years that there's been a decline. Let's not celebrate yet, though—the USDA is expecting a 3.6 percent rebound next year after COVID-19 is in the rearview mirror, likely due to the advent of a vaccine. But don't get too enamored with vaccines; our experiences with influenza show that obese individuals don't generate an adequate antibody response and remain susceptible to infection.

Bottom line is: processed food kills. Normally it kills the old-fashioned way, slowly, by causing chronic disease. But chronic disease puts you at risk for acute disease as well. Real Food won't prevent you from becoming infected with COVID-19, but it can certainly help you to survive it. Way safer than drinking disinfectant.

CHAPTER 14

=====

What and How Adults Eat

It's very clear that most American adults haven't processed the public health message that not all foods are equal in fomenting NCDs, in part because they are still stuck in calorie mode. They've not yet transitioned to insulin mode. Every diet that reduces insulin burden by improving insulin sensitivity (see Chapters 7 and 8) reduces the burden of metabolic disease and allows adipocytes to give up their stored fat, thus promoting weight loss. They also improve leptin sensitivity at the brain (see Chapter 7), making you feel full and reducing total food intake. Conversely, all caloric restriction diets lead to reduction in leptin levels within eighteen hours of starting, signaling brain starvation, and putting defense mechanisms into gear to maintain adipocyte storage. The difference between success and failure for both obesity and NCD reversal is whether you get insulin down and keep it down (see Chapter 9).

The "Secret" to Weight Loss

As many as forty-five million American adults (23 percent) go on a diet to lose weight every year. The ads are pervasive. "New Year, New You!" "Beach season is coming, are you ready?" Judging from the 40 percent adult obesity rate, which continues to climb, not many are successful. Nonetheless, everybody touts their own diet. Vegan, Ornish, keto, paleo, Mediterranean, Japanese—there are studies galore to document that each and every one of these diets fare better than the Standard American Diet. However, there's virtually no data to document that one outperforms another.

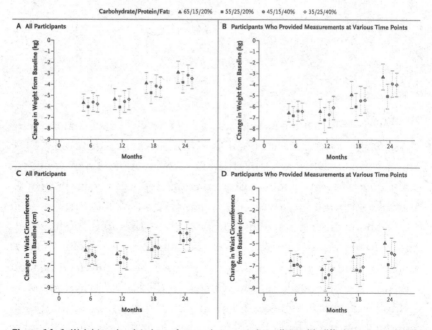

Figure 14–1: Weight and waist circumference loss on various diets with differing macronutrient composition, from 35 percent to 65 percent carbohydrate 3. The a) mean change in weight and b) mean change in waist circumference for each diet at each time point is essentially the same, suggesting that all four diets were equivalent. However, the standard errors of the mean (SEM, the "I-bars") demonstrate a wide distribution of response to each diet, suggesting that some subjects responded well to each diet, while others did not. This suggests that the authors' interpretation that all diets are the same is incorrect; rather that different diets work for different people.

A 2009 study from Frank Sacks at Harvard School of Public Health argues that dietary composition is irrelevant. Over two years, he assigned dieters to different percentages of carbohydrate vs. fat. On average, they all fared the same; the *New York Times* proclaimed, "Study Zeroes In on Calories, Not Diet, for Loss." I think the authors and the media both oversold this—just look at the data in **Fig. 14-1**.

It's true—the mean weight loss was the same for each group at the same time. However, that's not the message that should be gleaned from these data. Rather, we should focus on how the weight nadir occurred at six months, and after that, weight gain returned; none of the diets led to durable results. Furthermore, the standard error around the mean for every diet and every time point was quite wide. This means that for any given diet, some people benefited greatly, while others didn't benefit at all. The authors didn't generate any *a priori* data necessary to distinguish who was who; that is, who responded to which diet, or why. Last, we note that the diet with the lowest percent carbohydrate was only at 35 percent. In order for low-carb diets to be effective, you have to bring the insulin level way down so that the adipocytes can release their stored fat, or in the case of the keto diet, turn off insulin almost completely. There's no way that a 35 percent carbohydrate diet will do that—in other words, the low-carb diet that Sacks studied wasn't really low-carb; it was in fact middle-carb.

Similarly, in an attempt to determine which diet was best, Christopher Gardner's 2007 A to Z Weight Loss Study evaluated four separate diets—the Atkins (high-fat, low-carb), LEARN (low-calorie), Ornish (very-low-fat, high-fiber), and Zone (low–processed carbs, lean protein). This study demonstrated two things: all diets worked, but only for two months. At that point they stopped working, because people on all four diets had regressed to the mean. In other words, most people weren't vigilant enough to actually stay on it, and they slowly slipped back into their original eating habits. Gardner followed this up with his 2018 DIETFITS study, which looked at a low-fat diet (48 percent carb, 29 percent fat vs. should be less than 20 percent fat) versus a low-carb diet (30 percent carb, 45 percent fat, vs. should be less than

25 percent carb). Despite these limitations, he showed that on average, it didn't matter which diet you were on—low-fat or low-carb. If you ate Real Food and didn't revert back to processed food, on average you lost equal amounts of weight. It's important to note that both of these diets had two good things in common—low-sugar and high-fiber.

You have to take into account other disease states and genetics to determine which diet is best for any specific person. For instance, if you have familial hypercholesterolemia (one in five hundred people) or familial hyperchylomicronemia (also known as type 5 hyperlipoproteinemia; one in twenty thousand people), you need a low-fat diet *and* a statin, or your risk for heart disease jumps markedly, irrespective of what your weight does. Conversely, if you're insulin resistant (one in two people), you likely need to restrict refined carbohydrate and sugar in order to reduce four of the eight subcellular pathologies (glycation, oxidative stress, mitochondrial dysfunction, and insulin resistance). However, if you already have type 2 diabetes (one in ten people), you might have to eschew carbohydrate completely for a time, or possibly engage in intermittent fasting (see below). But the real issue, irrespective of carbs vs. fat in any diet, is processed food vs. Real Food.

You have a spectrum of macronutrient compositions to choose from, from one end to the other: vegan, Ornish, flexitarian, pescatarian, Japanese, Mediterranean, low-carb, paleo, keto. They all work, if you're eating Real Food. Real Food is low-sugar and high-fiber, which lowers insulin; it *protects the liver and feeds the gut.* The caveat is that each of us has different genetic predispositions, intestinal microbiota, and livers, so it's likely that there are specific diets that will work better for some and not for others.

The Rise and Fall of the Formula Diet and Drug Industries

The only diet that doesn't work, never worked, and never will work is the processed food version of the low-fat diet. Remember SnackWell's low-fat cookies? No one lost weight because they were laden with sugar and you ate the whole box thinking they weren't *that* bad for you. Remember: low-fat means processed food with high-sugar and low-fiber, which floods the liver and starves the gut. Clearly, low-fat products didn't perform as advertised—they were supposed to reduce heart disease and obesity, but instead they increased both, and added type 2 diabetes and fatty liver disease into the mix.

This didn't matter to the food industry because profits soared. The reduction of dietary fat meant food needed to be processed, which gave them an entrée to substitute sugar, with all of its metabolic and brain perturbations. Then, instead of examining our faulty thinking, society blamed the already distressed patient. They had no diet to turn to, so they glommed onto the no-food diet—partial meal replacement programs like SlimFast, Medifast, and, most recently, Soylent. Some of these use a corn syrup base—and virtually all of them drive up insulin. Despite the testimonials you see on TV, the controlled trials say they don't work. In fact, a meta-analysis demonstrated a mean weight loss at one year of about sixteen pounds, only five pounds better than a very-low-calorie diet. These substitutions don't get the insulin down—even when these formula diets contain slow-digesting starch instead of rapidly absorbed sugar. Glucose tolerance and insulin resistance worsens likely because these formulas lack the fiber to reduce early gut absorption (see Chapters 11 and 12).

But nobody wants to diet, and everybody wants a pill. So how have diet drugs fared? The best of the bunch, phentermine-topiramate, resulted in a mean twenty-pound weight loss over placebo after one year. That being said, adverse events plague these drugs. Orlistat leads to severe gastrointestinal symptoms; liraglutide and naltrexone-bupropion are both associated with the highest level of adverse event–related treatment discontinuation; and fenfluramine, sibutramine, rimonabant, and lorcaserin all had to be removed from the market because of side effects. Not an enviable track record, especially when you consider the fact that none of them actually cause weight loss because they don't get the insulin down either. In fact, the only drug that consistently induces weight loss without significant side effects is metformin—because it increases AMP-kinase (see Chapter 8) and improves mitochondrial function. It *does* get the insulin down. I employed metformin in obese children with great effect, but it works best in those with the highest insulin levels because that's what it treats, and only if they eat real food.

But the Elderly Need to Gain

In contrast to the general public, there's one group of adults who are desperately trying to gain weight—the elderly. It's normal for people to lose some weight as they age, but by sixty-five about half of them are clinically malnourished. Yet despite this weight loss they are at greater risk for NCDs.

What causes weight loss *and* metabolic disease? A lot of things, including the nine Ds: depression, dementia, diarrhea, dentition, dysgeusia (inability to taste), drugs, dysphagia (inability to swallow), disease (like heart failure), and the most important, immune dysfunction, in particular inflammation. The inflammatory cytokine Interleukin-1 circulates and acts like leptin at the hypothalamus, which means telling the brain that there's enough energy on board, therefore cutting back on appetite even as the patient loses weight (this is the reason people with high fevers become anorectic). Therefore, to maintain appetite, keeping inflammation at a minimum is essential for good nutrition, especially in the elderly. In turn, that means cutting out the sugar and processed food. Weight-bearing exercise and blood flow restriction (see Chapter 8) can also go a long way to salvaging muscle mass.

The New Battle Royale: Keto vs. Vegan

Without doubt, this section has been the hardest to write, because it's the most politically charged of all. The opponents on both sides of this debate are polarized to say the least. Meat and fat have problems (just not because of saturated fat); refined carbohydrate and sugar also have problems (just not because of glycemic index). Each side will pick apart the other's argument while ignoring the weaknesses of their own, because both diets are missing things that the other contains.

Keto and vegan are more alike than they are different, but both can be abused. Either diet works for some, but not for all. Both diets are difficult to stay on without some sort of monitoring and/or supplementation. I don't have a horse in this race, and I don't have a diet to sell you. I'm just going to put the science out there, and readers can decide for themselves.

Keto

Compared to the Standard American Diet of 45 percent carbohydrate, 40 percent fat, and 15 percent protein, a low-carb, high-fat (LCHF) diet like Atkins is 25 percent carbohydrate, 60 percent fat, and 15 percent protein. The *ketogenic diet* is even more extreme—a very-high-fat, very-low-carb diet consisting of mostly butter, eggs, cream, bacon, and green vegetables, to provide a dietary composition of 10 percent carbohydrate, 70 percent fat, and 20 percent protein. Say goodbye to Italian dinner.

The keto diet has been shown to result in significant and durable weight loss, improvement in insulin sensitivity in a majority of obese people, and diabetes reversal with medication discontinuation in a majority of patients.

Most people, when faced with a life of no bread, no pasta, no sugar, say *no way*. This diet may be extreme, but it has sound principles. Explorer Vilhjalmur Stefansson was shipwrecked in the Arctic for fifteen months and forced to eat nothing but caribou and whale blubber. When he returned to the US, he felt healthier than before. Many years later, to prove the point, he and his colleague checked themselves into New York's Bellevue Hospital and ate only meat for one year—they were healthier than the investigators, at least with the diagnostic tests available at the time.

The science has now been researched extensively, and the keto diet works through two mechanisms. The first is that in the relative absence of carbohydrate and insulin, the adipocyte will release fatty acids into the bloodstream, which go to the liver and are turned into ketones (e.g., beta-hydroxybutyrate) to be used for energy in the rest of the body, especially the brain. The liver kicks in to utilize any stored liver fat, and reduces fatty liver, insulin resistance, and insulin levels. The reduction in insulin improves leptin resistance, which reduces appetite. Insulin reduction will also occur with the less stringent LCHF diet. The second mechanism is beta-hydroxybutyrate itself, which is a signaling molecule that is measured in the urine or breath to determine if you're in ketosis. It tells the liver mitochondria to increase the production of sirtuin-1, which activates AMP-kinase and reduces mTOR, increasing metabolic rate, and induces autophagy (see Chapters 7 and 8). Further, beta-hydroxybutyrate alters the gut microbiome by reducing inflammatory cells and responses in the intestine. Last, beta-hydroxybutyrate also increases the synthesis of brain-derived neurotrophic factor (BDNF), which makes neurons grow and protects against dementia. This is why the keto diet has found favor among various Alzheimer's researchers.

Sounds pretty darn good, especially if you're metabolically ill—what's the downside? It's really hard to stay in ketosis. After two months, most ketogenic diets aren't ketogenic anymore because people aren't that diligent. In addition, keto adherents tend to be low in selenium, magnesium, phosphorus, and vitamins B and C (however, they don't have to be if they consume enough fiber in the form of leafy greens, as the micronutrients travel with the fiber). Newfangled ketone ester drinks are now on the market to try to biohack your body's system by adding ketones to your bloodstream, but they don't change your insulin, and as of yet there are no data that they can mitigate chronic disease states.

Vegan and Other Plant-Based Diets

There are many reasons to be vegan, including: cost, religion, animal welfare, and environment (although not as much as you think; see Chapter 25). But what about metabolic health? Note that a vegan diet is not a low-fat diet, as olive oil, nuts, and avocados have plenty of saturated and unsaturated fats. That being said, several vegan diets have been promulgated to improve metabolic health. The Adventist Health Study (see Chapter 4) showed that vegans, lacto-ovo vegetarians, and pescatarians all had improved risk profiles compared with nonvegetarians (that is, those on the Standard American Diet), but adherents of each of these were not different from each other. Another diet with clear and robust data promoted by Dean Ornish (full disclosure, Dean is a friend) is an extremely low-fat and low-animal-product diet, but is all Real Food providing very large amounts of fiber. To be clear, Ornish advocates for both diet and stress reduction, which plays a unique role in reducing cortisol, thereby improving insulin sensitivity. So is it the diet or the stress reduction that is the primary therapy? We still don't know.

Although vegans assume they eat healthy, in fact the biggest problem with a vegan or plant-based diet is processed food abuse. After all, Coca-Cola, Doritos, French fries, and Oreos are all vegan. In addition, a standard vegan diet is low in iron, omega-3s, vitamin B_{12}, and tryptophan (although you can supplement); if you're deficient in any of these essential vitamins, you might have to turn to eggs or fish, which isn't easy if you're vegan. In response, some have adopted the *flexitarian diet*, which allows for occasional meat and animal products (maybe once a week) in an otherwise vegan or vegetarian diet plan. As long as it's a non-processed food plan, this may be the best of both worlds.

It should be pointed out that there are no studies that compare biomarkers or events between vegan and keto diets. Each one is better than processed food, but we don't know which is better than the other, or in whom. Likely, the data in Chapter 9 can identify you as being insulin resistant or an insulin secretor, which should help you refine your own diet.

Artificial Meat

The whole food/plant-based craze has gone viral—at least on social media (see Chapter 25). Yet a recent Gallup poll shows that vegetarianism has reduced from 6 to 5 percent of Americans, while veganism has increased from 2 to 3 percent of Americans, meaning some vegetarians are going *full monty* vegan. It's not clear how many meat-eaters have converted to veganism, but one study says 84 percent of "born-again" vegans revert back to eating meat.

Nonetheless, Beyond Meat and the Impossible Burger are the hottest items on the menu—the companies can't keep up with demand. The question is, are these substitutions healthier for you? The companies don't provide direct health information, and they haven't been around long enough to assess data on purported benefits. Instead, we must look at what's in them. Each patty contains four main ingredients: water, pea protein isolate (not exactly Real Food), canola oil, and refined coconut oil. Better than saturated fat? Maybe, as canola oil, a polyunsaturated fatty acid (PUFA), lowers visceral (belly) fat. However, most canola oil is partially hydrogenated for shelf stability, and can more easily be turned into *trans*-fat upon heating (see Chapter 18). These plant-based patties contain potato starch, natural flavor, yeast extract, and beet juice extract, but minimal fiber. And finally, the secret ingredient in Impossible's patties to give it that meaty taste is heme (the same iron-containing compound found in blood and muscle) in the form of soy leghemoglobin; this meets 30 percent of your daily iron quota. However, this compound can also cause oxidative stress when overabsorbed (as seen in insulin resistance), leading to liver inflammation. While the FDA did approve this agent in 2019 as safe, they did so based on only twenty-eight days of human exposure, which is hardly enough to be sure. Plus, these patties pack the same caloric punch and the same insulin response as a regular hamburger.

All in all, while these veggie burgers might seem healthier for *your conscience*, it's not immediately apparent whether they're healthier for *you*. And, as you will see in Chapter 25, it's not immediately apparent that they are healthier for the *planet*.

The No-Eating Diet

Of course, there's another way to get insulin down—don't eat! This is only mildly tongue-in-cheek; there's something to this. Caloric restriction (CR) and intermittent fasting (IF) have become hot tickets in the nutrition field. Caloric restriction has been around forever—it's the basis of most New Year's resolutions. The goal is to make the liver think it's energy depleted by restricting calories (usually by about 25 percent). Your liver will stimulate its AMP-kinase, which will make new and fresh mitochondria, inhibit mTOR (the enzyme that determines cellular life and death; see Chapter 8), and ramp up autophagy—all good. This should lower your insulin, thus promoting weight loss—but there's one catch. Your leptin! If engaged in caloric restriction, your leptin level will decline within one day, your brain will immediately sense starvation, and your body will lower its sympathetic nervous system output in order to conserve energy (body temperature and physical activity go down). You will feel tired and irritable, and you will be painfully hungry. One scientist friend of mine put it this way—"Caloric restriction—you don't live longer, it just feels that way." Also, as we now know, *a calorie is not a calorie*, so restricting all calories the same will not lead to beneficial results. And those ads and resolutions come up every year because it's nearly impossible to maintain.

Is there anything more sustainable? Instead of restricting calories, you can just restrict meals. Intermittent fasting (IF) is a less painful way of jacking up the same subcellular processes. By depriving your liver of calories for fourteen to sixteen hours per day, IF gives it a chance to activate AMP-kinase, suppress mTOR, increase autophagy, chew up some of the liver fat that's been stored, improve insulin resistance, and lower your insulin—the same outcomes that low-carb and ketogenic diets achieve. IF has also been shown to promote weight loss, blood glucose control, reduced inflammation, improvements in memory and stress resistance, slowed aging, and longer life span. Each of these benefits is a manifestation of improvement in insulin sensitivity. In this way, your leptin won't drop so fast that you feel awful; and since insulin blocks leptin signaling, the lower your insulin levels go, the better your brain can see the leptin. This means your sympathetic nervous ratchets up, and you burn faster. All in all, most people find IF easier to adhere to long-term, and it's better for you.

Furthermore, IF comes in several flavors. The most common is early time-restricted feeding (eTRF)—a form of daily IF where dinner is eaten in the afternoon—which helps to improve people's ability to switch between burning carbohydrates for energy to burning fat for energy, an aspect of metabolism known as *metabolic flexibility*. People squeeze all their meals into an eight-to ten-hour period, followed by a fourteen-to-sixteen-hour overnight fast. Although eTRF doesn't affect how many calories participants burn, it does lower levels of the hunger hormone ghrelin and improve some aspects of appetite. It also increases fat burning over the twenty-four-hour day, particularly in the liver. A 2015 systematic review of forty studies showed that the various forms of IF were effective for weight loss, with a typical loss of seven to eleven pounds over ten weeks (on par with caloric restriction results).

My question is: why do people need to intermittently fast at all? Well, 45 percent of the population has liver fat that they need to burn off. However, if you ate a Real Food diet, the fiber in the food would've formed a gel in your duodenum, and you wouldn't be absorbing excess refined carbohydrates and sugar into the portal system. Your liver would be protected and never have generated that fat in the first place; therefore, you would have no need to burn it off. It's not that IF is bad (after all, we did it for millennia when food was scarce), but if you ate Real Food in the first place, it wouldn't be necessary.

Supplemental Earnings?

Go into a health food store, and the shelves are stocked floor to ceiling with big tubs of various dietary supplements. You've got your fats (e.g., omega-3s), your fat blockers (e.g., white kidney bean extract), your proteins (e.g., BCAAs), your protein blockers (green tea), your carbohydrates (e.g., polycose), your carbohydrate blockers (e.g., garcinia cambogia), your vitamins, your micronutrients, and your extracts. The nutraceutical industry is a $210 billion business in the US alone. Some people swear by them for various reasons, and I'm not going to try to change their minds, or yours. In truth, I take omega-3s, vitamin

C, and vitamin D. But do they work for the pathologies of metabolic syndrome?

There are two primary caveats to using supplements for metabolic syndrome: a supplement can be used to treat a deficiency, but not an excess; and a supplement will work only if it can be absorbed and transported into the cell. Different aspects of our eight subcellular pathologies (see Chapter 7) are due to excess, while others are due to deficiency:

1. **Glycation.** This is due to carbohydrate excess and can't be stopped just with a supplement.

2. **Oxidative stress.** Oxygen radicals must be quenched by antioxidants or they will do damage. Many studies demonstrate negative correlations between blood levels of antioxidants and metabolic syndrome. But this can't be fixed by just adding a supplement. Furthermore, supplementation with other antioxidants, such as vitamin E, has been linked to increased rates of mortality.

3. **Mitochondrial dysfunction.** Mitochondrial "boosters" are currently de rigueur. And if they worked, they would be a big win. But they don't get where they need to go. For instance, coenzyme Q10 is often used as a blood lipid treatment. But consumption of CoQ10 doesn't mean it is transported into the mitochondria. Meta-analyses show no effects of CoQ10 supplementation on lipids.

4. **Insulin resistance.** Lots of compounds, such as alpha-lipoic acid, chromium, berberine, bergamot, and resveratrol, show promise in animals. However, when the rubber hits the road, the human data don't support their use, because insulin resistance is due to nutrient excess, not nutrient deficiency.

5. **Membrane integrity.** Here, we see beneficial effects of omega-3 fatty acids (see Chapter 19), because of their role in suppressing inflammation,

improving insulin sensitivity, reducing triglyceride levels, and improving cognitive function. Omega-3s work because they are correcting a deficiency in the Western diet.

6. **Inflammation.** Polyphenols, such as curcumin, are thought to be valuable, as they would be correcting a nutrient deficiency; however, the scientific data has been anything but conclusive. One anti-inflammatory that holds promise is vitamin D, which has specific beneficial effects on the immune system via a set of toll-like receptors. These receptors reduce inflammatory mediators associated with infection, which can result in improved glycemic control. Vitamin D is also finding a primary place in the battle against COVID-19, because it is correcting a deficiency.

7. **Epigenetics.** Folate has been added to your bread in the grocery store to provide the recommended daily allowance, because our processed food diet meant that we were woefully deficient. Pregnant women, people on chemotherapy, and those with specific malabsorption or autoimmune conditions need more. They need to take a supplement. For the rest of us, further folate supplementation isn't necessary or beneficial in treating metabolic syndrome.

8. **Autophagy.** Spermidine, a polyamine found in cheese and mushrooms, can improve cardiovascular and cancer risk in animals. However, thus far no formulation has boosted levels enough to get it into the liver of humans. But the best way to increase spermidine in the blood is to change the gut microbiota, which is done with a prebiotic.

Real Food supplies all of these supplements in their natural state, whereas processed food is devoid of them. The simple act of food processing removes most of the micronutrients native to certain foods, as well as their fiber (think the germ of the wheat kernel; see Chapter 19). After all, many micronutrients travel in the fiber fraction. Furthermore, various items added during the processing of food, such as sugar and other preservatives, are even more toxic that we think. Many of the micronutrients are decimated by processing. While it's enticing to think that we could put them back into our bodies with a pill, the data doesn't support the use of most of our current nutraceutical armamentarium. In fact, nutraceutical use has been associated with a slightly higher rate of mortality, which doesn't necessarily mean that they're causal, but we don't know. Remember, disease A plus treatment B still equals death (see Chapter 6). Why not just eat Real Food?

Probiotic or Prebiotic?

As long as we're on supplements, let's talk about if they're affecting you or your gut microbiome. In Chapter 11, I stressed the importance of *feeding the gut.* The latest research shows that the bacteria in your gut have a mind of their own; they want to be fed, and if they're not, they'll release neuroactive factors that change your behavior. Also, by not feeding the good bacteria, the bad bacteria proliferate and release inflammatory mediators that cause disease.

The recognition of the pivotal role of the gut microbiome has turned medicine on its head. Now you've got people going around chanting, "*Bacteroides* is good; *Firmicutes* is bad." Every supplement company is offering their own proprietary probiotic guaranteed to fix your microbiome. But why is your microbiome broken in the first place? Maybe the caesarean section that delivered you at birth deprived your gut of beneficial vaginal flora. Maybe it was the antibiotics your doctor gave you for your ear infection when you were a toddler, or the antacid you took when you were twenty. Maybe it's the antibiotics in your meat (see Chapter 20) or maybe it's the diet sweeteners in the soda you drink to wash it down. We don't know why we have a sick microbiome, but we do.

So let's repopulate your unhappy gut with a probiotic. Probiotics are living bacteria; logic says that if you eat them, they should multiply and grow. But they don't. If they did, you wouldn't have to keep taking them. Processed food has made the intestinal environment inhospitable, and the good bacteria can't live in that environment. It would be like sending humans to Mars with no atmosphere. It doesn't matter how many you keep sending, they're not going to survive (unless they're Matt Damon). You have to *feed your gut*, and processed food starves it. More processing means more functional intestinal problems, more autoimmune disease, and more metabolic syndrome. Probiotics can't fix this because they can't survive in the subsequent environment.

There's a more effective way to make sure those good bacteria set up shop: a prebiotic, which will alter the gut environment, and permit those probiotics to take. The simplest and most effective isn't found in a supplement—but in dietary fiber. The microbiome will change for the better within two days of adopting a high-fiber diet. Add a probiotic with a prebiotic, and now maybe those bacteria will take because you're changing your intestinal habitat. However, you have to continue to support the new environment by eating Real Food.

Food Allergies

Cow's milk. Eggs. Peanuts. Shellfish. What was sustenance for some has now turned deadly for others. There are more than 170 foods that can trigger an allergic response, and these allergies have increased by 50 percent in just fourteen years. ER admission rates for anaphylactic shock have doubled. Why is this happening?

Almost all foodstuffs have various unique proteins, or antigens, on their surfaces. The enzymes in the intestine break these proteins down completely into their component amino acids, which are then absorbed and go to the liver. But if a protein gains access to the bloodstream before it's completely dismantled, its structure will be recognized by the immune system as foreign and will generate an immune response. The intestine normally serves as a barrier between the outside world where foreign proteins don't cause trouble and the inside world where amino acids don't; but there are checkpoints in the intestine, called tight junctions. These junctions are manned by a class of proteins called *zonulins* (think: border crossing official), which keep foreign invaders on the other side of the barrier. The Western diet, and particularly fructose, changes the energy status within the intestinal cell, leading to zonulin dysfunction. These tight junctions becoming porous (think: border patrol agent taking a smoke break, and someone cutting a hole in the fence). Your immune system jumps into the fray to fight off those pieces of undigested food that have breached the barrier, and those antibodies could activate your white blood cells that release histamine, leading to a food allergy. Take, for example, if you weren't allergic to chocolate or eggs or shellfish at birth, but developed an allergy along the way. Once that clone of cells attacks something that's leaked out— remember leaky gut?—it will attack it forever.

The Gluten-free Craze

Owing to William Davis's *Wheat Belly* (2011) and David Perlmutter's *Grain Brain* (2013), gluten-free is now mainstream. But is gluten the problem? Given how delicious bread and pastries are, there must be a reason that people are shying away from baked goods. It is true that 1 in 132 children in America has celiac disease, which is an allergy to either glutenin or gliadin, the two proteins that make up gluten (many of them also have type 1 diabetes, as autoimmune diseases tend to congregate in the same patient). Furthermore, the majority of these people aren't even aware of their condition. These kids and adults actually need a gluten-free diet—wheat, barley, and rye elimination. But that doesn't explain why 72 percent (triple the number since 2009) of the adults who are gluten-free don't have bona fide celiac disease. The new pseudo-medical term is *non-celiac gluten sensitivity* (NCGS). Full disclosure—I'm one of them. But I'm not *gluten-free*—I'm *wheat-free*. For five years, I had undiagnosed gastrointestinal troubles, and my gastroenterologist checked me for celiac disease three separate times— always negative. He first put me on rifaximin (an antibiotic to sterilize my gut), then a low-fermentable oligo-, di-, mono-saccharides and polyols (FODMAP) diet—to no avail.

In 2018, I finally learned why. Dr. Stefano Guandalini of the University of Chicago, one of the world's foremost celiac disease researchers, explained this disorder to me. Wheat is a complex organism—it's hexaploid (six nuclei) instead of diploid (two nuclei). It's been selectively bred to cultivate certain traits—among them higher gluten content, which means better bread because gluten is "sticky" and therefore rises better, making a fluffier loaf. Wheat also has seven hundred different proteins you could have an intolerance to—only two of them are the ones in gluten. The other 698 are just as capable of generating an immune reaction. This is why there's no biomarker in the blood for it; there are too many suspects. For example, if you take white blood cells from a celiac patient, put them in a petri dish, and throw either wheat, barley, rye, or purified gluten in as well, they'll go bonkers. But if you take white blood cells from a patient with wheat intolerance and test them, they'll react to the wheat but do nothing in response to the barley, rye, or purified gluten. Dr. Guandalini wants to rename this condition *non-celiac wheat intolerance* (NCWI), because these people can have a beer (made with barley)—and I do, without any problem.

The New Era of Personalized Nutrition—Ready for Prime Time?

What's become clear is that different people have different metabolic responses to different foods. One diet doesn't fit all. An Israeli group used continuous glucose monitors (CGMs), a device you wear, to predict which foods people should eat and which ones they should avoid. In doing so, they improved their weight and metabolic status short-term. This is a great step forward. There's also a current wave of interest among biohackers in wearing a CGM to reduce glucose excursions. Does it help? Not yet, because what we've also learned is that glucose fluctuations only describe one piece of the puzzle. To truly implement personalized nutrition, we also have to know how much insulin your pancreas releases, how much triglyceride your intestine and your liver make in response to those foods, and how your intestinal microbiota changed. As I've said many times already, the insulin response is even more important for metabolic health than the glucose response. Companies are working on a real-time insulin and triglyceride monitor, and others are honing their microbiome analysis capacities, but these new technologies aren't yet ready for widespread use.

Given the dramatic reduction in health span, the increase in health-care costs (see Chapter 1), and the lack of rational medications or monitoring strategies for the diseases of metabolic syndrome (see Chapter 2), it would seem to me that anything that can mitigate those eight subcellular pathologies, and synchronize those three enzymes, ought to be in high demand. However, adults are just the tip of the iceberg. The next two chapters will demonstrate how adolescents, children, toddlers, infants, and fetuses are uniquely susceptible to processed food, and at the most formative critical windows of development. Froot Loops, anyone?

CHAPTER 15

═══

What and How Children and Adolescents Eat

The leprechaun is right—Lucky Charms are "magically delicious." Yellow stars, green clovers, orange moons, pink hearts. Why are there marshmallows in the box? Because kids love them? Sure, but they also love Honey Bunches of Oats, Cracklin' Oat Bran, and Cap'n Crunch. Because they're colorful? Trix, Froot Loops, and Fruity Pebbles are also colorful. The real reason is because oats cost more than marshmallows. The marshmallows take up room in the box, which decreases the cost of ingredients per box, yet the company gets to charge more per unit. A great business strategy.

As a pediatric endocrinologist over forty years, I watched children grow—vertically at first, but now horizontally. My clinical practice started in 1980, so I saw the natural histories of the obesity and metabolic syndrome epidemics in real time. The only thing that changed faster than kids' waistlines was their diets. Bananas were replaced as the snack of choice by Gatorade, Go-Gurt, and granola bars.

Breakfast Is a Dangerous Meal

Breakfast is considered by most nutrition experts to be the most important meal of the day (this is arguably just a holdover from the AND's Lenna Cooper channeling John Harvey Kellogg (see Chapter 4)). To its credit, breakfast does get your kid's brain going in the morning. It increases the thermic effect of food, which is worth about 10 percent of your energy expenditure, and it suppresses ghrelin (the hunger hormone) so you won't overeat at lunch. But for children, it's easy to turn to what is fast and cheap, and what they can pour themselves. Cold cereal. Instant oatmeal. Granola bars. Protein bars. Yogurt smoothies. All marketed to kids and their parents and all laden with sugar. Consider Raisin Bran. Just raisins and bran, right? There are 16 grams of sugar in a serving, but the raisins only account for 8. That's because the raisins are all dipped in a sugar solution (they're white, not purple—see the book jacket cover!) to make them much sweeter. And if you think Cracklin' Oat Bran or Honey Bunches of Oats are any healthier, think again. The food industry knows how to market to kids—sports figures, celebrities, characters and mascots, cartoons, premiums, cross-promotion toys, collectibles, kids' clubs, internet games, and contests.

Sadly, as the National Diet and Nutrition Survey found, what you're really doing is giving your children a huge sugar load, half of their daily intake on average. Breakfast cereal averages a whopping 12 grams of added sugar in a typical serving. In 2011, the Environmental Working Group (EWG) identified 17 breakfast cereals marketed to children in which added sugar constituted more than 50 percent of calories, and 177 with 40 percent or more. Top of the list—Kellogg's Honey Smacks, at 56 percent sugar. Despite the notoriety of that disclosure, the EWG follow-up study in 2014 noted that not one of these breakfast cereals had reduced its sugar content. In 2018, the industry revised its 2011 thresholds for added sugar, but amazingly, the upper limit for breakfast *increased* from less than 10 grams to less than 12 grams.

How did companies pull that off? Because the kids wouldn't like it as much and they'd sell less product.

Yogurt is another example of a corporate ploy to ply our kids with sugar. Plain yogurt has 7 grams of sugar, all lactose (milk sugar), which isn't a problem, although not much help. Consider a carton of pomegranate yogurt, which has 19 grams of total sugar. Thus, each pomegranate yogurt has 12 grams of added sugar. Plus, the industry hides these facts well; there are 262 different names for sugar. By choosing different sugars as the fifth, sixth, seventh, and eighth ingredients, it can rapidly add up to be the dominant ingredient.

The American Heart Association recommends limiting kids to 3 to 4 teaspoons of added sugar per day. Yet a typical school breakfast consists of a bowl of Froot Loops and a glass of orange juice; that's already 11 teaspoons of sugar. Dr. Terence Kealey, dean of the University of Buckingham in the UK, penned a book in 2018 called *Breakfast Is a Dangerous Meal*. I had the opportunity to corner him at a meeting, and I got this modification: "Our kids' *current* breakfast is a dangerous meal." To that I can agree wholeheartedly.

Any food is a dessert if any form of sugar is one of the first three ingredients. Trader Joe's Beef and Broccoli (32 grams of sugar) is a dessert. Chinese chicken salad is a dessert. We, and especially our kids, are eating and drinking dessert all day long. It captivates our brain's reward center (see Chapter 21), similar to drugs, so kids get hooked on sugar early. This creates a tidal wave of chronic diseases so nefarious and insidious that our healthcare system isn't prepared for the flood of children with type 2 diabetes and liver disease who will be sick for decades. Tell a cocaine addict to lay off their drug of choice—see how far that gets you. About as far as telling a kid to cut the cookies.

Don't get me wrong. We all love dessert. How could you not? Sweet was the signal to our ancestors that a foodstuff was safe to eat, because there are no foods that are both sweet and acutely poisonous. But dessert should be safe, and rare. Just like Halloween, overdoing it also has a predictable output—a huge tummy ache.

Got Milk? Good, Now Let It Go . . .

So what about milk? Kids drink low-fat chocolate (and strawberry) milk at school. Why? Because we took the fat out in the 1980s to conform to the Dietary Guidelines and the kids no longer drank it. They needed to add sugar to make it palatable, though in doing so they're increasing risk of metabolic syndrome. But do we need milk at all, and how much?

For decades, we've been praising the benefits of dairy, in terms of growth, strong muscles, bones, and teeth. But these recommendations have recently come under increased scrutiny. We thought that everything in cow's milk was good for growing kids—calcium, vitamin D, protein, phosphorus—except for the saturated fat, and so we made nonfat and low-fat options. But the saturated fat in whole milk, due to its odd-chain fatty acids and phospholipid content, is actually protective in preventing diabetes and heart disease. Furthermore, milk is one of the products we definitely want to be processed. Pasteurization of milk is what kills the tuberculosis bacteria; irradiation of milk is what converts the 7-dehydrocholesterol in milk to vitamin D. You do need all of these things, but you don't necessarily need cow's milk to get them (though milk does increase kids' height and bone density). You could just as easily get your vitamin D from playing outside, and calcium from fish, leafy greens, and almonds.

No wonder people are rethinking the role of dairy in nutrition, suggesting that it not be its own dietary food group anymore. The USDA's insistence upon drinking milk is to support the dairy farmers, not you and your kids. Milk doesn't necessarily deserve the health halo the dairy industry bestowed upon it, but it doesn't deserve the pitchfork either. Cow's milk has been vilified for everything from eczema to type 1 diabetes to autism, but there are no cause-and-effect studies to prove it.

What about cancer? T. Colin Campbell's voluminous tome *The China Study* (2006) attempted to look epidemiologically at the difference between Chinese and American health, and determined that milk is a primary driver of chronic disease (especially cancer). In fact, this book isolated the bovine milk protein casein as the toxic factor.

There are a number of reasons to be skeptical of this view, including the types of statistical analyses that were performed to prove it. In fact, the stronger associations with cancer were sugar and alcohol—but these were ignored. Having said that, a meta-analysis does seem to support a slight positive correlation between whole milk consumption and prostate cancer in men, but cause and effect cannot be established. Nonetheless, as dairy saturated fat appears to be protective against cardiovascular disease and diabetes, it would seem to me either promotion or demonization of cow's milk (excluding the additives) seems quite inappropriate. Like a relationship on Facebook, it's complicated.

Lunch Is No Better

The Healthy, Hunger-Free Kids Act passed by Congress in 2010 raised the national per-pupil lunch expenditure from $2.80 to $2.86—not enough to even cover the cost of a carrot. Instead of upping the dollar amount, Representative Robert Aderholt (R-AL) and the House Committee on Appropriations in 2014 decided to gut the ridiculously low bar they themselves had previously set, by allowing schools to opt out of the federal nutrition standards. But in 2017, USDA Secretary Sonny Perdue, viewing discarded vegetables as waste, diluted these standards down even further. "Schools need flexibility in menu planning . . . it's clear that many still face challenges incorporating some of the meal pattern requirements. Schools want to offer food that students actually want to eat. It doesn't do any good to serve nutritious meals if they wind up in the trash can." Guess what kids find most appetizing?

A recent article in the *New York Times* highlighted the angst that parents currently feel about feeding their children. In response to both the obesity and eating disorders epidemics that have targeted children, the *intuitive eating* movement was born, embraced by culturists and some nutritionists as a healthier way of eating. Intuitive eating allows kids to eat whatever they want whenever they want. If obesity were about hunger, then this might be a rational modality. But eating is sometimes done in response to reward or stress, and kids often turn to sugar. As I said in Chapter 2, weight and BMI are often irrelevant to health, and there's no place for fat-shaming in our society. But these intuitive eaters have taken the issue too far the other way, by refusing to demonize any food or ingredient—they still fallaciously believe *a calorie is a calorie.*

No Wonder Kids Can't Function in School

The National School Breakfast Program has 25 percent of America's children enrolled, and the National School Lunch Program has 39 percent of children enrolled. The federal government caps the amount of fat and salt in breakfasts and lunches, setting the minimum standards for servings of fruit, vegetables, grains, milk, and meat. However, they've also designated pizza as a vegetable and hash browns as a fruit (see Chapter 24). And there's no official limit for sugar.

The brain is the biggest utilizer of energy, consuming 20 percent of all the glucose in your bloodstream at any given moment. Considering your brain weighs just three pounds, or 2 percent of your body weight, that's a very big draw. But what does the brain do with fructose? Remember, the intestine and liver will clear the majority of fructose, but if you overwhelm their capacities with a 20-ounce soft drink, a sizeable portion gets into the brain. Fructose alters brain metabolism in fundamental ways—not in neurons *per se*, but in *astrocytes* (the cells that nourish the neurons). And it's not feeding those cells, but rather driving two of the eight subcellular pathologies (glycation and oxidative stress). However, some of the ill effects of fructose in the brain can be counteracted by consuming more omega-3s.

Furthermore, fructose scrambles two trophic (growth) factors that help the brain develop and organize connections. Leptin is a fat-derived hormone that does a couple of different things. In Chapter 7, I discussed the impact of leptin on metabolic syndrome, but it also has a direct impact on brain development and cognition. Fructose, by inducing insulin resistance and hyperinsulinemia, blocks leptin's actions to permit neurons to branch and connect, leading to numerous cognitive deficits. Furthermore, fructose inhibits the functioning of a second protein, brain-derived neurotrophic factor (BDNF; the protein induced by exercise, see Chapter 10), which helps lay down new connections in the hippocampus (the memory center). Fructose is the proof in the pudding—*you can't outrun a bad diet.*

Three Impacts of Sugar on Your Kid's Brain

At school, every day is some kid's birthday; and unfortunately, that means that every day is a birthday party (PARENTS—PLEASE DON'T CONTRIBUTE TO THIS PRACTICE BY BRINGING CUP-CAKES TO SCHOOL!). Teachers know that once the sugar flows, the education stops, so the cupcakes are reserved for the end of the day. Sugar alters kids' brain function in three ways—behavior, cognition, and affect.

Behavior

Sugared beverages are clearly linked to behavioral problems in children, to irritability in preschoolers, and to violent behavior in middle-schoolers. However, thus far this remains correlation, not causation, and it's clear that not every kid who eats a Snickers bar turns into the Tasmanian devil. Sugar can run the gamut of irritability, from anxiety to sloth.

If you give a normal-weight five-year-old kid a cookie, what happens? He bounces off walls. Parents recognize this as the "sugar high," but it's actually the negative feedback system of energy balance at work. The cookie stimulated insulin release, which drove energy into fat tissue, which released leptin, which reached the hypothalamus, which activated the sympathetic nervous system, which led to increased energy expenditure, including involuntary contraction of muscles, aka fidgeting—all to maintain energy neutrality. But, the strange thing is, if you give an *obese* five-year-old kid a cookie, he's in the pantry looking for more cookies, and then back on the couch—because this kid's brain is leptin resistant. There is no sugar high.

Any study that looks at sugar and acute behavioral change has to look at leptin and insulin levels, too—but none of them have. Likely, it's processed food in general, the combination of sugar plus artificial flavors and colors to enhance sugar's effects.

Cognition

More and more young people are developing metabolic syndrome earlier. Adolescents with metabolic syndrome demonstrate cognitive decline and greater impulsivity. When you scan them, they exhibit white matter lesions, smaller hippocampi (the memory center), and re-duced prefrontal cortex mass (the executive function center). While not proven, such brain changes in the prefrontal cortex may be the under-lying cause of distractibility and the development of attention deficit disorder in children.

It won't be a shock to you that kids who eat processed food do less well in school. But is that correlation or causation? Is it the food, or could it just as easily be neglect, family stress, poverty, or genetics? One UK study changed the food in primary school in one county, using other neighboring counties as the control. The investigators found significant improvements in English and science, and the added bonus of a 14 per-cent reduction in school absences. It's a pretty good bet that changing the school food didn't change the home environment—but also a pretty good indication that the change in the food made a difference.

Affect

There's a reason that the WHO and the USDA have provided upper limits of sugar—because dietary sugar fries your kids' liver and brain, just like alcohol. Alcohol provides calories (7 kcal/gram), but it's not nutrition. There's no biochemical reaction that requires it. When con-sumed chronically and in high doses, alcohol is toxic, unrelated to its calories or effects on weight. Not everyone who is exposed gets ad-dicted, but enough do to warrant taxation and restriction of access, especially to children. Clearly, alcohol isn't food—but it's dangerous, because it's both toxic and abused.

Dietary sugar is composed of two molecules: glucose and fructose. Fructose, while an energy source (4 kcal/gram), is otherwise vestigial to humans; again, there's no biochemical reaction that requires it. However, fructose is metabolized in the liver in exactly the same way as alcohol. That's why, when consumed chronically and in high doses, fructose is similarly toxic and abused, unrelated to its calories or effects on weight. That's why our children now get the diseases of alcohol (type 2 diabetes, fatty liver disease), without ever taking a drink.

So which comes first? The diet, the biochemistry, or the behavior? This isn't an academic exercise—identifying the initial lesion between diet and brain function has enormous implications for both prevention and treatment. And it's true, we only have snapshots in time; we don't have the longitudinal or imaging studies to answer this question directly. But if our animal models are any indication, we should recognize that it's a two-way effect. Diet can alter biochemistry, which can alter behavior; but biochemistry can also alter behavior, which can also alter diet. The moral of the story is: when you see a change in behavior, think of the change in biochemistry, and then fix the diet accordingly.

I remember in the late 1960s when the first McDonald's was built in my neighborhood. I couldn't wait for it to open. Now I take singular delight in watching them close. In fact, in April 2013, I debated Jim Skinner, former CEO of McDonald's, who had moved on to become chairman of the board of Walgreens. He started out espousing "personal choice"; by the end, he was all about "public health." Even he couldn't deny the obvious.

It's a minefield out there; step in the wrong place, and you blow up (figuratively and literally). Our fast food society has placed undue stress on kids today, and it's taking its toll physically, mentally, and behaviorally. But teach the children, and someday they'll vote—with their dollars, with their ballots, and with their forks.

CHAPTER 16

What and How Fetuses, Infants, and Toddlers Eat

Babies are quite obviously different from adults. They have no teeth, sensitive tummies, and sometimes develop colic. They also have to be burped, and their main source of nourishment is breast milk. However, not every woman can breastfeed—both for medical and economic reasons—and that's OK. Formula was invented for this reason. However, there's also cow's milk, goat's milk, tea, and numerous other substitutes and concoctions to choose from—none of which are recommended by the American Academy of Pediatrics—and some of those are laden with sugar, salt, and the wrong kinds of fats.

Baby Vegans

In 1983, I moved to San Francisco for my pediatric endocrine fellowship. I had no idea what awaited me in the pediatric ICU: three toddlers, eighteen months old, all on ventilators in congestive heart failure because their parents had placed them on a macrobiotic diet. These ostensibly well-meaning parents were trying to prevent their children from succumbing to the "toxins" associated with meats, oils, and dairy products, so instead they fed their tots grains, cereals, vegetables, and, of course, tater tots. As a result, their hearts ballooned and couldn't pump from the lack of iron, vitamin D, and calcium.

We're currently seeing a resurgence in this practice. Vegan diets are all the rage in adults (see Chapter 12), and some parents are pushing it on their babies for ethical reasons, or because they've bought into pseudo-science hype. Some are saying to themselves, why should I give my kids dietary fat—the liver will make it from carbohydrate as needed. Wouldn't naturally occurring fats be healthier than the saturated fats in the Standard American Diet?

It's true that the liver can manufacture fat from carbohydrate—a process known as *de novo* lipogenesis (see Chapter 2). Indeed, our research team at UCSF and Touro University study this process. However, the liver only makes *palmitate*, the 16-carbon saturated free fatty acid that can do damage (see Chapter 12), but no other kinds—none of the monounsaturated, polyunsaturated, or omega-3 fatty acids necessary for the growing brains and bodies of infants. The vegan diet, by its very nature, is deficient in the fats necessary for babies.

In fact, parents from Florida to Belgium have been brought up on charges of neglect due to feeding their babies a standard vegan diet. The Royal Academy of Medicine of Belgium just published a legal opinion that argued it's unethical to subject children to a vegan diet because it doesn't include the animal proteins containing vital essential amino acids necessary to promote growth and prevent health problems. The worst part is that some pediatricians will defer to parents' preferences on infant feeding so as to not rock the boat. They should know better. This boat needs rocking.

Baby Brains

Babies also have different metabolic needs than adults. For one, they have a rapidly growing brain. A newborn has a brain 33 percent the size of an adult; yet it increases by almost 1 percent per day—by three months of age, it has increased 64 percent from birth, and is now 55 percent the size of an adult brain. Since the brain is composed of 60 percent fat, there's a lot that has to be laid down in a very short period of time, which means there has to be a lot of fat in the diet. But not just any fat.

We're talking omega-3s (see Chapter 19), which are essential fatty acids—fetuses must get them from their mothers, and babies must eat a lot of them very quickly. They come in two flavors: eicosapentaenoic acid (EPA) and docosahexaenoic acid (DHA). Because of their three double-bonds, omega-3s are more flexible, meaning they bend in different directions. For this reason, they're incorporated into cell membranes, especially neuronal membranes, where they increase fluidity (meaning they allow for easy cell deformation without rupture). This prevents cell aging and early cell death. Omega-3s also reduce inflammation at the nerve terminal, allowing for better neural transmission. Furthermore, omega-3s can be turned into *endocannabinoids* (ECs)—the brain's version of marijuana, which helps heighten mood by alleviating anxiety. And that heightened stress is predetermined even before they are born. Lack of omega-3s during pregnancy in rats messes with insulin signaling and brain growth factor levels in the offspring, leading to increased anxiety. Conversely, omega-3s help repair the damage to neuronal membranes caused by toxins such as fructose. Omega-3s are so important to neonatal development that formula companies started supplementing with them back in 2003.

So where do all those omega-3s come from? Breast milk is chock-full of them. But if mom is omega-3 deficient, there are immediate implications for all of us. First of all, what do we tell pregnant women not to eat? Seafood, out of concern for mercury poisoning. However, in the UK it's been proven that maternal seafood consumption predicts improved neurodevelopmental outcomes in children. So are we making more trouble than we're solving by advising against it?

In the absence of Real Food, obstetricians can skirt the issue by giving the pregnant mom omega-3 supplements, fixing the deficiency.

This provides a double bonus—the moms' risk for depression is reduced, and the kids' neurodevelopmental outcomes are improved.

Sugar Babies 1

Omega-3s aren't all that babies' brains need. Mother's, cow's, and other mammalian milks contain a special sugar called lactose, which is composed of two molecules—glucose and galactose bound together. You hear a lot about lactose because many people lack the enzyme that breaks the bond between the two molecules, a condition called lactose intolerance; affected individuals experience diarrhea, pain, and gas in response to milk or dairy consumption.

However, you don't hear much about galactose. When an adult consumes galactose, it goes straight to the liver and is converted immediately to glucose. Many adults don't drink milk, and adults have no need for galactose. So why does it exist? Why is it important? Why is it exclusively in mammalian milk?

Milk is food for babies; and babies, even more than children or adults, need to grow two parts of the body—the brain and the immune system. Galactose is an essential component of certain fats in the brain called *cerebrosides* and *ceramides*. Furthermore, the mammary gland is the only part of the human body that can make galactose, in order to properly feed the infant. But then is lactose-free formula a good idea? Parents often blame cow's-milk formula or the lactose it contains for their babies' feeding problems, fussiness, and other subjective symptoms. Currently, soy-based lactose-free formula is now 25 percent of all US formula sales. Is that good for all babies? A recent study showed breast-fed infants scored slightly higher on the mental development index than formula-fed infants at six and twelve months of age. They also showed higher psychomotor development index scores than soy-based lactose-free formula-fed infants.

Galactose is also important in the development of both the innate and adaptive immune systems. A rare, genetic inability of the liver to turn galactose into glucose, called *galactosemia*, is also associated with immune problems. Many of these babies die of neonatal meningitis. If they survive the newborn period, they exhibit moderate cognitive deficits—although it's not clear if it's a function of withholding of galactose or of the disease itself. The point is that galactose is necessary for babies but not adults. A trial of lactose-free formula is often the first maneuver a doctor attempts for a fussy baby; it shouldn't be. Talk with your doctor before you make the switch.

Sugar Babies 2

Then there's that other sugar—fructose. Remember, there's no biochemical reaction in any animal cell on the planet that requires fructose. So what happens when fructose enters a fetus? For a long time, it's been assumed that the placenta protects the fetus from mom's many missteps, but we now know this is false—otherwise we wouldn't have crack- or opiate-addicted newborns.

It turns out that fructose has effects on fetuses as well. If a pregnant mom drinks a Coke, the fructose crosses the placenta and the fetus gets a huge bolus (large amount), which has been shown to stimulate the liver to make even more free palmitate. In addition, the taste receptors on the tongue develop at thirty weeks' gestation—way before the first taste of juice—meaning the fetus is sensing the fructose in the amniotic fluid. So yes, you can be addicted to soda at birth.

Project Viva examined the associations between pregnancy, cognition, and childhood sugar consumption in the form of sugar sweetened beverages, other beverages (diet soda, juice), and fruit. Among 1,234 mother-child pairs enrolled, a mean maternal sucrose consumption of 50 grams/day—consistent with the upper limit of current USDA guidelines—negatively impacted mid-childhood cognitive testing. Also of note, prenatal *diet* soda consumption was shown to negatively impact mid-childhood verbal scores as well.

Furthermore, cutting the umbilical cord only compounds the problem. Doctors used to think that fructose didn't cross from the mother into the breast milk, but we now know that the only thing standing between mom's 20-ounce Coke and the baby is mom's intestine and liver. The amount of fructose that makes it into the breast milk correlates directly with the degree of weight and fat mass increase in six-month-old infants.

Eighty-three percent of American infants start out breastfeeding, but that percentage is cut to 60 percent by three months, a function of race, education, poverty, and culture. A whole lot of infants are consuming some type of formula, either solely or as a supplement to breast milk. In fact, the formula industry is a behemoth and expected to gross $103 billion by 2026. The industry would like us to think that formula is as good for babies as is breast milk—but does the truth live up to the hype?

A review of lactose-free infant formulas documents a dietary composition of half corn syrup solids and half sucrose, for a total of 10.3 percent of calories coming from sugar. While we don't yet know if this is enough to lead to metabolic disturbances in infants, it certainly is in older children. In fact, based on EU guidelines, several US FDA-approved lactose-free formulas are illegal in Europe.

Of course, infants eventually graduate from breast milk or formula up to baby food. Why? Because the marketers want them to. Was there always baby food? The first commercial baby food was marketed in the Netherlands in 1901 and in the US in the early 1920s. Gerber was founded in 1927, and Beech-Nut and Pablum (dried baby food) in 1931. Annually, the Gerber baby contest garners millions of submissions and views on social media—a brilliant marketing ploy. But what did babies eat before 1901?

Back then, adult food was macerated and churned into chunky pastes, which is still what babies consume in many other countries. In order to get babies to eat the commercial stuff, manufacturers had to make it "appealing"—so they added sugar. Lots of it. The problem is that obese infants taste sugar less well than normal-weight infants, so the industry needed to add a greater amount for those infants to register their approval—just as they do for adults. But no matter—even thirty days of exposure can turn a sugar-ambivalent baby into a sugar-liker. It's in the industry's best interest to keep adding sugar so that the infant will only want to eat sweet foods—that *they* make. In fact, you have to introduce a savory food to an infant a median of thirteen times before they'll accept it. That's a lot of "here comes the choo-choo." On the other hand, how many times do you have to introduce a sweet food to an infant before they'll accept it? Just once.

In 2015, the U.S. Centers for Disease Control and Prevention examined the nutritional information of 1,074 infant and toddler food products. It found 32 percent of toddler dinners, the majority of child-oriented snacks, and infant-aimed juices contained at least one source of added sugar. And 35 percent of all the calories in those foods or drinks came from sugar. Worse yet, a laboratory analysis of baby foods documents that their added sugar content is even higher than what's reported on the Nutrition Facts label. Maybe the reason is that there are 262 different names for added sugar, so the industry can sneak it in without you even noticing?

And then they're hooked. By the time they hit six months of age, 60 percent of US infants consume some daily added sugars. After six months, that number jumps to 98 percent. The American Heart Association, UK Royal College of Paediatrics and Child Health, and the WHO all say that babies and toddlers shouldn't be consuming any added sugar, and have all argued for mandatory guidelines on the sugar content of toddler foods to encourage reformulation. As a result, the newest 2020 Dietary Guidelines Advisory Committee (see Chapter 24) has written a section on infants and toddlers. We'll see if their guidance makes it into the final document. However, to their credit, some food companies have publicly acknowledged the added sugar problem and are now reporting their practices on the Nutrition Facts label. All in all, commercial baby food is a minefield. If you can't make your own, just remember this one piece of advice: avoid any food that comes in a pouch.

Baby Teeth

It seems so obvious—sugar rots kids' teeth. Well, it rots babies' teeth, too. In fact, early childhood caries in infants and toddlers are rampant today. If you think babies aren't drinking sweet drinks (fruit juice, sports drinks, soda), think again. Giving a baby soda has a negative social connotation, but they're often given juice—and guess what? Same amount of sugar, no difference. UK dental epidemiologist Aubrey Sheiham showed that the dose of sugar times the chronicity of exposure predicts the onset of dental caries in children. By three years old (traditionally the time of a child's first visit to the dentist), one-third of all toddlers already have dental caries. To stop this concerning trend, the American Dental Association and the American Academy of Pediatric Dentistry have recently ratcheted down their age recommendations to start oral health exams under the age of one year. While I was working as a pediatrician at UCSF, one ancillary disease that I treated was bottle-rot, the complete breakdown of the upper and lower incisors due to the constant presence of juice in a baby bottle. This is the greatest reason for chronic pain in children, and many of them were afraid to smile because of the humiliation—even at age three.

Baby Overjet

Ever wondered why beards came into fashion in the 1980s? Facial hair style trends come and go (mustaches, sideburns, muttonchops), but beards came and stayed. Don Johnson from *Miami Vice* (1984) popularized stubble, but this fad didn't recede—it only grew stronger. Though hipsters have repopularized the trend, one reason some men grow beards is to hide a weak chin. Dentists know it as *retrognathia*; you might know it as *overjet*. Similarly, *malocclusion* (not enough room for all the teeth in the mouth) has increased in the population over the last forty years; this was determined by looking at rates of orthodontia, even after controlling for financial concerns, which exhibit an increase in patient load between 1987 and 2004 (the years when children born in the late 1970s and 1980s would be fitted for braces). Why? Because sucking on mother's nipple is far better than sucking on a plastic one. The infant has to suck harder to make a seal, and this action strengthens and grows the sixteen muscles of the tongue. The well-developed tongue then applies continuous pressure against the hard palate of infants so that it's broad and flat (mimicking the shape of the tongue), thereby creating a larger space in the mouth and a wider airway. A low, lazy tongue means that the palate narrows and develops a high arch.

Thumbs and pacifiers can vault the palate, keeping it narrow, and lead to future dental and airway issues. The position of the tongue and the vaulting of the palate is the difference between nose-breathers and mouth-breathers. The tongue has to be elevated in the palate for us to be nose breathers, and sucking on mother's nipple instead of a plastic one reduces the risk for mouth breathing and overjet in later life.

The problem mounts further in toddlerhood because of pureed baby food. What and how did babies eat after weaning off the breast before there was commercial baby food? As we explored earlier, they ate what their parents ate, and they gummed it to death. As a result, they got very strong mastication muscles (masseter, temporalis, and pterygoids), necessary to grow the jaw and increase the airway size. However, we've now abdicated this practice for defibertized and pureed baby food, because it's yummier (added sugar), easier, and faster, and there's a lower risk of choking.

Sadly, these associations between food, jaw growth, and sleep apnea have been known for at least a century. In 1921 Dr. LeRoy Johnson, dean of the Harvard Dental School, stated, "The face has evolved with the functions of mastication and respiration." Nonetheless, the pureed baby food market continues to grow even today. While there are many new entrants vying for market share into what had been a closed oligopoly (Gerber, Abbott, Beech-Nut, Carnation), the problem remains.

Furthermore, this isn't just a cosmetic issue, it's a metabolic one, too. Retrognathia, overjet, malocclusion, and a small airway set children and adults up for the development of obstructive sleep apnea (OSA), hypoxia (lack of oxygen), enzyme dyssynchrony (see Chapter 8), the eight subcellular pathologies (see Chapter 7), and obesity and metabolic syndrome in early childhood. As a kid gains weight, fat is deposited in the tongue, soft palate, and lateral pharyngeal walls, which results in enlargement of these tissues, narrowing the airway even further and contributing to the development of OSA. The OSA feeds the obesity and the obesity feeds the OSA. It's this vicious cycle that can lead to metabolic syndrome. Today, 85 percent of sleep disordered breathing in children goes undiagnosed, and 24 percent of ADHD is really sleep disordered breathing that has been misdiagnosed. Is your kid snoring? It may be cute, but it's not normal. Tell your dentist.

Malocclusion is also the reason more wisdom teeth are being extracted. The jaw doesn't grow enough, so there isn't enough room for the third molars. Wisdom teeth are a biomarker, or sign and symptom of the problem started by a plastic nipple or pacifier. But when dentists take them out, the jaw and oral airway collapse even further. In fact, you could develop OSA after wisdom teeth extraction.

Real Food for Babies—and Pregnant Moms

Food has evolved. Unfortunately, babies have not. Now they are regressing—because the food doesn't match their anatomy, physiology, or biochemistry. But babies have no choice, they have no control of their diet; and worse yet, they had no control over mother's diet while they were gestating. As a society, we're suffering the damage and aftermath of feeding pregnant women processed food and feeding our children commercial formula and pureed baby food, setting them up for cognitive and medical problems. None of these can be undone with a simple pill. We're slaves to our genes, our epigenes, and our upbringing, and by the time we realize it, it's too late to fix. But we could fix the food, and it's never too late to start.

Part IV

(Processed) Food Fight

CHAPTER 17

Food Classifications

If there's a single theme that pervades this book, it's that the problem isn't *what's in the food*, but rather *what's been done to the food*. Parts II and III dealt with nutrition, and now in Part IV we're on to food science, and why it matters.

As an MIT undergraduate in the 1970s, I majored in nutrition and food science—"Food 'n' Nuts" as it was affectionately called—and was exposed to both sides of this equation. Does food science provide better nutrition? Or does it detract? Back then I studied under Nevin Scrimshaw, Hamish Munro, and Vernon Young—luminaries in the vitamin and protein fields who successfully researched and treated nutrient deficiencies. They were convinced it's *what's in the food* versus *what's missing*, and if we can just add nutrients, so much the better. They were right—just not for everyone.

But the food industry was happy to oblige my professors, as it gave them yet another selling point and front-of-package claim (see Chapter 24). It has been this kind of thinking, as well as the calorie hypothesis, that's led to much of our ignorance and incompetency around food. It's why consumers have no idea why America and the world continues its inexorable downward health spiral.

Processed food is defined by seven engineering criteria:

1. mass produced

2. consistent batch to batch

3. consistent country to country

4. uses specialized ingredients from specialized companies

5. consists of pre-frozen macronutrients

6. must stay emulsified so that the fat and water do not layer out

7. must have a long shelf life or freezer life

It's *exactly* these engineering issues that make processed food toxic to human physiology by promoting the eight subcellular pathologies of Chapter 7. We will deal with all of these in the rest of Part IV.

First, let's review the public classification systems used to convey nutrition information/disinformation.

Pamphlets, Pyramids, and Plates

The USDA is the primary sanctioned outlet for nutrition education. Its classification system started in 1902 with a brochure written by none other than Wilbur Atwater (see Chapter 4), entitled *Principles of Nutrition and Nutritive Value of Food*, in which he introduced the concept of calories to the American public. By 1917, the USDA issued *Food for Young Children*, a brochure providing guidance to parents trying to navigate the new foodscape that evolved from the Industrial Revolution, which then morphed into a revised brochure for adults titled *How to Select Foods*. The national bouts of malnutrition and star-vation during the Depression and the Dust Bowl of the 1930s caused the USDA to invest in the "science" of nutrition. John Steinbeck got it when he wrote about a woman whose baby died, and instead breast-fed a starving old man in *The Grapes of Wrath* (1939). By 1940, the USDA developed its guidance into the seven food groups (that is, car-bohydrates, fats, dietary fiber, minerals, proteins, vitamins, and water). Notice that dietary fiber was its own food group prior to World War II. Why was that? Through the experience with malnutrition, the USDA knew about the importance of green vegetables for general health, and so fiber was considered an integral part of a balanced diet.

However, over the course of the war and with food rationing, the American dairy and meat industries saw consumption dwindle. Then, after the war ended, they wanted to drum up business, so they made a push to gain relevance. This resulted in further refinement of the USDA food classification in 1956, which yielded the four basic food groups (dairy, meat, fruits and vegetables, breads and cereals; the one I learned in elementary school), in which dairy and meat both occupied prominent positions. Gone was any mention of fiber as a necessary nu-trient. Furthermore, it was at this time that fruit juice was classified as a fruit by the USDA, further gutting any fiber requirement.

The USDA Food Wheel of 1984 was the first classification system after the first Dietary Guidelines for Americans in 1980, which were strictly based on calories. This morphed into the 1992 Food Pyramid, with bread and grains at the base, because they were the least calori-cally dense of the macronutrients. Oils and sweets were placed at the top, because they were the most calorically dense (to be clear, sugar has the same caloric density as starch and protein at 4.1 kcal/gm, but sweets are usually a mixture of sugar *and* fat). The USDA followed up in 2005 with MyPyramid, which started favoring certain foods over others. But how did it become a pyramid in the first place?

It turns out that the USDA didn't invent the food pyramid, Sweden did. Sweden's was scrapped, but the USDA adopted it anyway, because its 1980s policies of agricultural monoculture had generated a glut of cheap refined carbohydrate, which served as the base of the pyramid. USDA nutritionists had initially settled on 5 to 9 servings of fresh fruits and vegetables and 3 to 4 servings of whole grains per day, putting refined carbohydrate (like crackers) at the top. However, when the actual pyramid was revealed, the numbers were quite different: 2 to 3 servings of fruits and vegetables and 6 to 11 of all types of carbohydrate, including crackers. The nutritionists said "eat less," but the pyramid said "avoid too much," which is basically saying, "don't eat more."

Who orchestrated this sleight of hand? The Reagan administration—which also advocated that ketchup was a vegetable. One of the originators of the Food Pyramid, Luise Light, is quoted as saying: "Ultimately, the food industry dictates the government's food advice, shaping the nutrition agenda delivered to the public. In fact, to the food industry, the purpose of food guides is to persuade consumers that all foods (especially those that they're selling) fit into a healthful diet."

The Food Pyramid came under immediate fire, even from those within government. In response to the growing obesity crisis, the USDA was forced to back away from it, and in 2011 introduced MyPlate, which endorsed the low-fat myth. To its credit, at least MyPlate didn't tout refined carbohydrates; however, its low-fat imperative continues to miss the point and it somehow still categorizes fruit juice and fruit and veggie straws as a vegetable. The evidence base for any and all of these classification systems is spotty at best and nonexistent at worst. The USDA has promoted the corporate takeover of the American Diet by ultra-processed food—which was, in fact, their intent.

The Distinction between Calories and Food

Ultra-processed food now accounts for 70 percent of the items in the supermarket, the majority of the food consumed in the US. It also accounts for 85 percent of the fare produced by the top twenty-five food manufacturers, providing 60 percent of all of our energy intake. It provides 90 percent of the added sugar in the diet. But if it's just about calories, why should we care where the calories come from?

As I'm hoping to convince you: it's not about the calories. The only way to understand the role of food processing is to hammer home the difference between calories and food. Alcohol is calories, but not food. *Trans*-fats are calories, but not food. Furthermore, the point I've tried to make from the very first page of this book is that sugar is calories, but not food (see Chapter 21). Therefore, using the same logic, ultra-processed food is not food.

Nutrition Facts or Fictions?

The FDA is in charge of the Nutrition Facts label. The question is, does it alert people to any dangers inside the package? Does it tell you what's been done to the food? Or whether that food is healthy or not? Has that label made any difference to anyone's health?

An educated consumer can spot certain code words on things that were *added* (see Chapter 20). For instance, the one thing on a food label that's actually been shown to predict the development of disease were the words "partially hydrogenated." Of course, this is code for *trans*-fats. Despite good data demonstrating the toxicity of *trans*-fats as early as 1957, it wasn't until 2006 that the FDA altered the Nutrition Facts label to list *trans*-fats separately. The problem is that the current food label can't tell you what's been *adulterated* (see Chapter 18) or *subtracted* (see Chapter 19).

Unfortunately for us, despite continued talk about revamping the US Nutrition Facts label to highlight individual components of food, there's no movement to address the degree of food processing. However, other countries have gotten on the bandwagon. Two classification systems are worth mentioning. Hopefully, publicizing their success can move the needle on this side of the pond.

They Know the Nutri-Score

Nutri-Score is a French invention introduced by Santé Publique France, based on the work of pioneering physician and nutritionist Serge

Hercberg and the UK's Food Standards Agency nutrient profiling system. Nutri-Score is a front-of-package five-level color-coded labeling system that awards points for healthy food components (e.g., fiber, fruits and vegetables, and protein), while subtracting points for problematic components (e.g., total sugar, sodium).

While Nutri-Score is light years ahead of the US system, I do have several issues as to its algorithm. First of all, it negatively weights calories and saturated fat, therefore assuming all saturated fats are the same, and it lists total rather than added sugar. It also doesn't address food processing directly, though because it highlights fiber and sugar in its calculations, some of the effects of industrial processing are captured within the score. At a population level, Nutri-Score correlates with risk for NCDs, but individual prospective data is still needed for validation.

This classification system was six years in the making. One of the reasons it took so long is because Big Food Europe saw it as a major threat to business as usual. They pulled out all the stops to try to sink this effort at the industry, governmental, and European Food Safety Authority levels. They even went so far as to design an entirely different front-of-package food classification system to compete with Nutri-Score, called the Evolved Nutrition Label (ENL), which quantified calories, total fat, saturated fat, total sugar, and salt. Ultimately, Big Food Europe couldn't agree on whether foods should be listed per serving or per 100 grams. For instance, Ferrero Rocher's Nutella spread, which is 90 percent sugar and 10 percent fat, would get a green light based on a 1 tablespoon serving, but a red light for 100 grams! Ultimately, the ENL system was deep-sixed by the industry, and instead Nutri-Score has been adopted voluntarily by much of Western Europe (except Italy, where pasta is still king).

Super NOVA

Perhaps the most innovative (and in my opinion useful) food classification system comes out of Brazil. The brainchild of São Paulo public health nutritionist Carlos Monteiro, the NOVA system is a giant step forward in how food should be viewed because it assumes all food is inherently good and ascribes different levels to the degree of processing. At an ecological (population) level, the NOVA system has been validated using the UK dataset, and thus far the system has correlated with prevalence of disease much better than the US Nutrition Facts label.

NOVA divides food into four groups: 1) unprocessed or minimally processed foods (such as fresh or frozen vegetables and fruits; plain nuts; pulses, grains, flours, and pasta; eggs; pasteurized milk and plain yogurt; chilled or frozen meat, etc.—these should be the basis of the diet); 2) processed culinary ingredients (substances extracted from group 1 foods or from nature, such as oils and fats, sugar, and salt—to be used in small amounts in the conversion of group 1 foods into dishes and meals); 3) processed foods (group 1 foods added of substances from group 2, such as freshly made breads and cheeses—to be consumed, also in small amounts, as part of dishes and meals based on group 1 foods); and 4) ultra-processed foods (formulation of several ingredients, most of exclusive industrial use, such as soft drinks, sweet or savory snacks, reconstituted meat products, "instant" meals, and industrial desserts—to be avoided). Thus all four categories include processed food.

What You Are, and How They Did It

In his iconic tome *The Physiology of Taste, or Meditations on Transcendental Gastronomy* (1826), the first nutritionist and gastronome Jean Anthelme Brillat-Savarin famously said, "Tell me what you eat and I will tell you what you are." Along the way, this was contracted by others to the diminutive "You are what you eat." Based on nutritional biochemistry and physiology, I've known for over a decade that this wasn't true. In *Fat Chance* (2012), I popularized an alternative mantra, "You are what *you do with* what you eat." I got it wrong back then, too. I must now refine it yet again to "You are what *they did* with what you eat." This is actually close to Brillat-Savarin's original intent. What we are is a mess caused by food processing, and we're suffering from the eight subcellular pathologies because of it. Chapters 18 to 22 will show you what you are, and how they did it.

CHAPTER 18

———

Food Adulterations

Food is food all over the world, right? Not exactly. Not every plot of land is the same, not every farm grows crops the same, not every ranch feeds animals the same, and not every chef cooks the same. You shouldn't be surprised to know that your health could differ as well, not due to conscious food subtractions (removal of nutrients in food processing; see Chapter 19) or food additions (items put into processed food; see Chapter 20), but rather due to food adulterations that result in untoward food quality and propensity for chronic metabolic disease. While any and all of these factors can alter plants and animals grown organically as well, they're most prevalent in relation to ultra-processed food.

Toxins and Heavy Metals

Environmental toxins build up in animals and plants, unleashing their metabolic havoc inside us. Although ostensibly they're not *added* by the industry, some are the by-products of industrial chemical and food processing. For instance, mercury contamination of seafood is a well-documented problem. The FDA says, "Nearly all fish and shellfish contain traces of methyl mercury. However, larger fish that have lived longer have the highest levels of methyl mercury because they've had more time to accumulate it. These large fish (swordfish, shark, king mackerel, and tilefish) pose the greatest risk." Where did the mercury come from in the first place? Thermometers? Maybe. But mercury is also a by-product of various technological "advances," including the processing of corn into high-fructose corn syrup.

Of course, there are many other toxins in the water that concentrate in the fat of animals, such as PCBs and dioxins. You might be lured into complacency thinking that eating plants instead of fish or animals would fix this problem, but you would be wrong. Heavy metals concentrate in underground and aboveground plant parts, inhibiting the process of photosynthesis. To avoid toxicity, plants have developed specific mechanisms by which toxic elements are excluded, retained

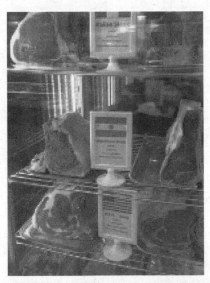

Fig 18–1: Cuts of Italian, Argentinean, and US beef. Picture taken through a restaurant window in Rome, Italy, 2016. The Italian and Argentinean beef is homogeneous, while the US beef is marbled, a sign of fat deposition in the muscle, insulin resistance, and metabolic syndrome.

at root level, or transformed into physiologically tolerant forms—for them, not for us. For instance, arsenic, cadmium, chromium, mercury, antimony, and lead have been found in American rice and in forty-five prepackaged juices, according to *Consumer Reports*. Particularly high levels have also been found in processed baby food. All in all, food processing results in heavy metal runoff, which finds its way into our food supply.

Branched-Chain Amino Acids (BCAAs)

Take a look at **Fig. 18-1**. If you're a carnivore, each of these cuts of meat should make you salivate. They're all delicious, but they're not the same. Take a good hard look. What do you see?

The Italian and Argentinean cows were raised on grass from birth to slaughter in eighteen months. The meat is pink and homogeneous. These steaks taste phenomenal, but they're a little on the tough side. The US cow, on the other hand, was raised on corn from birth to slaughter in six months. Corn fattens them up faster, so they can go to market sooner—good for cash flow. American cattle ranchers prize their beef for being so tender you can cut it with a butter knife. You can see the fat, the marbling; this is *intramyocellular lipid*, meaning fat inside the muscle. That's insulin resistance.

How does corn perform this magic? It's replete in valine, leucine, and isoleucine, known collectively as *branched-chain amino acids*, or BCAAs. These are essential amino acids; you must eat them. They collectively account for 20 percent of the amino acids found in human muscle. BCAAs are also what's in protein powder, consumed by bodybuilders in order to augment muscle mass. If you're a bodybuilder, you need lots of them. But what if you're not? What if you're a mere mortal, and you consume more BCAAs than your muscles need? The excess travels to the liver to be metabolized for energy. There, the amino group is removed by an enzyme called *branched-chain amino-acyl transferase* (BCAAT), where they're turned into organic acids like oxaloacetate. They then enter the mitochondria either for burning or to be turned into liver fat. Like fructose, this can predispose people to insulin resistance.

Christopher Newgard at Duke University School of Medicine has demonstrated that patients with metabolic syndrome exhibit higher levels of these amino acids in the bloodstream. Newgard also showed that animals who clear BCAAs faster are protected from metabolic disease. In other words, industrial feeding of animals is making both the animals and the humans sick at the same time. Furthermore, countries whose cattle are pastured have a lower prevalence of nonalcoholic fatty liver disease, while those that import American beef have a higher rate.

Omega-6 Fatty Acids

The advent of the cholesterol hypothesis of heart disease in the 1970s (see Chapters 2 and 12) brought about wide changes in our dietary predilections. Butter was out, but not frying. Eggs were out, but not chocolate cake. What could we fry foods in and substitute as a binder for baking, all at low cost? This was the advent of industrial monoculture; Iowa and Nebraska are now awash with corn and soybeans as far as the eye can see.

A rapid switch to seed oils occurred in the 1980s—and our diet became replete in omega-6 fatty acids through industrial processing of corn and soybean oils. This was only made worse by industrial corn feeding of cows, chicken, and fish, increasing the omega-6 content of their diet, and therefore of ours. Overall, our consumption of omega-6s tripled in the twentieth century. As a result, the concentration of linoleic acid (the main dietary omega-6 fatty acid) in our adipose tissue increased from 9 percent in 1959 to 21 percent in 2008.

The problem is that omega-6 fatty acids are pro-inflammatory (see Chapter 7). They're the precursors to arachidonic acid, the molecule that gives rise to a bunch of inflammatory mediators, such as prostaglandins, leukotrienes, and thromboxanes. These chemicals are desirable when you're fighting off a foreign invader like an infection, but not when you're fighting a blood vessel blockage. Nutritionists talk about our omega-6 to omega-3 ratio as an index of inflammation balance; it's supposed to be 1:1. On a processed food diet, this rises to 20:1. The good news is that grass-fed animals have lower levels of omega-6s and higher levels of omega-3s, so consuming less processed options can bring your ratio closer to 3:1 (see Chapter 19).

Cooking Your Goose

Perhaps the most neglected but insidious adulterations are what we do ourselves in the process of cooking. To be sure, this isn't strictly a processed food problem, but some components in processed food provide more opportunity for these dangerous chemicals to be formed during cooking. Here are four that you make right in your own kitchen.

Trans-fats

Yes, you heard that right. *Trans*-fats are very low in Real Food, but you can make them right on your stove from any unsaturated fat. In fact, you can turn one of the healthiest fats in your kitchen (olive oil) into the deadliest (*trans*-fat) with just extra heat. The reason? Unsaturated fats have *cis*-double bonds (see **Fig. 7-3c**). If you heat an unsaturated fat past its smoking point, that *cis*-double bond can isomerize (flip) into a *trans*-double bond, and voilà—a *trans*-fat (see **Fig. 7-3b**). As an example, a recent study fried some falafel in canola oil at high temperature, and then mixed the spent oil into rat feed; those rats that ate spent canola oil had a higher incidence of colon tumors and gut inflammation than those who ate canola oil cooked at lower temperatures. The lower the oil's smoking point, the easier it is to turn it into a *trans*-fat. Extra virgin olive oil has the lowest smoking point of all the fats, at 160°C (320°F).

The exception to this smoking point rule: saturated fat—because there are no double bonds and therefore nothing to isomerize. Even though lard got a bad name as a saturated fat, it's way safer to fry in than any other oil.

This *cis*-fat to *trans*-fat conversion is probably one of the biggest

conundrums in trying to sort out nutritional epidemiologic data, because investigators can't measure how hot the stove is in each kitchen.

Polycyclic Aromatic Hydrocarbons (PAHs)

There's no doubt that PAHs, which are found in coal and gasoline,
lead to cancer. This has been known since the 1930s, when scientists
painted coal tar on rats (see Chapter 6) to elicit tumors. Essentially,
PAHs bind to DNA bases, generating oxygen radicals, which can cause
cellular mutations. Of course, PAHs from vehicle exhaust and tire erosion promote lung disease and various cancers, but barbecuing or
even smoking your meat leads to PAH formation as well. A set of studies showed that charcoal briquettes generate PAHs released into the
air even without meat on the grill (propane doesn't), and then it worsens with chargrilling meat, which has definitely been shown to lead to
DNA mutations and cancer. Chargrilling vegetables also causes PAH
formation, albeit at a lower level. Though grilling is definitely one of
America's favorite pastimes—I'm a grill-master extraordinaire—the
PAH problem can become an issue. More grilling means more risk, so
as with almost everything in this book, moderation is key.

Dietary Advanced Glycation End Products (Dietary AGEs) and Acrylamide

Glycation (see Chapter 7) occurs naturally in the body and in food—
especially in response to heat. Have you ever made slow cooker caramel? You take white sweetened condensed milk in a can, heat it very
hot, and you get brown caramel. This is because the heat drives the
Maillard reaction to cause the glucose and fructose to bind to the milk
proteins, which makes AGEs. This happens in many processed foods,
because heating is a method for killing bacterial contaminants.

Until recently, dietary AGEs found in processed food were thought
to be benign. However, recent studies show that they are absorbed
through the intestine, enter the bloodstream, and then bind to receptors for AGEs (called RAGEs—yes, really) on liver cells, which drives

a molecular signal for mitochondria to stop burning and promote fat accumulation instead. My colleagues at Touro University looked at the blood level of RAGEs in teenagers, and found that they were higher in those who were obese. Furthermore, the level of RAGEs in those adolescents correlated with the degree of blood vessel damage, suggesting that they are not exactly benign. Another recent study looked at the diets of seventy-eight thousand women versus the risk of breast cancer over an eleven-year period; those who consumed the most dietary AGEs had a 30 percent increased risk of developing breast cancer. Neither of these correlative studies prove causation, nor do they prove that the RAGEs came specifically from processed food, but given the fact that many processed foods undergo flash heating to reduce risk for bacterial contamination, it seems probable that the food processing is contributing both to dietary AGEs and to our burden of chronic disease.

One particular dietary AGE, called *acrylamide*, has garnered the most attention. It is formed when carbohydrate and fat meet at high temperature. It's one of the things we love about French fries—that great crunch. Acrylamide is also a by-product of the coffee roasting process. Dietary acrylamide is absorbed, carried to the liver, and turned into a compound called *glycidamide*, which is a potent carcinogen. One study showed that one-third of cancers tested showed alterations in the cancer genome associated with this compound, which can only be made from food. Furthermore, a recent meta-analysis associated acrylamide exposure with premenopausal breast and uterine cancer. None of these studies reach the threshold of causation to prove that those AGEs are actually causing damage. But when you look at the data, there is enough prospective correlation for concern.

3-Monochloropropanediol (3-MCPD) Fatty Acid Esters

These bad boys occur in processed food when a free fatty acid (in fat) meets a chloride ion (in salt) during the procedure of flash heating at 204°C (400°F) or greater. They are particularly toxic to the kidney and testis, but may also have effects on the liver and other organs. The European Food Safety Authority (EFSA) has put an upper limit on the amounts in foods, but the FDA has only issued a guidance, not a limit.

Raw Data

To cook or not to cook? Raw restaurants have been popping up in trendy urban areas, primarily with a vegan menu. Ostensibly, eating raw food is better for nutrition, since heating can destroy as much as 50 percent of vitamins B and C. But of course, this has to be balanced against the inactivation of any viruses or bacteria during cooking. Perhaps fermentation (e.g., kimchi, sauerkraut, miso, tempeh, kombucha) is the best of both worlds. Some like the slightly sour taste, and the bacteria tend to be benign and can help improve microbiome diversity. Furthermore, the production of lactic acid during the fermentation process provides natural food preservation, and apparently vitamin and mineral availability can be greater after fermentation, possibly due to the degradation of phytic acid, which can inhibit intestinal vitamin absorption. Ah, but two caveats . . . processed food won't ferment. And frozen yogurt doesn't count—if the label doesn't say "live cultures," it's just dessert.

It's not *what's in the food*, it's *what's been done to the food* that matters. Nowhere is this mantra more clear than in this chapter, which documents what's been done to the food—by us—irrespective of any food conglomerate. But that's cupcakes compared to the secret recipes that the industry has been cooking up for you.

CHAPTER 19

Food Subtractions

R eal Food is chock-full of all sorts of health-promoting biochemical bonuses. Why in the world would Big Food want to strip it of its inherent nutritional value? Well, for one, the micronutrients themselves aren't all that tasty, and two, these compounds are metabolically active. Upon exposure to oxygen they either lose potency or turn rancid, or both.

Let's take wheat as an example. Once upon a time, people stoneground wheat kernels and made a rustic bread out of the pulverized semi-smooth flour (today that would be an artisanal loaf that costs about $15, if you can find it). But once the wheat was ground, it couldn't be stored. Why not? Well, each wheat kernel is made of three parts: on the outside is the bran, composed of soluble and insoluble fiber that coats the kernel; inside there's the endosperm, which is pure starch or what makes white flour; and, last, there's the germ, which is where the nucleic acids, polyphenols, flavonoids, vitamins, antioxidants, and other micronutrients reside (this is the goodie bag). I remember as a kid every day my mother reaching into the fridge to grab the Kretschmer

Wheat Germ and forcing a tablespoon down my gullet, to my great displeasure. I found it pretty nasty, but it was kept in the fridge so it wouldn't get even nastier. The micronutrients in wheat germ are amines, purines, and phenolic acids, all of which can be easily oxidized to quinones, which render them both nonnutritive and disgusting. But if during the milling, you separate the fiber and the germ from the starch, you can keep the starch in five-pound bags forever without spoilage. Good for depreciation; good for business; bad for nutrition. This is just a sample of what's wrong with processed food. Let's look at the specifics.

Fiber One or Fiber Zero

Stephen Jones is a geneticist and director of the Bread Lab at Washington State University, a think tank and baking laboratory where scientists, bakers, chefs, farmers, maltsters, brewers, distillers, and millers congregate to experiment with flavor, nutrition, and functionality of wheats, barley, and other grains (which sounds better than Disneyland!). What do all grains share? Bran, endosperm, and germ. Jones demonstrated that, during the process of milling, between 20 and 30 percent of the weight of the grain is the husk, the fiber. That's a lot of waste—if you waste it.

As discussed in Chapter 12, fiber is perhaps the single most important nutrient for health, because it both *protects the liver* and *feeds the gut*. Yet it's the nutrient you don't absorb, because the fiber isn't for you, it's for your gut bacteria. *You* have to consume it to make *them* happy. You're not eating for two—but for a hundred trillion.

Remember (see Chapter 12), there are two kinds of fiber: soluble (e.g., pectins that hold jelly together) and insoluble (e.g., cellulose, the stringy stuff in celery). You need both, and the geometry of each, in order to both *protect the liver* and *feed the gut*. Of course, you can mill the kernel, but now the protective husk has been breached; the starch is out and readily available for digestion and absorption, thus raising the glucose and insulin response. The processed food industry can claim that their product is whole grain because it started with whole grain, but it's not *what's in the food*, rather it's *what's been done to the food* that really counts.

Got Your Juices Flowing?

When intact, the fiber in Real Food does double duty in both *protecting the liver* and *feeding the gut*. The best fiber is the combination of both soluble and insoluble fiber, and that's pretty much everything that comes out of the ground—until it's processed.

What can be done? Insoluble fiber doesn't freeze well. I'll prove it to you. Take an orange, put it in the freezer overnight. Take it out the next morning, and let it thaw. Then try to eat it. It's not an orange anymore. It's turned to mush. The ice crystals have macerated the cell walls of the orange, so that upon thawing, the water rushes in, destroying the texture of the orange. Of course, Big Food knows this. So what do they do? They squeeze it and freeze it. Now it lasts forever and there's no depreciation. They've turned an orange into a commodity, that is, storable food.

The question is, was anything lost nutritionally in the process of juicing? The answer is an emphatic yes—all of the insoluble fiber is now gone. The soluble fiber alone still has some benefit; orange juice moves the food through the intestine faster (to generate the satiety signal sooner), and the soluble fiber can be converted to short-chain fatty acids. But those benefits pale in comparison to the suppression of the insulin response associated with the combination of the two. Remember, it doesn't matter where the fructose comes from—fruit, sugar cane, beets—without the fiber, it all has the same metabolic effect on your body.

Furthermore, juice is as egregious a delivery vehicle for sugar as is soda. Studies of juice consumption show increased risk of diabetes and heart disease even after controlling for calories, while whole fruit demonstrates protection. It's the processing that causes the problems. Our ancestors didn't have the health complications associated with fructose because they ate the whole fruit.

Don't believe it? This will make it clear—metabolically, is applesauce more like apples or apple juice? It turns out from a glycemic excursion standpoint, applesauce is like apple juice. It might feed the gut, but it's not protecting the liver.

What about smoothies? The blades of the Vitamix, Breville, or Magic Bullet shear the insoluble fiber to smithereens, same as juice. As a result, the fiber can't assemble the latticework for the gel in the duodenum—so it's not protecting the liver from the onslaught of the sugar in the fruit smoothie. In fact, the European Society for Paediatric Gastroenterology, Hepatology and Nutrition has suggested refraining from giving smoothies to children. On the other hand, if it's a green vegetable smoothie, then there's nothing to protect the liver from, so have at it.

Why can't you just supplement with fiber? After all, there are enough Fiber One bars, oatmeal cookies, and Metamucil for everyone. Except it doesn't work like that. Metamucil is a soluble fiber (psyllium), but has no insoluble fiber. Furthermore, thus far Metamucil hasn't succeeded as a stand-alone therapy for type 2 diabetes. It has been shown to improve cholesterol and insulin, but only after a healthy diet was instituted. It did nothing to reverse the effects of a bad diet, and the FDA refused to approve even a qualified health claim.

Raiding the Goodie Bag

The bran surrounding the wheat kernel provides one kind of health benefit, while the germ confers a second. It's a little goodie bag filled with cofactors needed to keep the eight subcellular pathologies (see Chapter 7) at bay. When you make bread or any grain product, our current methods of processing strip away all the good stuff. A recent study from the Global Burden of Disease group has determined that processed food is bad for health for two reasons: the stuff in the processed food causes damage; and processed food crowds out Real Food from the diet, resulting in a paucity of the stuff that could prevent the damage.

Antioxidants such as vitamins C and E, carotenoids, and alpha-lipoic acid within the germ are also removed during processing, which are then thrown away along with the fiber fraction or are diverted to nutritional supplement companies who isolate and sell them under their own brand. Not enough antioxidants in the diet means oxygen radicals run amuck, putting the cell at risk for dysfunction and death, which can later manifest as chronic disease.

Unquenched oxygen radicals disrupt necessary protein folding within the cell, which leads to metabolic havoc. In the pancreas, if you can't fold your insulin molecules, you get insulin deficiency; in the liver, you get insulin resistance. Without antioxidants, the liver is at risk from oxygen radicals, and inflammation ensues. The lack of Real Food means the lack of fiber, vitamins, polyphenols, polyamines, flavonoids, and other antioxidants that normally keep those eight subcellular pathways running smoothly.

Selective Outbreeding

Over the last fifty years, we've used selective breeding of crops so that they're sweeter, but some nutritionists are concerned that we've outbred the micronutrients. Examining this claim can be somewhat difficult, as much of the research has been done by the food industry, which as we've discussed has a vested interest in the outcome.

Let's look at tomatoes as an example. The pigment in them is the antioxidant lycopene, a precursor to vitamin A, which has been credited with improving heart health and eyesight, as well as reducing cancer risk. However, the more sugar and sweeter the tomato, the less lycopene there is. Processing kicks it down another notch, because heating the lycopene molecule causes oxidation and isomerization from the all-*trans* (active) form to the all-*cis* (inactive) form. Same is true for grapes—the higher the sugar, the lower the vitamin C.

Grass and Omega-3s

Omega-3s are fish oil, not snake oil. Omega-3s might just be the healthiest thing you can put in your mouth. There are two kinds—docosahexaenoic (DHA) and eicosapentaenoic acids (EPA)—both of which reduce the inflammatory response in the fat cell and prevent the release of free fatty acids (see Chapter 12). This keeps them from hitting the liver, where they would be packaged into triglyceride. It's also why omega-3s can prevent heart disease, but only in those people with high triglycerides at baseline, because they're omega-3 deficient to start with.

Even more important is the effect of omega-3s on the brain, which is why EPA and DHA have both been added to baby formula (see Chapter 16). Breast milk is chock-full of them, provided mom has been eating them herself. Omega-3s also indirectly affect serotonin release from nerve terminals throughout the brain. When the area surrounding the nerve terminal releasing serotonin is inflamed, it inhibits serotonin release, which may explain why people whose bodies and brains are undergoing inflammation tend to be so irritable, even if they're taking an SSRI or other antidepressant. In fact, one study found that a Mediterranean diet improved symptoms of depression, and in another fish alone reversed depression. Omega-3 supplementation can also reduce risk for depression in children and adults, and can serve as an adjunct to antidepressants. Last, administration of omega-3s, with Real Food or a supplement, to patients with recurrent self-harm (e.g., cutting, picking, scratching, burning; the ultimate expression of anxiety) showed a reduction in suicidality, depression, and daily stress. A recent trial gave omega-3s along with minerals to eleven-year-old kids with oppositional defiant disorder (the kids who routinely find themselves in the principal's office), and within three months their aggression was reduced. Omega-3s are not a magic bullet to cure all of our ills, but a lack of them seems to cause general havoc on our brains and bodies. Real Food is the best way to ingest them, but supplements can also work to fix the deficiency.

So, where are omega-3s in the diet? Normally they're found in fish, but not just any fish—*wild* fish. When omega-3s are made by algae, wild fish eat the algae, and in turn we eat the fish. However, farmed fish eat corn—filled with omega-6s and branched-chain amino acids (see Chapter 18). You can also get omega-3s from eggs, but only from pasture-raised chickens, because they're eating grass as opposed to corn feed. Just check out **Fig. 19-1**, which shows the difference between an egg yolk from a chicken that was pasture-raised versus one that was factory-raised. This extends to meat as well. Pasture-raised is omega-3 rich. And if you're vegan, flax is your best bet.

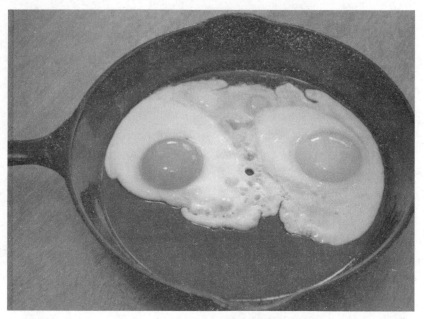

Figure 19–1: An egg from a pasture-raised chicken with high omega-3s (left) has a deep orange–colored yolk vs. a standard feedlot chicken with low omega-3s (right) has a pale yellow–colored yolk.

Egg-static

While all amino acids are important, tryptophan is the most important, because it's the hardest to come by. It's an essential amino acid, which means the only source is your diet. It's highest in eggs, poultry, and fish. Furthermore, it's the only amino acid that can be converted by the brain into serotonin, which as we discussed above is the happiness/ anti-anxiety/anti-depression/pro-sleep neurotransmitter.

Eggs aren't often included in processed foods because they curdle with time, go rancid when not refrigerated, and enough people are allergic to them. Fish isn't usually a big seller as an ingredient in processed food, in part because certain fish don't freeze well and most people want to see the catch to determine how fresh it is. Nuts also have tryptophan, and spinach and soy have a little as well. But what about a tryptophan pill? It will definitely increase your blood level, but not without a bunch of side effects.

Anyone who eats Real Food can get all the goodies delineated in this chapter, which will *protect the liver* and *feed the gut*. However, processed food is missing all of these, and four out of five Americans are deficient in the nutrients that contribute to a functioning immune system (vitamins A, C, D, E, and zinc). How do you argue with Real Food? Big Food can and does, because processed food tastes better, and they've got you hooked.

===

CHAPTER 20

Food Additions

The ultra-processed food industry adds chemicals at various points. They may add it to the animal while it's maturing to prevent infection, or they may add it to the plant while it's growing to prevent infestation. They may also add chemicals to the food during processing for flavor, color, texture, and/or preservation. In any case, when they add it to the animal or plant or food, they add it to you as well. Many of these chemicals act directly on those eight subcellular pathologies (see Chapter 7) to increase your burden of chronic disease; I'll point out those pathologies as we go.

Germ Theory

Bet you never thought of a rural farm as a clean place, but they are, because the manure feeds the plants by fixing nitrogen and bacteria into the soil where they belong. Conversely, concentrated animal feeding operations (CAFOs; see Chapter 25) aren't clean, as there's no soil for the manure to fix the nitrogen, and no grass for the animal to eat to maintain a healthy intestinal microbiome. Feedlot animals eating corn are not only carbohydrate- and BCAA-overloaded, but they're also micronutrient malnourished, which leaves them open to infection. Furthermore, pathogenic bacteria can take hold in the unsanitary conditions of confined feedlots, so animals are routinely given low doses of antibiotics to prevent sickness, promote rapid growth, and therefore maintain cash flow. Of the antibiotics sold in 2014, 80 percent were for use on livestock and poultry; only 20 percent were for human use. Those antibiotics given to animals survive slaughter and processing, and are then delivered to our intestines. This results in two human health hazards that are now playing out: metabolic syndrome, and antibiotic resistance in bacteria that can cause illness. The last two decades have seen an emergence of drug-resistant organisms that are now affecting people and altering the bacterial flora of the human gut. As discussed earlier, intestinal dysbiosis occurs when the "bad bacteria" like *Firmicutes* outgrow the "good bacteria" like *Bacteroides*. These bad bacteria can attack the intestinal epithelial cells to cause leaky gut, which drives systemic inflammation and contributes to metabolic syndrome (see Chapter 7). The FDA has urged stricter limits for antibiotics in livestock and use has dropped 38 percent between 2015 and 2018. However, lots of serious challenges remain.

To top it all off, a new sugar-loving bacterium inhabits our intestine, and apparently we invented it. *Clostridioides difficile* is a nasty denizen usually held at bay by the "good" bacteria. However, hospitalized people receive big-time antibiotics, which kill off the good guys in the intestine and allow the *C. difficile* to run rampant. This has resulted in a completely new strain (more than 5 percent DNA difference) that's become specifically adapted to the high sugar content of processed food—so maybe this will become an equal opportunity offender, and not just inside hospitals.

It's a Jungle Out There . . .

When you're trying to keep food cheap, maintaining crop yield is paramount. But nature has other ideas. Insects, weeds, rodents, and fungi also call the American farm "home." Even today, a species of locust threatens the entire African food supply. Toxicologists of the twentieth century did a bang-up job on finding chemicals to control these pests. But what they didn't do very well was assess their toxicities to humans.

Dichloro-diphenyl-trichloroethane (DDT)

Pesticides have been around since World War II, with the advent of DDT, an estrogenic compound that inhibits the insect life cycle and protects crops. The trouble is that it inhibits our life cycle as well, and promotes cancer in estrogen-responsive tissues. This was the basis of Rachel Carson's *Silent Spring* (1962), and the tipping point of the environmental revolution. Even though DDT was officially banned by the EPA in 1972, it's never really disappeared and remains one of the *persistent organic pollutants*, or POPs. It's still in the environment, and its breakdown product DDE is still found in babies today. It's been linked to reducing mitochondrial metabolism and promoting insulin resistance.

Glyphosate

Understandably, the food industry needed a new pesticide right away, so it introduced glyphosate (Roundup) in 1974. It was such a big seller that by 2014, 826 million kilograms were sprayed worldwide annually. From a strictly agricultural standpoint, glyphosate has been a panacea, as it controls all manners of weed growth. To improve glyphosate's actions, Monsanto genetically engineered corn and soy (the primary components in commodity foods) to be Roundup Ready, specifically so that their growth wouldn't be inhibited and yields would be further increased. Here's the problem: chemically, the active ingredient in glyphosate (N-phosphonomethyl-glycine) is a derivative of glycine, the smallest amino acid found in proteins. The glyphosate is taken up by the plant, incorporated into the structure of newly formed plant proteins in lieu of glycine (not human proteins), and inhibits the enzymatic pathways that can turn simple carbohydrates into complex aromatic amino acids (phenylalanine, tyrosine, tryptophan). Remember, phenylalanine and tryptophan are essential amino acids, which means you have to eat them, and tyrosine comes from phenylalanine—meaning glyphosate-treated crops are going to be low in these amino acids necessary to make the neurotransmitters serotonin, dopamine, and norepinephrine.

Glyphosate has also been shown to contaminate all different kinds of crops. From a nutritional standpoint this can be problematic, especially for vegans who don't have an alternative source for these amino acids, but ultimately it's a problem for all of us. Remember, the bacteria in our gut are plants. Therefore, glyphosate affects the microbiome, which could contribute to leaky gut and subsequent inflammation. Although glyphosate has been implicated by some in the rise of celiac disease and cancer, this remains correlation, not causation. In animal studies, glyphosate also appears to alter methylation (see Chapter 7), which leads to epigenetic changes and obesity in subsequent offspring.

Similar to the subterfuge of Big Tobacco, Monsanto knew as early as 1985 that glyphosate had carcinogenic potential in animals, but did nothing about it. Finally, the data became overwhelming, and in 2015 the WHO reclassified glyphosate as a probable carcinogen in humans. Since then, US courts have fielded forty-two thousand class action lawsuits against the industrial giant Bayer, which bought Monsanto in 2018. These concerns have been minimized by some scientists, and the upper limit for clinical toxicity has been increased from 6 to 100 by others—the only issue is that these scientists take money from Monsanto.

There's been a call among academics to reassess the entire glyphosate toxicity profile, but the industry continues to resist. In 2020, Bayer settled all its glyphosate class actions suits for a mere $10 billion, and they're still selling it worldwide.

Atrazine

This herbicide has been in use since 1958, in particular for corn. Atrazine (Buctril) inhibits photosynthesis, the primary energy pathway in plants. We humans don't do photosynthesis, so it should be safe for us, right? Atrazine is a known teratogen (causes birth defects) in amphibians, so it's affecting more than just plants. It's also been shown to induce mitochondrial dysfunction and insulin resistance, diabetes, and methylation, influencing epigenetics. While Syngenta has always publicly maintained that atrazine is safe as used, it nonetheless paid $105 million in 2012 to settle a class action lawsuit alleging that it had contaminated Midwestern towns' water supplies, having admitted no wrongdoing. Apparently the Trump administration agreed with Syngenta, as the EPA discarded the provisions of the Food Quality Protection Act (1996) to give atrazine a clean bill of health in September 2020. Many other pesticides have been shown to have detrimental effects on human mitochondria and insulin resistance. Perhaps even more concerning is that some of these pesticides may be acting like selective antibiotics, killing off both the animal's microbiome and our own, letting the bad methane-producing bacteria take its place (see Chapter 25). This can result in leaky gut, inflammation, insulin resistance—and climate change.

Flavor Enhancers

Today, everyone expects bold flavors from their food. Scratch cooks can add spices. But processed food companies have to appeal to a wide array of palates, and many of those spices lose potency on the shelf. The industry has instead developed flavor enhancers to pique the palate of processed food consumers. Unfortunately, they have effects past the tongue that can promote chronic disease.

Diacetyl

Diacetyl is used as a butter flavoring in microwave popcorn and butterscotch. It easily decomposes to acetaldehyde, which is a known lung and liver toxin. Diacetyl is also associated with a severe and irreversible respiratory condition called *bronchiolitis obliterans*, which leads to inflammation and permanent scarring of the airways. In 2000, a microwave popcorn plant tested its employees, and 25 percent had compromised lung function. There was little or no response to medical treatment, and several of the workers, some only in their thirties, ended up on waiting lists for lung transplants. Breathing microwave popcorn is bad for you, although no one has yet shown that eating microwave popcorn is bad for you, unless you also have diverticulitis (inflammation of the colon), in which case you'll have a flare and never do it again.

Potassium Bromate

Potassium bromate is used to strengthen bread and cracker dough, helping it rise during baking. It's listed as a known carcinogen by the state of California, and a possible carcinogen by the International Agency for Research on Cancer. The process of baking converts most of the potassium bromate to benign potassium bromide, but not necessarily all of it. The UK, Canada, and the EU have all banned potassium bromate; the FDA issued an advisory in 1991, but the US still allows its use.

Natural Flavors

Did you ever wonder what a "natural" or "artificial" flavor was? Aside from salt, sugar, and water, natural or artificial flavor is the most commonly listed item, appearing on one out of seven food ingredient lists on the Nutrition Facts label. But what are they exactly? They're chemicals, and the company doesn't have to tell you what's in it, and the FDA doesn't require them to. Since most flavors are nonpolar, it usually means there's an emulsifier (e.g., polysorbate 80), a solvent (e.g., propylene glycol), and a preservative (e.g., butylated hydroxyanisole; BHA), although it could be several of one hundred different items. The companies that make flavors also make fragrances. In general, the dose is small, so disease is unlikely—unless you have an allergy. But we don't know for sure.

Emulsifiers

Lecithin (chocolate), polysorbate 80 (shortening), carboxymethylcellulose (salad dressing), and carrageenan (ice cream) are added to foods to maintain food consistency upon storage. After all, who wants clumpy ice cream? These molecules have one polar end and another nonpolar end, so they're able to bind fat and water together to keep them from separating. However, emulsifiers are also detergents, and can strip away the mucin layer that sits on top of and protects intestinal epithelial cells from the bacteria, thus predisposing individuals to intestinal disease, food allergy, or leaky gut. Thus far, however, the FDA states they haven't found cause for human concern.

Don't Talk to Me, I'm Hormonal

Hormones are super important (spoken as an endocrinologist)—without them, the human species would die out. But what happens when extra hormones hit the food supply? In the case of the estrogenic pesticide DDT, it led to cancers. Unfortunately, we have not learned our lesson. Numerous hormones are used throughout the food supply to boost yield or prevent spoilage, but with numerous untoward side effects.

Bovine Growth Hormone

Recombinant bovine somatotropin (rBST; aka bovine growth hormone) is given to cows used for both dairy and beef production. It could influence human health in two ways.

Dairy and cancer risk. rBST induces a hormone called IGF-1, which boosts a cow's milk production by 15 percent—a boon to dairy farmers. IGF-1 is also a growth factor associated with human breast and prostate cancer. The concern is whether bovine IGF-1 present in milk is absorbed across the human intestine, predisposing milk drinkers to increased risk for cancer. The data demonstrates that milk drinkers do have a slightly increased blood IGF-1 level, but it's not clear that this came from the milk itself, as almond milk consumers also have higher blood IGF-1 levels. Thus far, there hasn't been any convincing epidemiologic evidence of an increase in human cancers from drinking milk. Today, the US is the third largest dairy exporter, annually shipping 2.2 million tons of milk powders, cheese, butterfat, whey, and lactose across the world. Considering the countries to which we sell our milk also have increased risk for metabolic syndrome and autoimmune disease, could this be a contributor? The good news is that rBST use has declined; in 2002, 22.3 percent of dairy cows were injected, but that number today is close to 10 percent.

Beef and inflammation. The one thing we're sure of is that rBST increases udder tissue inflammation and infection in the cow, which requires increased use of antibiotics for the animals. In 1999, the European Union's Scientific Committee on Veterinary Measures Relating to Public Health said in a press release that six commonly used growth hormones had the potential to cause "endocrine, developmental, immunological, neurobiological, immunotoxic, genotoxic, and carcinogenic effects." The EU subsequently banned imports of US beef because of scientific concerns about hormones. The US government successfully challenged the ban in the World Trade Organization.

Estrogen

In 1979, the island of Puerto Rico experienced an epidemic of early breast development in children, both in girls *and* boys. As it turns out, enterprising farmers were spiking the chickens with estrogen to increase their breast size, so they could sell the meat at a profit. If this were an isolated incident, you could just chalk it up to foolish avarice. But virtually the same thing happened again in 2002 at a Netherlands animal feed company. They used the contraceptive agents medroxyprogesterone acetate and estradiol in the feed marketed to thousands of farmers. Suddenly, young Dutch girls and boys were sprouting breasts. This caused a lot of damage in pig farming and the feed sector; lots of farmers went bankrupt. The Dutch government knew of the risks for cancer, diabetes, depression, obesity, cardiovascular disease, and immune and birth defects, yet instead of initiating a legal remedy, they concealed the threat and covered up the incident for years.

There are many other estrogenic compounds floating around our environment, because it doesn't take much for any molecule to be an estrogen—and the estrogen receptor is the most promiscuous of them all, binding to many classes of compounds, which is why everything seems to cause breast cancer. One common chemical is bisphenol A (BPA), added to baby bottles, cash register printer receipts, and food. It's not added *directly* to the food, rather it's *indirectly* added to the interior of the can, in order to protect the food from taking up metals and to retard spoilage. BPA seeps in anyway, and high levels in the blood correlate with obesity and insulin resistance (similar to that seen with DDT/DDE). Another class of compound called parabens is used as a preservative in cosmetics and lipstick, and in certain foods such as tortillas and muffins. They can alter the expression of genes, including those in breast cancer cells, and contribute to impaired fertility in women. My UC Berkeley colleagues and I even showed that parabens can advance the timing of puberty in girls.

You're So Well Preserved—for Your Age

How long should food last on the shelf? It could rot, or it could mold, or it could go stale. But it doesn't—witness the miraculously preserved twenty-year-old Hostess Twinkie and the ten-year-old McDonald's cheeseburger, both stars on YouTube. Chalk it up to the chemicals the industry uses to preserve food. But, like formaldehyde, that doesn't mean you want to ingest it; it might preserve your insides, too.

Butylated Hydroxyanisole (BHA) and Butylated Hydroxytoluene (BHT)

These are standard preservatives for chips and meats. However, the International Agency for Research on Cancer categorizes BHA as a possible human carcinogen, and it's listed as a known carcinogen under California's Proposition 65. These designations are based on consistent evidence that BHA and BHT causes tumors in animals—but data in humans are hard to come by.

Propyl Gallate

Propyl gallate is a preservative in products that contain fats, such as sausage, vegetable oil, soup bases, and even chewing gum. There's some evidence that suggests it may also have estrogenic activity. It's been implicated in a rat model of Parkinson's disease, but not with any human disease at this point.

Nitrates and Nitrites

Nitrates and nitrites are the preservatives in cured meats, such as bacon, salami, sausages, and hot dogs. Although they can prolong a food's shelf life and give it an attractive hue, they're directly implicated in human disease. Nitrates turn into nitrites, which react with amino acids to form *nitrosamines*, which then react with nitrogen to form *nitrosoureas*. These are among the most potent carcinogens around and are associated with virtually every cancer of the alimentary tract: stomach, intestine, and colon. In 2010, the WHO declared nitrates as probable human carcinogens, and there are now regulations as to how many can be added to your cured meats, though we still don't know what a safe amount actually is.

Trans-fats

Trans-fats were probably the single most important reason for the advent and success of processed food. Invented in 1911, the first *trans*-fat, called Crisco, hit the market, and by 1920 virtually every bakery product sold in America was laced with it, since it acts as a preservative and a hardening agent. *Trans*-fats can't go rancid, because the *trans*-double bond can't be oxidized by bacteria, as they don't possess the enzyme to cleave it. The problem is that our mitochondria are refurbished and repurposed bacteria—they even have their own DNA—meaning they don't produce the enzyme either, so *trans*-fats line our arteries and generate oxygen radicals, leading to metabolic syndrome.

Gandhi said, "First they ignore you, then they laugh at you, then they fight you, then you win." The first glimpse of the danger of *trans*-fats came in 1957, when an immigrant German biochemist at the University of Illinois named Fred Kummerow demonstrated their presence in arterial plaques of rats. This finding was ignored for thirty years, until corroboration in 1988. It was then that Kummerow launched a scientific campaign against *trans*-fats, and he was laughed at until 2006, when the FDA agreed that the science was strong enough to warrant a warning label on foods. Kummerow filed a petition with the FDA to ban *trans*-fats, while Big Food was kicking and screaming. He was ninety-nine years old when he sued the FDA in 2013, and finally *trans*-fats were taken off the generally recognized as safe (GRAS) list (see Chapter 24).

Nitrates and *trans*-fats are the only items that have ever been removed from the FDA GRAS list, so you know they *must* be bad (see Chapter 24).

Sugar—It's a Flavor Enhancer *and* a Preservative *and* an Endocrine Disruptor, and Oh So Much More

Attempting to avoid all the above chemicals is the reason that organic has taken off in the past decade. Many of the products in boxes and jars bought at Whole Foods have "organic" front and center on the package. But from a danger standpoint, they pale in comparison to the one chemical that's added indiscriminately to 74 percent of the foods in the grocery store and has been specifically added to ultra-processed foods, organic or not, to increase palatability so you will buy more (see Chapter 21).

The processed food industry vociferously argues that sugar is a required and necessary ingredient in their recipes. And that's true, because if it weren't for the sugar, you wouldn't eat it, and their profits would dwindle. Here are five of the industry's pro-sugar arguments, and why it's good for them and bad for you.

1. **Sugar adds bulk.** Kellogg's Honey Smacks are 56 percent sugar. 'Nuff said?

2. **Sugar makes food brown.** Indeed, we love the brown color and caramel taste. Chapter 7 introduced the Maillard, glycation, browning, or aging

reaction. Every time this reaction occurs, it throws off an oxygen radical that can damage the cell.

3. **Sugar raises the boiling point.** This allows for caramelization to occur, which like we said is very tasty, but again this is just the Maillard reaction, which, over time, can cause your cells to age. There's also data to suggest that fructose could "caramelize" your hippocampus, which might contribute to memory decline.

4. **Sugar is a humectant (attracts and maintains moisture).** How soon does fresh bakery bread become stale? Maybe two days? How about grocery store commercial bread? More like three weeks. Ever wonder why? In commercial bread, the baker adds sugar to take the place of water, known as water activity. Sugar doesn't evaporate, but instead takes up space in the bread while holding onto water during baking so the loaf stays moist.

5. **Sugar is a preservative.** Have you ever left a soda at room temperature? Of course, after the carbonation escapes, it goes flat. But do bacteria or yeast ever grow in it? Never.

Oh, and by the way, sugar is addictive. They don't want you to know, they'll deny, deny, deny; the same way the tobacco industry executives testified in Congress, "I believe that nicotine is not addictive." Read on to examine the evidence.

＝＝＝

CHAPTER 21

Food Addictions

There's no doubt that we eat more than we used to. But why? We have a negative feedback system in our brains called *leptin*, which, until fifty years ago, told us that we had enough energy to burn, and therefore prevented us from overeating. However, as I explained in Chapter 2, insulin blocks leptin signaling (leptin resistance) at the hypothalamus, mimicking brain starvation, which causes us to overeat in an attempt to drive the leptin level higher. That being said, if insulin and leptin were the only problems, then we would overeat all types of foods—but we don't usually overconsume fruits, vegetables, or beans/legumes/lentils. No, the foods we overeat are all found as components of fast food.

Often we're not consuming food just because we're hungry. It's become the easy "reward" and a balm for chronic stress. Which begs the question: is fast food addictive, and if so, what about it is addictive? Recent revelations in popular literature have alluded to this signature aspect of the Western diet, driving excessive consumption. Addiction is one of those bandied-about terms that changes meaning based on context.

So what do scientists mean? Very simple—there's *liking*, there's *wanting*, and then there's *needing*. Addiction occurs when you need a stimulus and there are physiological, behavioral, and/or social consequences. Scientists have validated the Yale Food Addiction Scale (YFAS), which demonstrates that specific foods possess addictive properties. Furthermore, a pediatric YFAS argues that food addiction is common, especially among obese children.

Yet, not everyone subscribes to the idea that specific foods or ingredients can function in this way. For instance, a group of academics in Europe called NeuroFAST doesn't accept the concept of food addiction; they prefer to label it as "eating addiction." In contrast to the YFAS, this group has proffered its own eating addiction scale in which all foods are treated similarly. NeuroFAST claims that it's not the food, but rather the behavior that distinguishes the phenomenon.

This isn't just a semantic argument—if it's about the food, then the food industry bears some culpability; but if it's about eating, then it's your fault and the industry gets off scot-free. NeuroFAST also states that even though specific foods can generate a reward signal in the brain, they still can't be considered addictive because food is essential to survival. How could something essential be addictive? After all, nicotine, alcohol, heroin, and cocaine are not essential (although alcohol is debatable, especially after the nightly news).

From their website, in their own words:

In humans, there is no evidence that a specific food, food ingredient or food additive causes a substance based type of addiction (the only currently known exception is caffeine) . . . Within this context we specifically point out that we do not consider alcoholic beverages as food . . .

So NeuroFAST acknowledges caffeine's addictive properties, but they separate it from food. NeuroFAST also recognizes alcohol as addictive, but they also separate it from food. Why? Natural yeasts constantly ferment fruit while still on the vine or tree, causing it to ripen, yet NeuroFAST says that purified alcohol isn't a food. Rather, alcohol is a drug—we used to give it to women to stop premature labor. Once it's processed and purified, its properties change.

New Definition, New Rules

So what is it about processed food that makes it addictive? First, let's define addiction.

In the past, the concept of food addiction was eschewed by the American Psychiatric Association (APA), but the *DSM-IV* published in 1994 categorized "substance use disorder" as requiring both tolerance and withdrawal, but no foodstuff (apart from caffeine or alcohol) elicited withdrawal. However, as the public health difficulties stemming from addiction expanded, the definition did as well. The *DSM-5* published in 2013 reclassified the criteria so as to include "behavioral addictions" such as gambling, video games, social media, and pornography. In the extreme, these behaviors can activate the same reward pathways as heroin, cocaine, and nicotine, but don't have the same physiologic effects that lead to withdrawal. All you need now for addiction is tolerance and dependence (engaging despite conscious knowledge and recognition of their detriment), with resultant misery. Thus, a revised set of criteria was proffered by the APA, including:

1. Craving or a strong desire to use;

2. Recurrent use resulting in a failure to fulfill major role obligations (work, school, home);

3. Recurrent use in physically hazardous situations (e.g., driving);

4. Use despite social or interpersonal problems caused or exacerbated by use;

5.   Taking the substance or engaging in the behavior in larger amounts or over a longer period than intended;

6.   Attempts to quit or cut down;

7.   Time spent seeking or recovering from use;

8.   Interference with life activities;

9.   Use despite negative consequences.

Our UCSF research group has explored the question of addiction to specific components of food by using the opiate antagonist naltrexone, which blocks the reward system and is often prescribed for other addictions including alcoholism. From these studies, we've defined a phenomenon called *reward eating drive* (RED), which induces people to consume "tasty" foods unrelated to hunger or caloric needs. In a series of clinical research experiments, we showed that some people experience a loss of control with certain foods, and those that do tend to binge on high-sugar/high-fat foods (think chocolate cake). This aberrant behavior is driven by dysfunction of the reward system.

Fast Food Nation

Americans are fast food junkies—up to 37 percent of adults eat some form of it every day. Fast food is highly processed, nearly all fiber and nutrients have been stripped, and it's designed to tickle your taste buds in colorful packaging.

Is it just the calories, or is there something specific about fast food that generates the addictive response? Fast food contains four specific chemicals that have been examined for addictive qualities: salt, fat, caffeine, and sugar. Let's look at the data that supports or refutes each one.

Salt

In humans, salt intake has traditionally been conceived as a learned preference rather than as an addiction. Four-to-six-month-old infants establish a salt preference based on the sodium content of breast milk, water used to mix formula, and diet. Fast foods are relatively high in salt, energy density, and caloric intake. On the other hand, studies show that people can reset their preference for less salty items. This has been demonstrated in adolescents deprived of salty pizza and hypertensive adults who were retrained to consume a lower sodium diet over eight to twelve weeks.

Furthermore, salt intake is tightly regulated. For example, patients with a pediatric disease called *salt-losing congenital adrenal hyperplasia* (which I specialized in treating) lack the hormone that retains salt by acting on the kidneys. These kids urinate salt constantly, taking water with it, leading to low blood pressure and eventually shock. They drink the pickle juice right out of the jar. But when we give them back the missing hormone, called fludrocortisone, this craving stops.

Last, the UK government engaged in a secret mass campaign with food manufacturers to reduce public salt consumption, and saw a 40 percent reduction in hypertension and stroke without signs of addiction. Why aren't we doing that in the US?

Fat

The high fat content of fast food is vital to its rewarding properties. There may be a high-fat phenotype among some people, characterized by a preference for specific high-fat foods and weak satiety in response to them, which acts as a risk factor for obesity. However, it's unlikely for most people, who get full from drinking whole milk as opposed to low-fat. So-called high-fat foods preferred by people are almost always also high in carbohydrate (e.g., potato chips, pizza, donuts)—then add sugar, and preference for high-fat foods goes up even more. Conversely, if you take the carbs out and just eat the fat (as in low-carb and ketogenic diets), people eat less.

Caffeine

Caffeine is a model drug of dependence, meaning it meets all the criteria for addiction in children, adolescents, and adults. People not only become tolerant of caffeine, but also experience physiological withdrawal when they try to kick it. However, in today's fast-paced world, we've leaned even more into caffeine and as a result are sleep-deprived. To add insult to injury, most people ingesting caffeine do so with sugar—look at Red Bull, Coca-Cola, and low-fat vanilla lattes with two extra pumps of syrup. Starbucks and its signature Mocha Frappuccino have gone global. These drinks provide impetus for caffeine-dependent customers to frequent fast food franchises to get even more of their fix.

Sugar

Other than caffeine, the foodstuff with the highest score on the YFAS is sugar. In fact, adding a soda to a fast food meal increases the sugar content tenfold; multivariate analysis demonstrates that only soft drink intake, not animal products, is correlated with changes in BMI. Sugar has also been used for its analgesic effect in neonatal circumcision, suggesting a link between sugar and opioid tone in the brain's reward center. Some, but not all, self-identified food addicts describe sugar withdrawal as feeling "irritable," "shaky," "anxious," and "depressed," symptoms also seen in opiate withdrawal. Other studies demonstrate the transference of addiction from one toxic addictive substance to caffeine, nicotine, and/or sugar—meaning sometimes when you stop smoking, you start drinking. Sometimes when you stop drinking, you start eating. All of these behaviors activate the same dopamine reward system.

Human imaging studies also support the contention that sugar, and specifically the fructose molecule, is addictive. Fat activates sensory areas where you experience mouthfeel, while sugar activates the limbic system, the emotional part of the brain, where you experience reward. Taking the sugar molecule apart, glucose and fructose activate different parts of the brain, with fructose specifically lighting up the reward center. Sucrose establishes hardwired pathways for craving in these areas that can be identified by fMRI. Furthermore, the effects of fructose on dopamine are attenuated in obese adolescents, suggesting that they have fewer receptors due to tolerance.

Animal studies also show that sugar, and specifically the fructose molecule, is addictive. Sugar administration induces behavioral alterations consistent with dependence (i.e., bingeing, withdrawal, craving, and cross-sensitization to other drugs of abuse, consistent with addiction). Indeed, sweetness surpasses cocaine as a reward in rats. In fact, addicting rats to opioids makes them binge on fructose instead, because of alterations in the reward center, and especially in adolescent rats. All in all, while sugar doesn't exhibit the *DSM-IV* standards of tolerance and withdrawal, it sure as hell meets the *DSM-5* standards of tolerance and dependence. So, whatever criteria you decide to use, it's now obvious—sugar is addictive and many of us are junkies.

Is Sugar a Gateway Drug?

The prevalence of substance use disorders, such as opioids, has risen steadily. Could these people be primed for reward early on? And could sugar be their experience of this feeling? We know that sugar activates opioid pathways in the brain, even in newborns. We also know that certain genetic traits increase risk for both sugar seeking and drug addiction. While these are correlation, not causation, it's not too far a stretch to imagine that some people are more susceptible to the addictive effects of sugar than others. This is similar to what is seen in alcohol—40 percent of Americans are teetotalers, 40 percent are social drinkers, 10 percent have a binge drinking problem, and 10 percent are bona fide alcoholics. We don't know the percentage of people who are addicted to sugar, but how many people say, "I have a horrible sweet tooth"?

So let's say you're one of these sugar-addicted people. Maybe you employ lots of restraint to stay away from the obvious triggers—soda, cakes, ice cream. But you still have to eat. What if food has sugar mixed or baked right into it, and you don't even know it? Sugar is added to food as sucrose, high-fructose corn syrup (HFCS), honey, maple syrup, or agave. Can you break an addiction if the addictive substance is so pervasive that it's in everything? In general, each sugar molecule is assumed to consist of half fructose, half glucose, although this percentage has recently come into question when an analysis of store-bought sodas in Los Angeles revealed a fructose content as high as 65 percent. The ultra-processed food category (see Chapter 17) is where 65 percent of the sugar in our diet lives—and it's all been added. In fact, there's only one place added sugar is not—Real Food.

The hedonic nature of sugar is also revealed by examining its economics. For instance, coffee is price-inelastic (i.e., increasing price doesn't reduce consumption). For example, when prices jumped in 2014 due to decreased supply, Starbucks sales didn't budge an inch. As consumables go, soft drinks are the second most price inelastic, just below fast food. Raise the price 10 percent (e.g., with taxes), and consumption drops only 7.6 percent, mostly among the poor, as we saw in Mexico.

Food or Food Additive?

So how do we reconcile these two conflicting ideas of food addiction vs. eating addiction? It would appear that of the consumables prevalent in the Western diet, only sugar and caffeine have hedonic properties, that is, increasing food consumption independent of energy need. But if sugar is a food, meeting an energy need and necessary for survival, how could it qualify as being addictive?

First, as discussed in Chapter 12, sugar isn't necessary for survival. Second, does sugar legally qualify as food? Without appearing too lawyerly, it depends on how you define the word "food." The Food, Drug, and Cosmetic Act (FDCA, 1938) 321.201(f) defines the term "food" as: (1) articles used for **food** or drink for man or other animals, (2) chewing gum, and (3) articles used for components of any such article. The first rule of vocabulary is that you are not allowed to use the word in the definition. The *Merriam-Webster Dictionary* defines "food" as: "a material consisting essentially of protein, carbohydrate, and fat used in the body of an organism to sustain growth, repair, and vital processes and to furnish energy." Fructose supplies energy, so that makes it a food, right? But can you name an energy source that isn't nutrition by any dietitian's estimation, for which there is no biochemical reaction in the human body that requires it, and that causes disease when consumed chronically and at high dose implying addiction? Answer— alcohol. It has calories (7 kcal/gm), but it's clearly not nutrition. When consumed chronically and in high dose, alcohol is toxic, unrelated to its calories or effects on weight. Not everyone who is exposed gets addicted, but enough do to warrant public health interventions. Clearly, alcohol is *not* a food. Similarly, sugar isn't a food, as it's also not essential for animal life, causes damage in chronically high dosage, and a sizable percentage of the population is addicted.

It's All in the Processing

It's true that certain foods are necessary for survival—while others aren't. We need essential nutrients that our body can't make out of other nutrients, but there are only five classes: 1) essential amino acids (nine out of the possible twenty found in proteins); 2) essential fatty acids (such as omega-3s and linoleic acid); 3) vitamins; 4) minerals; and 5) fiber. Furthermore, none of these essential nutrients are remotely addictive. Of the hedonic substances found in food, only alcohol, caffeine, and sugar are addictive—and these are food additives, not foods in themselves.

When you process and purify something, you change its properties. Coca leaves are medicinal in Bolivia, but cocaine is a drug. Opium poppies were medicinal, but heroin is a drug. Caffeine is found in coffee (medicinal for many), but concentrated caffeine (e.g., in weight loss remedies) is a drug. In ancient times, sugar was a spice. Through the Industrial Revolution, it was a condiment. Now that it's processed and purified, it's a drug. How is this any different from refined sugar? Refined sucrose is the same compound found in fruit, but the fiber has been removed, and it's been crystallized for purity. This process of purification turns sugar from food into drug, just like alcohol and caffeine. And just like these addictive consumables, sugar is a food additive. The minute the dose exceeds the liver's capacity to clear and metabolize it, it's in the brain, driving reward in all people, and addiction in some. And it's being added by Big Food to 74 percent of the food supply, because when they add it, we buy more.

CHAPTER 22

═══

Food Fraud

When asked to comment on food fraud, an executive of a well-known food manufacturer said, "We don't want our company name and the words 'food fraud' in the same sentence." Right. Don't ask, don't tell. This is the food industry's dirty little secret, and they'll do anything to keep it that way, because all food companies trade on trust. This also means there aren't good data on food fraud—we really only hear about it when someone gets caught.

We could literally be consuming anything and everything known to man—I'm sure some things not even known to man!—and remain completely oblivious to it. It's estimated that 20 percent of the seafood sold is mislabeled, and the records show that 1.7 lawsuits per week are filed in the Northern District of California for some form of food fraud.

Still think your food is what you thought it was? OK, here's your reality check—is the farmed salmon really pink, or is it the food dye astaxanthin? Is the fish farmed in sewage water? Is the milk powder in a chocolate bar mixed with detergent or melamine? Is the olive oil really cooking oil dyed green or even recycled and cleansed motor oil? Is your sushi really the fish advertised on the menu or some other species that you've never heard of? Is that veal cutlet really veal or that lamb gyro really lamb? Are there only tea leaves in that tea bag? Is that ground coffee really 100 percent ground-up coffee beans or was something else mixed in? How about the spices? You're constantly being cheated without even knowing it—and sure, sometimes it doesn't matter, but other times it will cause you to inadvertently compromise your buying, religious, and health practices. Not to mention it will always compromise your wallet.

Guilty of Passing Bad Food . . .

Food fraud is literally defined as "misrepresentation as to the state of the food." There are six different forms of it and some engender health risks while others don't, but they all share three things in common— alteration of the food itself, lying to the consumer, and a profit motive. A seventh version, called *misbranding* or misrepresentation as to the state of the *food label*, will be discussed in reference to the FDA in Chapter 24. Below are six examples of food fraud that reached your restaurant's or grocery store's shelves without your knowledge:

1. **Dilution/adulteration.** Something is added to the food to disguise or extend it. Milk is a common vehicle. In 2019 in India, milk was determined to have lower fat levels than advertised because the cows are inadequately fed. Another dilution is olive oil; it's estimated that up to 80 percent of Italian virgin olive oil is neither Italian nor virgin.

2. **Substitution.** It's common for restaurants or food stands to substitute something of lesser value in an attempt to reap a higher profit. Vendors in New York City got caught selling beef gyros or goat gyros advertised as lamb; this occurs more frequently when the meat is shredded and mixed together. Another common substitution occurs in fish sales, where one study demonstrated that 21 percent of the fish underwent substi-

tution, and that one out of every three establishments visited sold substituted seafood. Fish substitution is more likely to occur in restaurants (26 percent) than at grocery stores (12 percent). A common substitution occurs when tilapia (containing red dye), which costs $3.51 per pound, is swapped out for snapper, which costs about $15 per pound. Of the species tested, sea bass and snapper had the highest rates of mislabeling (55 percent and 42 percent, respectively). Much of the substituted seafood is labeled as a local favorite, while the truth is it may have been flown from halfway around the world.

3. **Intentional contamination/concealment.** A famous international case occurred in 2008, where melamine was found in infant formula and other dairy products. In China, the milk was being diluted by dairy producers so more of it could be sold. The dilution decreased the amount of protein in milk, so the dairy producer replaced the natural milk protein with melamine, a nitrogen-rich compound used to make kitchen countertops. When ingested, melamine causes kidney stones and kidney failure. The melamine in milk killed six infants and sickened over 300,000 people in China, but dairy products laced with melamine were exported around the world and made it to our shores. Luckily no one in the US died. Another example is Parmesan cheese. In 2012, cellulose, a by-product of wood digestion, was added to several brands; in fact, one brand didn't even have any cheese in the product at all.

4. **Country of origin.** Many food items are prized because they come from unique places. But what if that place isn't so unique? For instance, beer-battered pollock might come fresh from the waters of Alaska, or it might come frozen from a basin in China. More likely, the reason for this kind of fraud is to avoid paying duty on imported goods, such as alcohol.

5. **Organic.** You might think that buying organic would save you from fraud. You would be wrong. The markup on organic is enormous, anywhere from 25 percent for avocados to 65 percent for milk. Furthermore, there's a clear economic impetus to mark individual items as organic, as the only

way to be caught is through laboratory analysis. One fraudster netted $142 million for faking organic on the label, and then spent his ill-gotten gains on Las Vegas casinos and sexual escapades. He eventually committed suicide rather than go to jail.

6. **Counterfeiting.** Perhaps the most brazen of all food fraud occurs in the luxury space. Finding out that some high rollers were duped by the counterfeiting of rare wines and scotches may give you a moment of schadenfreude satisfaction, but this is a very alarming issue. If they can do that with something under that much scrutiny, imagine what they can do to you.

The Decline of the American Hive

Another frequent fraud is honey, which is in increasingly short supply. Yet paradoxically, American honey producers are sitting on millions of gallons of the stuff that they can't sell because imported honey is cheaper than American honey—because it's largely adulterated. If American farmers and food producers can't compete on price, then their businesses fail.

But honey matters, because it's one metric of a healthy bee population. Bees play a critical role in our environment. Bees produce honey and wax, but even more important, they're responsible for pollination. Without pollination, most of our crops won't survive. However, cheap imports from Asia and other parts of the world have made it such that it's no longer profitable for beekeepers in the US and Canada to produce honey, and there go the bees.

The people who buy honey from around the world and put it in bottles are called packers. Most packers blend foreign honey with domestic, but the foreign honey (especially that coming out of Asia) is adulterated. So perfectly good domestic honey is cut with several different kinds of sugars to dilute the product, many of which are not detectable by testing. Others are cleansing honey in such a way as to remove its nutritional components.

So even though American beekeepers produce 40 percent of the honey we consume, they also carry surpluses because the packers won't give them a fair price. The honest beekeepers are expected to compete with dishonest honey producers and exporters.

Food fraud is already negatively impacting us, economically and environmentally. We just don't know about it because of the forces at play to cover it up.

Big Food's Albatross

You might think food fraud would be the purview of just a few bad apples, but it's even more prevalent with processed food, where the source and identity of individual food components can be a "trade secret." Consumers demand an abundant and constant food supply, so Big Food sources ingredients from the cheapest suppliers from abroad. Garlic, soy, chiles, rice—all imported. It doesn't matter if the product is made in the US if the raw ingredients come from somewhere else. It is not unusual for processed foods to have five or more ingredients in them—for each additional ingredient, the chances of adulteration of that processed food increases to the 1.7 power. This is particularly true for the organic label on imported foods. Food producers in developing countries are entrusted with growing and purifying the raw materials with virtually no oversight. But why should Big Food care as long as it turns a profit, and no one gets acutely sick?

Don't Make a Federal Case Out of It

When it affects public health (think melamine), we expect our USDA and FDA to spring into action. But do they? Can they? The FDA has largely steered clear of the issues of processed food fraud because they don't have boots on the ground in every food-producing country in the world, and their charter is to ensure food is safe, not authentic.

When discovered, food fraud can sour trade relations. For instance, in 2013, horsemeat and pork were found in 33 percent of European products that were represented to contain only beef, sometimes a complete substitution. In response, most countries in Europe chartered their own food fraud units, or at the very minimum, nominated a person or group to take on the responsibility for investigating domestic cases. Nonetheless, corruption and graft abound. In the UK, the food industry plays nice with the regulators—that way, if they get caught, they can ante up a settlement and keep it out of the newspapers.

What distinguished the horsemeat fraud case of 2013 from the melamine fraud case of 2008 was geography, timing, and illness. Melamine was a China problem, but horsemeat was a Western problem. Serendipitously, the Global Food Safety Initiative (GFSI) conference was being held in Barcelona, Spain, in 2013, at the same time, and the food industry jumped on it. Their business is based on trust, which could be rapidly undermined if consumers really knew just how pervasive food fraud is.

Big Food, trade associations, and some academics remain in an unholy alliance to cover up and paper this over. How are they entitled to self-regulate when they're complicit in deceiving the public? But here's the real problem: why is Big Food more worried about consumers' trust regarding food fraud (which rarely kills), but less concerned about consumers' trust about processed food and NCDs (which kill millions)? Because it's easier for the public to understand and be horrified by horsemeat, rather than the science behind what will actually poison, addict, and kill them.

Food "Truthiness"

Big Food's approach to dealing with fraud has always been flawed—though isn't food fraud the responsibility of their food safety teams? The good news in the melamine case was that it was a problem both in food fraud *and* safety. It was the food safety leaders from Danone, Walmart, and Ahold who created the Food Fraud Think Tank, which reported directly to the board of directors of the GFSI. The Food Fraud Think Tank also consisted of INSCATECH, a US food fraud detection and prevention company; Eurofins, a food testing laboratory; and Professor John Spink of Michigan State University. The Food Fraud Think Tank was tasked with making recommendations to the GFSI Board of Directors as to how to handle food fraud going forward.

The Board of Directors represent the largest food producers, restaurant chains, and retailers in the world. In other words, is Big Food the fox in charge of the henhouse? Unfortunately, only about half of the companies on the board of GFSI felt it was their responsibility to even address fraud. The Food Fraud Think Tank made two recommendations: companies must conduct vulnerability assessments (which they did); and they also must develop food fraud control plans (which they didn't).

Who's in Charge? And Who's Responsible?

Right now, Big Food's methods for detecting and remediating food fraud rest with the corporate executives in charge of safety, who aren't fraud professionals. Rather, the food fraud professionals are those in charge of risk management, supply chain security, procurement, brand protection, and international law. They're trained to combat fraud, but corporate execs are under orders to buy food at the lowest possible price, with the magical expectation that the food they are buying is authentic and high quality. Every day they go to work inherently conflicted.

Big Food's procurement system is like the Wild West; they're at the mercy of other countries who supply us. But why does Big Food outsource in the first place? Sometimes it's because certain foods only grow in certain regions, such as spices, vanilla, olive oil, cocoa, and coffee. However, the climate in the US is diverse enough to grow almost everything here. California, Florida, and Hawaii can sustain cocoa, coffee, and vanilla plants in addition to most citrus fruits. In other regions of the US, foods like honey, corn, wheat, cherries, grapes, pears, apples, peaches, plums, tomatoes, carrots, lettuce, grains, and a host of other produce can be grown in abundance. It would just cost more than our current outsourcing.

Statistics vary slightly, but why does two-thirds of the apple juice in America come from China, and why does over 50 percent of orange juice and concentrate come from Brazil (especially since Brazil is dousing their oranges in glyphosate)? Why do we get milk powder from India, or seafood from Vietnam? Big Food has done the cost calculations down to the hundredth of a penny. Legitimate producers who grow or procure authentic food can't compete with cheap imports. Yet the added cost—meaning the health difference—may or may not be known, and may or may not be quantifiable. Just wait for the mistake that costs lives. It happened with Katrina, Sandy, and coronavirus. It will happen with food fraud. Consumers will demand explanations, and Big Food will finger-point at the USDA, who will finger-point at the FDA, who will finger-point right back. At the end of the day, consumers must realize how vulnerable they really are.

Food Sleuths

Testing for food fraud is very much in its infancy. DNA testing for seafood and meats is well established, but labs struggle when food is in liquid or ground-up form. If perpetrators are using an unidentified adulterant, the labs are blind to it. Furthermore, the more highly processed the food, the less likely that testing can detect the fraud.

There are only a handful of food testing laboratories around the world who do food authenticity testing. They use sophisticated technologies that can run in the millions of dollars, like nuclear magnetic resonance spectroscopy (NMR) to identify certain sugars, or liquid chromatography–mass spectrometry (LC-MS) to measure pesticides and antibiotics. These tools have great potential, but like most technology, they're only as good as the data that goes into them. Therein lies the problem. Without the intelligence about how food fraud is being committed, the tools are nothing more than expensive toys. Science can provide evidence, but intelligence is the key to providing cause, placement, and authenticity. Science alone cannot keep up with the criminals.

Since the horsemeat scandal of 2013, the UK has tried to share information with the US about food fraud. However, producers, retailers, academics, and law enforcement have conflicting interests, and don't trust one another. Laboratories are supposed to be independent of food industry funding, but they take dirty money anyway. Food testing labs must retain their independence, or risk losing their International Organization for Standardization certification. Some Big Food companies do want to solve the problem (after all, they're being cheated, too!), but it's a heavy lift. Consumers and governments must help, but education about what's actually going on has to come first.

Accentuate the Positive

When you mention food fraud, Big Food goes running. But when you mention food authenticity, they're all ears. My colleague Mitchell Weinberg of INSCATECH has developed an opt-in food authenticity certification program called GenuCert, and the first test case is GenuHoney. If a honey producer or packer wants to be certified, it must regularly undergo unannounced forensically based audits, where samples from hives and/or honey extraction equipment are taken and sent for analysis. In this way, beekeepers can be fairly compensated for their work and their product (as we said, the entire food system depends on bees!). Other items ripe for food authenticity certifications, and on INSCATECH's radar, include maple syrup, olive oil, dairy products, fish, beef, vanilla, and alcohol.

In the meantime, what can you, the consumer, do to protect your health and your wallet from food fraud? It's tough to say. But there are three precepts to remember:

1. The more ingredients, the more risk (e.g., salted peanuts have three ingredients, Oreos have eleven ingredients). Avoid highly processed food.

2. Buying organic may decrease your risk for cancer, but it increases the risk of fraud because fraudsters focus on organic due to the higher profit margin.

3. Buy from the supplier directly (e.g., the farmer or the farmer's market). Fewer middlemen mean fewer entities jacking up the price and people to hide behind, as well as more direct and face-to-face responsibility to the consumer.

We are years, perhaps decades, away from truly fraud-free food. However, trust in food authenticity is essential to remaking the food system. We need and must demand more transparency; this is going to take a cultural movement. Growers have to believe that they will get a fair price and not be undercut. Consumers have to believe they're getting what they want, and what they paid for. And manufacturers have to believe that they'll get in trouble if they ignore us.

Part V

Where Are the Food Police When You Need Them?

CHAPTER 23

The Party Line

As demonstrated in the film *Merchants of Doubt* (2014), the tobacco industry followed a consistent playbook for several decades to keep the world smoking. Ultimately, the science caught up with the industry, and the law caught up with everyone (even though the tobacco executives themselves weren't found to be personally culpable). However, it took forty-four years from the first report of tobacco and lung cancer to the Mississippi attorney general suing Big Tobacco for recoupment of Medicaid costs related to lung cancer. As dramatized in *Dark Waters* (2019), E. I. du Pont consistently stonewalled for nineteen years to avoid litigation regarding its use of perfluorooctanoic acid (PFOA or Teflon) in pots and pans. We learned the hard way that big money industries will do anything they can to turn a profit at whatever cost to lives, the environment, and society at large.

The sugar industry is one of the most egregious villains in the bunch. Based on our current recognition of sugar's toxicity and their responses to litigation thus far, one might assume that Big Sugar learned its tricks from Big Tobacco. But it's actually the other way around—the Sugar

Research Foundation was founded in 1943, and one of its executives, Dr. Robert Hockett, peddled his manipulation tactics to the Tobacco Industry Research Committee in 1954. In any case, the playbooks are almost identical—deny, deflect, distract, delay. The entire processed food industry has adopted this policy. Some tactics involve influencing scientists, others influence public opinion, and even more influence governments and the courts. The UCSF Industry Documents Library now hosts a food industry section open to the public, with a particular focus on sugar, which has been used by my colleagues to document the extent and magnitude of food industry subterfuge.

Influencing Scientists

"More doctors smoke Camels over any other cigarette . . ." This was just one of many advertising efforts of Big Tobacco to co-opt the public by co-opting scientists, as documented by Stanford research Robert Proctor in his book *Golden Holocaust* (2012). True to the corporate playbook, the processed food industry has similarly co-opted their most influential, but not necessarily knowledgeable, critics using four different strategies.

Distracting away from the real problem. As we explored in Chapter 10, we have the data to demonstrate that processed food is a primary causative factor for diabetes, fatty liver disease, heart disease, and tooth decay; correlative for cancer, dementia, hypertension, addiction to other substances, and depression; as well as plausible for autoimmune disease and anxiety. But when the food industry addresses these issues in public, they only refer to the "obesity epidemic." Until about 2010, they ignored the problem entirely, deflecting the issue back to the consumer and using the tobacco industry meme of "personal responsibility." When they couldn't deny culpability any longer, they chose to divert the public health conversation specifically toward obesity, for two reasons: because for them and the dietitians, it's still all about calories, and the public still believes it (hopefully I've done a good enough job with this book to finally *kill the calorie*). The data for sugar and obesity is also relatively weak, or at least it has been until recently.

One study showed that soda and desserts rank below French fries and potato chips as a cause of weight gain. You'll notice that all are processed foods and that French fries are generally consumed with loads of sugar-sweetened tomato ketchup and most flavored potato chips have lots of sugar, even if they aren't technically a dessert. This is the crux of the food industry's overarching message—if sugar is only *one* of *many* causes of obesity, then why pick on it specifically? The industry regurgitates its mantra that "a calorie is a calorie"; therefore it's about energy balance, gluttony and sloth, diet and exercise, and if you're fat, it's your fault. Yet, when weight and calories are factored out, the correlation between sugar consumption and diabetes becomes much stronger—in other words, the effect of other calories on weight gain dilutes out the specific effects of sugar on diabetes. In addition, there are countries where diabetes rates are astronomical while obesity rates are low—such as India, Pakistan, and China—yet their sugar consumption has increased by 15 percent in the past six years alone.

Of course, fast food is more than just sugar. Maybe it's the hamburgers, maybe it's the French fries, maybe it's the Filet-O-Fish sandwiches; it could even be the salad dressing. Roberto De Vogli at UC Davis wanted to know which component was the real culprit, so his team assembled the cash register receipts for eighteen years in all thirty-seven OECD countries (a mean feat to be sure), categorized what was consumed, and correlated each with weight gain over time. His research revealed it was the sugar-sweetened beverages that drove the weight gain over the processed animal- and plant-based products. Of course, this study was retrospective, not prospective, and it doesn't prove causation. Nonetheless, the sugar remains a constant.

To date, the food industry refuses to engage in a rational discussion about the role of added sugar in chronic metabolic diseases exclusive of its effects on obesity, because the message of obesity works for them. Or at least it worked for them until 2019, when the reason for this paradox was unraveled. It turns out that sugar has two effects on weight gain. One is an immediate function, where year by year consumption predicts year by year weight gain; the second function is what your mother ate before you were even born. As explored earlier, mother's consumption of sugar reaches across the placenta, goes to the liver to turn sugar into liver fat, and to the pancreas to make extra insulin, which drives fetal fat cell development. This is why obesity rates keep going up in the US, even though sugar consumption has dropped slightly in the last decade—the current generation is still paying for the previous generation's SpaghettiOs. That Coke wasn't just the "real thing" for you, but for your unborn kids, too.

Following the money. The sugar industry has a long history of co-opting scientists. My UCSF colleagues Cristin Kearns, Laura Schmidt, and Stanton Glantz have discovered the paper trail of influence by the Sugar Research Foundation. The foundation engaged in a coordinated disinformation effort to exonerate sugar and divert attention toward saturated fat as a cause of cardiovascular disease in 1967, and away from sugar as a cause of dental caries in 1971. Since then, sugar, high-fructose corn syrup, beverage, and processed food industry concerns have paid scientists to be complicit in marketing sugar as healthy, or at least benign. More recently, an analysis of Web of Science citations from 2008 to 2016 identified 779 articles with Coca-Cola conflicts of interest regarding funding. A subsequent comparison with Coca-Cola's own transparency website (established in 2016 after the *New York Times* exposé on the Global Energy Balance Network) identified 128 articles and 471 authors who weren't disclosed by Coca-Cola, as well 19 academic investigators who had direct email contact with the company. The question is whether academia and industry should be allowed to work together, especially if academia can be so easily co-opted by money.

Espousing the alternate view, Dr. John Sievenpiper of St. Michael's Hospital in Toronto, in the documentary *Sugar Coated* (2015), stated, "Academics, as much as people believe they are biased, they want to do good research, and if they can't get the money to answer important questions as they see them, in their labs and clinics, from the government, they'll look to other sources." But what if those sources have their own agendas?

Obfuscating scientific research. One would expect the totality of evidence on the detrimental effects of sugar to be reflected in systematic reviews or meta-analyses; however, many of these publications yield inconsistent results. It's a classic rewrite of the tobacco playbook. One problem is that many of these studies are funded by the food industry, with the intention of diluting the available data, specifically to paper over any significant effects. However, these inconsistencies are exposed completely when food industry sponsorship is taken into account. We shouldn't be surprised to find that studies funded by industry are 7.4 times more likely to show a favorable conclusion, and in cases when the data didn't fit the industry's narrative, they just deep-sixed it. The industry's influence in distorting public health messages even extends to institutions and organizations that have a responsibility to scientific integrity, such as the University of Sydney protecting scientists who used a faulty dataset in order to exonerate sugar as a cause of obesity.

Co-opting public health experts. For years as part of their public relations machinery, soft drink companies would push lack of physical activity as a cause of obesity. However, the evidence reveals that the impact of physical activity on chronic disease is minimal. You just can't outrun a bad diet. The beverage companies have sponsored a total of ninety-six public health efforts, with the proviso that they don't address soft drinks. For example, Dr. Brenda Fitzgerald, the recently disgraced director of the U.S. Centers for Disease Control, wouldn't divest her portfolio from tobacco stocks and had also taken money from Coca-Cola. Coca-Cola also bankrolled the now-defunct Global Energy Balance Network, a consortium of three academics "on the take" to promulgate lack of exercise as the cause of obesity. In their own words, "an energy balance framework is the only framework that makes sense in addressing obesity." Even Michelle Obama caved to food industry pressure in the president's second term, shifting her focus away from

the importance of a healthy diet exclusively toward promoting physical activity. Even the Academy of Nutrition and Dietetics (AND),
British Dietetic Association (BDA), and the Dieticians Association of
Australia (DAA) all receive annual contributions from food industry
concerns. After all, you shouldn't bite the hand that feeds you.

Influencing Public Opinion—the Meme of "Personal Responsibility"

The most egregious corollary to energy balance, which follows directly
from it, is the meme of "personal responsibility"—just another way of
saying "it's your fault that you're fat." It's an ideology that requires four
separate prerequisites to be in play: knowledge, access, affordability,
and externalities (or how your behavior impacts other people). If any
of the four are not met, then you can't invoke personal responsibility.

But who invented personal responsibility anyway? It's an ideology,
but is it a human right? Some people believe it was handed down by
God; after all, take the risks, suffer the consequences. Very American.
But where did this idea actually come from? The Declaration of Independence? The Constitution? The Magna Carta? Maybe Hammura-
bi's Code? No, this came from the tobacco industry, who embraced
this concept wholeheartedly in 1962 to deflect from corporate responsibility, and used it as a reason to keep on smoking. They were getting
killed on the science of lung cancer, and had to invent another reason
to keep people smoking. No one put that cigarette in your mouth, right?
No one lit it for you? You did all that on your own.

Then, Big Tobacco made it look cool—who didn't want to be or sleep
with the Marlboro Man? It's all personal responsibility—you smoked
it, you bought it. The food industry just co-opted this ideology. It still
markets well, because you don't have to smoke, but you do have to eat.
And you may as well enjoy it. But you don't have to eat poison. Let's dig
deeper into these personal responsibility prerequisites:

1. **Knowledge.** Can you trust the food industry to tell you when something
    is healthy or not? People have no idea what they're eating. The Nutri-

tion Labeling and Education Act of 1990 gave us our current food label, which was supposed to provide information to the consumer of what's in the food, but of course says nothing about what's been done to render it poisonous. The food label is currently unintelligible in part because the industry skirts the rules (see Chapter 17). What the public needs to know *(protect the liver, feed the gut)* is what's been done to the food—but that's exactly the information that's withheld.

2. **Access.** With 74 percent of foods in the supermarket containing added sugar, it has become almost unavoidable that you will, knowingly or unknowingly, consume contaminated food in your daily life. Processed foods are quick, easy, and have permeated workplaces, gyms, schools, and your refrigerator.

   People in poor neighborhoods live in "food deserts," without access to Real Food because grocery stores are hard to come by. But the problem of food deserts becomes magnified when those same areas are rife with fast food outlets and convenience stores that provide only processed items (because of shelf life and depreciation). Sometimes these are called "food swamps," the density of which predict obesity and chronic disease in poor populations even better than food deserts. And why not? You can drown in a swamp faster than you can starve in a desert.

3. **Affordability.** Assuming one wants to buy healthy food and has access to it, they have to be able to afford it. Analysis of the cost of food demonstrated that Real Food (fresh produce, eggs, and meat) was twice as expensive as processed food (Cheetos and Pop-Tarts) in 2002, and increased by 17 cents per pound of food per year over the next decade, as compared with processed food, which only increased 7 cents per pound per year. However, the cost of obesity to the individual ends up much higher. The amount of money that they pay directly for healthcare is double that of a person of normal weight.

   Furthermore, if you're working three jobs and have kids, then you need something quick and easy. Affordability is coming from a place of privilege not just in cost of food, but in time for menu planning, etc.

It's one of many social justice issues—if you don't have the time or the money to procure and prepare Real Food, what options do you have? And the processed food industry has positioned itself to perfectly fill the gap. Cheap food seems like a no-brainer—but not really.

4. **Externalities.** The belief that your actions can't harm anyone else needs reconsideration. For example, if you smoke, you not only hurt yourself, you hurt your employer, as the cost to that employer is $5,816 per year just to carry you. The cost to employers as a result of the obesity epidemic adds an extra $2,751 per employee. There are double the workers who are obese (45 percent) as there are smokers (23 percent)—never mind the costs of the diseases of metabolic syndrome. The medical costs of chronic metabolic disease due to processed food consumption will cause a doubling of social network costs in the next decade. In the US, Medicare will be bankrupt by 2029 and Social Security will be bankrupt by 2034, bankrupting healthcare systems around the world. There's the additional burden of diet-related harm experienced by children who are especially vulnerable to poor diet at critical developmental stages.

Clearly, the ideology of personal responsibility falls apart when we're dealing with public health problems. Let's take the last health-care personal responsibility issue as an example—HIV. Patient Zero was 1979, the term AIDS was coined in 1981, Robert Gallo and Luc Montagnier discovered the virus in 1984, and Surgeon General C. Everett Koop called attention to it in 1986. But when did HIV go from being a personal responsibility issue to a public health crisis?

On November 7, 1991, Magic Johnson declared he had HIV—and the whole world went, *"Wow,* this could happen to me." Up to that point, HIV was thought to infect homosexuals, hemophiliacs, and drug addicts. Easy enough to marginalize them. Then, all of a sudden, a straight basketball player contracts it, and the public does a 180-degree turn because it finally dawned on them that everyone is at risk. That's the nature of a public health crisis. Well, anyone can get the chronic diseases of type 2 diabetes or heart disease or Alzheimer's disease or cancer. Nonetheless, Big Food will continue to push the obesity argument to sell their products, and Big Pharma will back them up to sell theirs.

Influencing Government and the Courts

In the 1960s Ralph Nader and *Unsafe at Any Speed* (1965) spearheaded the American consumer movement. Environmentalism was gaining speed. Regulatory agencies like OSHA and the EPA were founded. Distrust of Big Business was at its peak. But then in the 1970s something happened. Big Industry, of which Big Food is a major player, started to wage a propaganda war in the halls of Congress and the Supreme Court to take back what they viewed was rightfully theirs. How did they do it?

1. **Disinformation campaigns and legislation.** In 1972, Sugar Information, Inc., ran a public disinformation campaign to deflect criticism from its product. The U.S. Federal Trade Commission (FTC) engaged in a damaging court battle, which shuttered their efforts. However, in the late 1970s, efforts to ban junk food marketing on television led to a corporate power struggle pressuring Congress to "declaw" the FTC (take away its enforcement powers), which eventually occurred in 1980; the FTC has never been heard from again.

   The 1970s also saw the rise of the American Legislative Exchange Council (ALEC), a bill mill that writes legislation beneficial to the oil, pharma, tobacco/alcohol, and food industries. Through contributions from affiliated groups and individuals, it effectively pays off congressmen to introduce these bills in order to make sure the playing field is not kept level, that these industries are protected. This goes all the way to the top. One example was the privatization of the FDA's Generally Recognized as Safe (GRAS) list in 1997 (see Chapter 24). Most recently, the Trump administration limited even more information on junk food labels at the bidding of Big Food.

2. **Trade organizations.** Trade organizations are sponsored by many companies within an industry to lobby and further the needs and profits of the industry as a whole. In the US, there's the American Beverage Association and National Restaurant Association. In the UK, the Food and Drink Federation performs similar functions. In Australia and New Zealand, there's the Sugar Research Advisory Service, renamed the Sugar Nutrition Resource Centre. The claim is that this is a scientific information service for health professionals, academics, and the media that aims to provide "an evidence-based view of the role of sugars in nutrition and health." It is fronted by academics and health professionals receiving money directly from the industry, and is blatantly pro-sugar.

When Nonprofits Profit

Perhaps the most egregious organization of all is the International Life Sciences Institute (ILSI). Its mission, according to its website, is "to provide science that improves human health and well-being and safeguards the environment." This organization, though nonprofit and private, is really a corporate lobby group. They say they're all about the science—but only the science the industry promulgates. ILSI has a $17 million budget, all funded by four hundred corporate members, including some of the biggest names in food processing (e.g., Coca-Cola, DuPont, PepsiCo, General Mills, and Danone). It pushes the benefits of food processing while ignoring any science that mentions its risks. Furthermore, under the auspices of being a scientific nonprofit, one of its true missions (if it chooses to accept it) is to infiltrate the agencies that could regulate them. Nowhere is this more clear than in China, where members of China's FDA are on the board of directors of ILSI. What could go wrong? China's food safety has been consistently called into question, but the conflicts of interest here are widespread.

Astroturf groups are "citizens" or nonprofit groups that mask their sponsors to appear as though they're grassroots organizations. The U.S. Center for Organizational Research and Education (CORE; formerly the Center for Consumer Freedom) is an organization with a name deliberately designed to divert attention away from industry connection. They claim to be "dedicated to protect consumer choices and promoting common sense." In fact, they're funded by the fast food, meat, alcohol, and tobacco industries.

The group was founded in the mid-1990s, using tobacco (Philip Morris donated $600,000) and restaurant industry money to oppose smoking restrictions in restaurants. Its founder, Richard Berman, also began the American Beverage Institute, which fights restrictions on alcohol use and raising the minimum wage. In a secretly recorded interview reported by the *New York Times*, Berman encouraged main players to attack those that oppose industry interests with threats that they could either "win ugly or lose pretty."

Across the pond, the Institute of Economic Affairs (IEA) is self-pronounced as "the UK's original free market think tank." They claim to be independent of any political party, group, or organization. But is this true? Last year they received £1.6 million ($2 million) from Big Tobacco, Coca-Cola, and sugar manufacturer Tate & Lyle. In July 2014, the IEA released a report arguing that lack of physical activity was driving the obesity epidemic rather than excess calories, and then another report (with no science) saying that research shows that sugar isn't the cause of diabetes. When questioned as to whether the organization takes money from the food industry, spokesman Christopher Snowdon replied that the question was "irrelevant." On the BBC, Snowdon recently suggested that those public health bodies calling for reduction of sugar, alcohol, and tobacco are responsible for increasing misery in society. Because who could be happy without a Captain and Coke in one hand and a cigarette in the other? Simultaneously, ignoring all medical information to the contrary, he suggested that we couldn't be healthier.

The food industry knows what it's doing. And I know, too, because I've been an expert witness in several lawsuits against the food industry. When a lawsuit goes forward, the attorneys on both sides engage in the process of *discovery*, which entitles each side to see the correspondence and emails of the other side. As a result, everyone knows what the defendant knew and when they knew it, as does the judge. The fact that lawsuits against the food industry aren't immediately thrown out and live to see a payday says that the courts now find that the industry is knowledgeable and culpable. **This is the second of our three immoral hazards**—creating a market to profit off the misery of others. And the processed food industry has done exactly that, profiting off poisoning their customers. And now those processed chickens are coming home to roost.

Inside Job

Not all food industry executives are heartless sociopaths. Some recognize the problem and want to fix it. For instance, Indra Nooyi, former CEO of PepsiCo (2006–2018), is from Madras, India, where diabetes rates have skyrocketed to 8.8 percent. She knows it's because of their "fun for you" food line, purveying Pepsi and Doritos.

Nooyi was on a mission to fix the food. In 2007, she hired Dr. Derek Yach away from the WHO to become senior vice president for Global Health and Agriculture Policy. Yach was a known public health expert, having taken on the tobacco industry during his tenure at the WHO. Many doubted Yach's intentions when he went to work for the "enemy," but nonetheless, Nooyi and Yach followed through in 2011 when they introduced the "good for you" line of products, including Nut Harvest and Quaker with significantly lower sugar. They proceeded to lose $349 million in one year because these products were sold alongside their competitors' sugary options, which the customers have been trained to prefer. The shareholders called for Nooyi's head on a spear because "she took her eye off the ball." No one has heard from the "good for you" line since. Nooyi didn't try again, and Yach bolted from PepsiCo in 2013.

Todd Putman was an executive for Coca-Cola, and while in the Amazon researching sites for placing Coke vending machines, he happened upon a seven-year-old with a Coke T-shirt and no teeth from chronic tooth decay. Putman flew back to Atlanta and quit; he now gives talks about the dangers of the processed food industry.

Finally, Campbell Soup CEO Denise Morrison (2011–2018) was also motivated to fix the problem from the inside, introducing healthier fare, but instead resigned abruptly. She had high hopes to turn Campbell's around, but ended up stuck with a portfolio of Goldfish crackers, Cape Cod potato chips, and Snyder's pretzels. Reducing sodium was a great way to reduce profits, when you go it alone. A cautionary tale for the rest of the industry, to be sure.

In response to sustainability goals in Europe, some supermarket chains have announced a shift to healthier products. However, "healthier" is in the eye of the beholder, as in one case, the director of merchandising watered down the effort by promoting chocolate and beer as the #1 and #2 items. Furthermore, as an inducement to eat healthier, they tried chilled cabinets at the checkout, with fruit and vegetables, muesli bars, nuts, etc. At one store in a low-income neighborhood, the removal of the impulse-buy confectionery lost the store 1,000 euros in one week—and that was the end of that experiment.

Hank Cardello, a former executive at Coca-Cola and chief strategist at the Hudson Institute, argues in his book *Stuffed* (2009) that the food industry has a problem, yet only the food industry can fix it. However, the simple fact of the matter is that no one inside the food industry can or will fix this, because of Wall Street, shareholders, and quarterly earnings reports. Nope, change is going to have to come from the outside.

CHAPTER 24

The USDA and the FDA Don't Kill People; Rather They Let Them Die

The food industry lying about the costs and benefits of processed food is no surprise, and my book *Fat Chance* (2012) and Marion Nestle's *Food Politics* (2003) and *Unsavory Truth* (2019) document many of their subterfuges. The fact that food companies employ lobbyists and liaisons and Washington bill mills is also no surprise. But what about governments? Do they lie?

The USDA is the political arm of the food industry, and the FDA is the political arm of the drug industry. The USDA is supposed to support American agriculture in all its guises and to all its consumers, including you. The FDA is supposed to make sure your food and drugs are safe and effective. Both organizations are supposed to be independent of the industries they regulate, yet they do their bidding. Known as "agency capture," both have a revolving door policy between government and industry about hiring and lobbying. Furthermore, the heads of both come from the private sector and return to it. They each have their own horses in the race and, sadly, yours has been scratched.

USDA and DGAC

Starting in 1977 with the McGovern Commission and every five years since, the USDA has issued successive sets of its Dietary Guidelines for Americans. The USDA's charter of 1862 entails two roles: to ensure a sufficient and reliable food supply; and to provide useful information on subjects related to agriculture. Therefore, one might rightfully question why the USDA is in charge of guidelines related to health in the first place. You can thank the Senate Select Subcommittee on Agriculture (remember, McGovern was from South Dakota), made up of a legislative Who's Who of midwestern states, which invited American agribusiness (located in those same states) to the table. The Farm Bill of 1977 expanded the USDA's role into providing dietary advice to the public, and in 1988 the House Committee on Appropriations codified the USDA as the lead agency for dietary advice.

Commensurate with the initial 1977 guidelines, American (and indeed global) health has declined, as measured by increasing obesity and chronic disease rates, as well as reduction in life span and health span. The percent of GDP spent on healthcare also rose from 7 percent to 17.9 percent. Those original 1977 guidelines have been exposed for the sham that they were—the McGovern Commission first issuing a missive to "eat less fat, salt, and sugar," but after concerted pressure from the food industry, changed to "eat more low-fat alternatives," which inherently meant people ate more sugar to make their food palatable.

Behind the pamphlets, pyramids, and plates is the political debate that occurs within the Dietary Guidelines Advisory Committee (DGAC), made up of thirteen academic and industry representatives, who meet every five years to review the latest research. After a year's deliberation, where they review all the clinical data available for the previous ten years, they submit a report to the USDA. To their credit, all of the activities and deliberations of the DGAC are completely transparent. What happens afterward isn't—functionaries within the USDA rewrite the guidelines, leaving aspects out that would anger or disadvantage the food industry.

I stood for candidacy for the DGAC in 2008. The previous 2005 DGAC committee chair, Dr. Janet King, was in favor of my candidacy, as were six academic organizations. But she warned me—what the DGAC said and what the USDA did with what they said were two completely different things. At the end of the day, DGAC is *advisory, not enforceable.* They have no teeth. And they're not allowed to complain to the USDA about it. The food industry appoints half the committee. Needless to say, I was not appointed.

Journalist Nina Teicholz investigated the DGAC's actions over the previous thirty-five years. In 2015 she penned an editorial in the *British Medical Journal* that the DGAC had systematically ignored large-scale clinical trial evidence, mostly funded by governments around the world (and therefore presumably independent), on more than seventy-five thousand people for up to twelve years. In 2017, the U.S. National Academies of Sciences, Engineering, and Medicine (NASEM) similarly concluded that the process for guidelines development wasn't using the best practices for conducting systematic reviews and "lacked scientific rigor." NASEM advised the USDA to adopt one of the international standards for systematic reviews of the science, and the USDA staff then announced in March 2019 that it planned to use a "modified" version of GRADE (Grading of Recommendations Assessment, Development and Evaluation). This is an internationally recognized methodological standard for reviewing scientific literature. However, the cofounder of the GRADE system, Dr. Gordon Guyatt, issued a public rebuke to the USDA, in which he pointed out that this modified version lacked the methodology to distinguish between high-quality and low-quality evidence: "This distinction between high- and low-quality evidence lies at the core of any rigorous evaluation of science and is at the heart of the GRADE methodology." Guyatt urged the USDA not even to use the name GRADE "because doing so would give the appearance of rigor where it did not exist."

I've already shown you the data (see Chapter 16) showing that the high sugar in baby food leads to dental caries and insulin resistance, while the low fiber leads to poor airway development. In 2019, the WHO agreed that baby foods are excessively high in sugar and inappropriately marketed. Therefore it was somewhat heartening to see that the 2020 DGAC incorporated these findings to argue for cessation of added sugar to baby food (although no mention of pureed foods was made). We will wait and see if the USDA stands up to Big Baby Food and accepts this advisory into the next Dietary Guidelines.

USDA and SNAP

American agribusiness produces 3,900 calories per person per day, but Americans can only eat 1,800 to 2,000 of them. Where does all the excess food go? The Supplemental Nutrition Assistance Program (SNAP; also known as food stamps), run by the USDA, is designed to "provide improved levels of nutrition among low-income households." It serves a population of forty-two million people, or one-eighth of America. Seventy percent of SNAP recipients are families with children, and seventy-five percent of their food expenditures are within the program. Considering our country makes twice as much food as we need, the fact that half of all households enrolled in the SNAP are food insecure is mind-boggling. Yet when it comes right down to it, SNAP recipients receive the equivalent of $1.40 per meal. This is just half of the $2.86 per meal allocated to students enrolled in the National School Lunch Program (NSLP; also run by the USDA), which is itself woefully inadequate.

Where does such a determination on expenditures come from? It's based on what the USDA considers a nutritionally adequate diet at minimal cost. We already know what the USDA considers adequate nutrition. Given that SNAP recipients are more likely to suffer from metabolic syndrome than the general population, it's hard to make the case that SNAP provides nutritionally adequate support. It's also worth noting that $321 billion (three-quarters of the total) of the $428 billion Farm Bill (see Chapter 26) is used for this and other nutrition programs ostensibly aimed to help low-income populations.

And get this—a long-hidden USDA report exposed by Anahad O'Connor of the *New York Times* revealed that 9 percent of those on SNAP food dollars go to sugar-sweetened beverages (SSBs) (as compared to 7 percent of the disadvantaged non-SNAP population), and that 40 percent of all purchases on SNAP were for SSBs. We don't provide alcohol on SNAP—and for good reason—but sugar does the same damage as alcohol (see Chapter 7), so isn't that a little disingenuous? Now, it's not that SNAP recipients drink more SSBs than those who aren't on SNAP—it's that everyone is drinking them, to their detriment.

So, 0.09 x $1.40 = 15 cents spent on soda per meal. That's a lot of soda SSBs, and a big chunk of SNAP. The US government spends $608.7 million on soft drinks and $110 million on juices, all of which drive more chronic disease. In fact, modeling studies suggest that banning sodas from SNAP purchases could prevent as many as 400,000 cases of obesity and diabetes. Yet in 2011, the US government denied a request from New York City disallowing food stamps to be spent on SSBs in order to curb the obesity epidemic, citing "personal responsibility" and arguing for more "incentive-based solutions."

Yet forty-two million people get their food from SNAP, which makes it a necessary lifeline between satiety and starvation. Which makes the Trump administration announcement that it was throwing three million of those forty-two million Americans off the SNAP rolls, and five hundred thousand kids out of the National School Breakfast and Lunch Programs, even more disastrous. What's needed is not to throw 10 percent of people off SNAP; what's needed is to throw 100 percent of SSBs off SNAP.

USDA and NSLP

Vegetable is defined as "a plant or part of a plant used as food." Apparently, Ronald Reagan knew this when he declared that ketchup was a vegetable, in order to cut the monetary subsidies to the National School Lunch Program (NSLP) in 1981. Yes, ketchup is made from tomatoes, which, last time I looked, are plants that are used as food. So I suppose Reagan was technically correct, except that tomatoes are fruits, so not really. The scientific question that confronts us, however, is how much processing must occur before a vegetable isn't a vegetable anymore?

A quick analysis of Heinz ketchup gives pause. Yes, tomato concentrate is listed as the first ingredient, then vinegar, and then high-fructose corn syrup (HFCS) and corn syrup are numbers three and four. When you look at the calories (20 kcal) versus the carbohydrate content of 5 grams (4 of which are sugar) multiplied by 4 calories/gram, you realize that tomatoes may be the plurality, but not the majority of the ingredients. Does that mean that ketchup isn't a vegetable? Well, by definition, corn and sugar cane are plants, so HFCS and corn syrup are vegetables; in fact, every carbon-containing compound that's not meat or dairy is by definition a vegetable. That includes ketchup, as well as the hemlock consumed by Socrates, and chewing tobacco consumed by Major League Baseball players.

And apparently, that includes pizza as well. In response to Michelle Obama's effort to improve nutrition and the passage of the Healthy, Hunger-Free Kids Act (HHFKA) of 2010, the pizza served in school cafeterias nationwide would have to be struck from the menu. But 70 percent of the frozen pizzas are manufactured by companies located in Minnesota, and so to rescue the Minnesota pizza industry, Senator Amy Klobuchar (yes, that Amy Klobuchar) got a special treatment for tomato paste—an eighth of a cup of tomato paste is now credited with as much nutritional value as half a cup of vegetables. It was even written into a congressional agriculture appropriations bill. As a result, pizza is cheese (dairy) plus vegetables and wheat (plant), tomato sauce (plant, including HFCS), and oil (derived from plants).

But all of these procedural machinations pale in comparison with what the Trump administration proposed in January 2020. The USDA conducted a study that showed when given a choice between pizza and French fries versus real vegetables on their cafeteria trays, kids waste the vegetables. This was of course stating the obvious. Therefore, Trump's secretary of agriculture, Sonny Perdue, cut the unnecessary cost of food waste by eliminating vegetables from school lunches nationwide. After all, when you were ten, would you choose the French fry or the carrot?

FDA and Food Safety

The FDA is supposed to guarantee the safety of our food supply. It's in their charter—the Food, Drug, and Cosmetic Act (FDCA) of 1938. But when it comes to food, the charter only provides for screening for *acute* toxicity—things that will make you keel over and die, like melamine in milk, botulism in vichyssoise, *E. coli* in apple cider, *Salmonella* in eggs, and *Listeria* in spinach. The FDA has done most of that pretty well, save for the occasional hamburger recall. But nowhere does the FDCA mention *chronic* toxicity, where one exposure isn't toxic but rather cumulative exposure will kill you. This loophole lets the food industry get away with all sorts of slow murder.

A perfect example is tobacco. Do cigarettes kill? Yes, but not one, and not today, and not even tomorrow; but ten thousand smoked over ten years just might. As a result, the FDA couldn't and didn't regulate tobacco, because it didn't fit under the heading of "acute toxicity." Even with all of FDA commissioner David Kessler's railing and lobbying, he couldn't bring Big Tobacco to heal, because *chronic* toxicity isn't in the FDA's charter (eventually tobacco finally did come under the FDA's regulatory framework, but only after Congress passed the Tobacco Control Act in 2009).

In 2012, I debated the food industry at the American Society for Nutrition (ostensibly independent, but really a forum for industry scientists), and David Klurfeld, national program leader (human nutrition) of the FDA, got to weigh in. In his own words, "There are currently insufficient data to justify a decision on regulation or taxation of sugar-containing foods . . . there is no credible evidence that added sugar or any single saccharide is toxic or addictive or contributes to any disease independently of a diet that provides <u>excess energy</u> other than dental caries." For Klurfeld and the FDA, it's still all about obesity and calories.

FDA and Food vs. Health Claims

That's not to say that the FDA has no authority; they do have some rules. A food company isn't allowed to "outright lie," meaning they can't say there are no peanuts when the food was processed on a machine that also processes peanuts. They can't claim something is gluten-free if it's made with wheat; they can't claim something is organic if it tests positive for glyphosate. Otherwise, though, the rules are fluid and the food industry frequently steps over the line. For example, the industry often subverts the FDA's regulatory guidance on leveling with the public by exploiting the distinctions between the FDA's two different kinds of claims—structure-function claims versus health claims.

A structure-function claim is anything on the food label that doesn't mention a disease. "Now with vitamin C," "Helps build strong bodies 12 ways," "good source of fiber," "calcium builds strong bones and teeth"—these are all examples of structure-function claims. They may implicitly invoke disease states, but they don't name them. For such a claim, the structure of the food is indirectly related to the function of the body. Structure-function claims imply health benefits without actually coming out and touting them. And sometimes the structure-function claim may have nothing to do with what is in the box or the wrapper; for example, putting "GMO-free" on water? One could argue that this is food propaganda, but it is entirely legal under FDA guidelines.

A health claim is different. A health claim mentions a specific disease or disease process. If a label for a calcium pill says "helps prevent osteoporosis" or a breakfast cereal says "helps reduce heart disease," this is where the FDA can automatically intervene to protect the public. These kinds of health claims are strictly monitored, regulated, and enforced by the FDA—if the company can't produce the studies to prove it, then the claim is stricken.

However, there is a big gray area between these two sets of claims. The food industry's spin doctors spend countless hours trying to figure out how to word the claim to get around the rules. And when they do, the FDA is impotent—but luckily the law isn't. For example, can Cocoa Krispies really "boost immunity" because it contains 25 percent of the recommended daily allowance of vitamin C? Doesn't "boost immunity" really mean "prevent infection"? This front-of-package claim occurred in 2009 in the middle of the H1N1 flu epidemic. The FDA was powerless, but the San Francisco City Attorney's office sent a cease and desist letter to David Mackay, CEO of Kellogg's, and the boxes were removed within a week. More recently, Kellogg's settled a private class action lawsuit about the front-of-package claim that Raisin Bran was "heart healthy" because it contained fiber. If it is heart healthy, doesn't that mean it can help "prevent heart disease"?

A new challenge is winding its way through the courts—what does "lightly sweetened" mean? How much sugar qualifies as "lightly"? Are Kellogg's Frosted Mini-Wheats or Frosted Flakes "lightly" sweetened, when the entire cereal is covered in frosting? And if sugar is added to water, is that enhancing the flavor of the water, or creating an entirely new taste?

But if all else fails, if you can't spin your way out of it, there's just plain snubbing the FDA altogether. One example is the flap over the term *evaporated cane juice* (ECJ). ECJ is what the industry uses to sweeten yogurt, because it's "juice" and therefore evinces a "health halo." FDA guidance sanctions ten—count 'em, ten—sweeteners (sucrose, high-fructose corn syrup, maple syrup, honey, agave, molasses, brown sugar, turbinado, muscovado, and demerara), but ECJ isn't one of them.

So, what do you get when you evaporate cane juice? You get sugar, plain and simple. The FDA has issued three separate guidances over the past decade on ceasing use of the term *ECJ* on the label, so as to not mislead the public; the most recent guidance was in 2016. Not one yogurt company has followed suit. Why does the industry flout the FDA's rules? Does the FDA have an enforcement arm? Well, yes, the Department of Justice. Do you think the DOJ would prosecute the food industry? Especially when the guy in the White House was a fast food junkie?

FDA and "Healthy"

One of the most egregious omissions of FDA guidance is to mask chronic toxicity of specific foods by allowing the food industry to lie to people about their products being "healthy." If something is healthy, doesn't that mean it prevents disease? What counts as healthy? Healthy is not a *health claim*, because there's no disease mentioned. Except what could be more of a health claim than healthy?

This is the kind of word play the industry banks on. Here's what the FDA calls "healthy" on its website: 1) is not low in total fat, but has a fat profile makeup of predominantly mono- and polyunsaturated fats; or 2) contains at least 10 percent of the Daily Value (DV) per reference amount customarily consumed (RACC) of potassium or vitamin D. In my view, no ultra-processed food can be healthy, because the (at least my) definition is *protect the liver, feed the gut.* Yet, by the criteria above, virtually any ultra-processed food that contains polyunsaturated fat, potassium, or vitamin D can be called healthy.

No label, packaging, or jingle can make an ultra-processed food healthy. Furthermore, you can't make processed food healthy by adding supplements. Conversely, Real Food, which is universally healthy, doesn't even have a label on which to make a structure-function or health claim. At the FDA, it's Alice in Wonderland, because up is down and down is up. But if the industry can claim that something is healthy, and it's not, and they know it's not; and if eating that food prevents you from choosing something that is healthy (because of share of stomach), doesn't that constitute a moral hazard? And if the federal government sanctions it, aren't they guilty of the same moral hazard?

It's not like the FDA is a monolith, either. There could be some movement on this issue in the near future, as KIND Bars have already changed what "healthy" means. Before 2015, the FDA labeled saturated fat as unhealthy, and in March 2015, the FDA sent a warning letter to KIND stating that it had mislabeled its products and misled consumers because they placed the moniker "healthy" on their bars. Because of too many almonds, they contained more than 1 gram of saturated fat per 40 grams of weight; more than 15 percent of its calories were derived from fat. In response, KIND filed a citizen's petition to the FDA to review its guidance on the question of "healthy." And they won. Saturated fat is no longer mentioned in the FDA's healthy definition. If KIND can do it, so can we.

Are any bars truly healthy? It's all relative I guess—KIND Bars have 2 grams of fiber and 5 to 12 grams added sugar, vs. CLIF Bars, which have 5 grams of fiber and 17 to 22 grams of added sugar. But it has absolutely nothing to do with almond count.

FDA and "Natural"

Another common and pernicious term is "natural." The term is highly confusing to consumers, many of whom conflate it with the word "organic," a term defined by law, while "natural" isn't. Others think it just means healthy; how could natural be bad? But then—is a Dole Fruit Bowl natural, even though it contains added ascorbic and citric acids, possibly synthetically produced? And what about foods with high-fructose corn syrup? That ingredient came from corn—which is technically "of nature"—but the finished product was made in a lab.

Refined sugar is no better. It's been acidified and bleached. But many would accept sugar as natural, despite everything we know about its effects on glycation, oxidative stress, inflammation, mitochondrial dysfunction, and insulin resistance—not to mention the gray area of "natural flavors," which usually just signifies added sugar. For example, there are 11 grams of sugar in a serving of Kashi Go Lean Crisp Toasted Berry Crumble Cereal, which claims to be naturally sweetened. However, dried cane syrup is the third ingredient (by weight), and both the cranberries and the blueberries are made with cane syrup. Is that still *natural* flavor? Natural means about as much as healthy does—nothing.

FDA and GRAS

Perhaps the worst FDA subterfuge is the Generally Recognized as Safe (GRAS) list. GRAS was developed as part of a congressional act in 1958 to streamline various food additives without specific FDA oversight. The government defines GRAS [U.S.C. 321(s)] as "generally recognized, among experts qualified by scientific training and experience to evaluate its safety, as having been adequately shown through scientific procedures (or, in the case of a substance used in food prior to January 1, 1958, through either scientific procedures or experience based on common use in food) to be safe under the conditions of its intended use." The important operative phrase here is "intended use." Intended use means a dose is assumed, including a maximum dose. As Paracelsus said in 1537, "the dose determines the poison." Nothing is safe at infinite dosage. Were the quantities of substances currently in processed food ever intended back in 1958? Even if Congress foresaw the rise of processed foods, GRAS was never meant to give the food industry free reign to add any substance in any amount to our food supply. GRAS provided a means to avoid the lengthy and expensive food additive approval process—but only for those common ingredients backed by scientific data and endorsed by qualified experts as safe. GRAS has let the food industry get away with slow murder.

And what is "intended use"? Sugar has been a condiment for at least twelve thousand years. However, prior to the eighteenth century, it was extremely rare, available only to kings and nobility, and not part of the average human diet. Its intended use was pretty paltry back then.

The invention of the pot still in the 1600s allowed for refining, and by the early nineteenth century, sugar became more available to the general populace (as did hard alcohol). Over the next 150 years, due to expansion of the baked goods, candy, and soft drink industries, sugar consumption slowly rose and finally stabilized at approximately 15 teaspoons a day. It was during this time that various forms of metabolic disease (diabetes, heart issues) became prevalent. In the 1980s, when the American Diet was revamped to reduce consumption of saturated fat, sugar (either sucrose, which is glucose-fructose bound together, or high-fructose corn syrup, which is glucose and fructose unbound) replaced the fat in processed foods due to taste and price. By 2000, sugar consumption in the US reached a median of 22 teaspoons per day; although in the last decade, reported intake dropped off about 12 percent (to 19.5 teaspoons per day), primarily as a reduction in sugar sweetened beverage (SSB) consumption. Nevertheless, consumption of added sugar by US adults remains triple over recommended limits (the WHO suggests 6 teaspoons per day—two-thirds of a can of Coca-Cola is the entire day's allotment).

Before 1997, a food company had to petition the FDA to get a substance on the GRAS list. Now it's privatized and there's no centralized list. All that's required is a meeting of scientists (paid by the company—talk about conflicts of interest) to sit in a room and declare a substance is GRAS. They don't even have to tell the FDA they did it. We know that at least three thousand items on the GRAS list have never undergone review; and it's estimated that for at least one thousand, the FDA wasn't even notified. How's that for disclosure and transparency?

Worse yet, the FDA doesn't systematically reconsider the safety of GRAS substances as new information becomes available. Even if it wanted to, it couldn't because it's been underfunded by Congress for decades. GRAS has simply become a back door for the food industry to add substances to our food supply without FDA approval.

Sugar is just one factor that drives weight gain and obesity. If other items also drive weight gain, and they are GRAS, by inference that means sugar is also GRAS. Except . . . sugar uniquely drives metabolic

disease apart from its calories. It's been known to increase serum triglyceride levels for at least forty years; yet the role of triglycerides in
heart disease always took a back seat to LDL (see Chapters 2 and
12). Recent data implicates added sugar as a cause of cardiovascular
mortality, even after controlling for total calories and obesity. Furthermore, in a recent prospective study, SSBs appear to uniquely contribute to risk for diabetes; every can of soda per day increases risk
for diabetes by 29 percent, even after controlling for total calories and
BMI. Furthermore, an econometric analysis of the Food and Agriculture Organization (FAO) statistics database (which logs food availability by country) demonstrates that for every extra 150 total calories per
person per day available within a country's border, diabetes prevalence
increased by 0.1 percent. If those 150 calories were sugar, diabetes
prevalence increased by 1.1 percent, exclusive of total calories or BMI.

Due to the increase in heart disease that's been experienced in the
US since the 1970s, there was data to support that sugar was a risk factor because it raised triglycerides. The FDA finally decided to examine
it, but the fix was in before it started. The resultant report, headed by
Dr. Walter Glinsmann (now a consultant to the Corn Refiners Association), assessed US data up to 1980 (prior to the advent of HFCS
in the diet) and was released in 1986. The average and peak doses in
the Glinsmann report were 51 (12 teaspoons) and 100 grams (23 teaspoons) per day, respectively. The data was cross-sectional from the
first National Health Examination Survey (NHES) of 1977, before the
ever-pervasiveness of HFCS. They didn't even classify fruit juice as a
source of sugar. In terms of the effects of sugar on obesity and heart disease, the results of this report were "inconclusive," meaning causation
couldn't be proved, and thus no changes were undertaken (it's important to note that diabetes wasn't assessed). If the same analysis were conducted today, it would be a slam dunk—but they haven't done it again.
I wonder why?

One way to reverse the food industry sugar glut is to remove fructose
from the GRAS list. In doing so, sugar would go from "food" to "food

additive." Fructose is an energy source, but it's not a nutrient. This will limit the amount of fructose allowed in any given processed food as well as require the food industry to list the amount and the percent contributed. The result will be the reduction of added sugar to virtually all processed foods. Such a reclassification would also increase awareness that certain substances, however sacrosanct in our culture (e.g., alcohol), may be determined to be toxic at higher doses, and also need to be reclassified, both legally and socially.

There's only one problem: while it's very easy to get a substance onto the GRAS list, it's very difficult to remove it. However, two items have been removed: nitrates and *trans*-fats. *Trans*-fats are particularly notable, because they were considered to be a standard food product as early at 1911, when Crisco was introduced into the American market. *Trans*-fat use peaked in the 1960s, along with the increase of cardiovascular disease. Then, when the saturated fat craze took hold in the 1970s, things got worse, as margarine (*trans*-fats with an emulsifier chaser—yum!) supplanted butter in the American ethos. Remember, "everything's better with Blue Bonnet on it." In 1988, the first paper linking *trans*-fats to heart disease was published, and from that time on, continued reports linked *trans*-fats to heart disease, stroke, and nonalcoholic fatty liver disease. Despite numerous calls for the removal of *trans*-fats from the American Diet, the food industry continued to protest and lobby the FDA for them to remain. In 2006, the FDA added *trans*-fats to the Nutrition Facts label, and on November 7, 2013 (twenty-five years after they were first determined to be toxic), *trans*-fats were removed from the FDA GRAS list. So it can be done.

Healthy. Natural. Generally Recognized as Safe. None of these are true. They're all spin, and inherently misleading because consumers purchase products under misconceptions about their origins, contents, and contributions to health. Plus USDA and FDA guidance on any of these issues have no teeth. When was the last time either agency prosecuted anything? Companies oppose banning the use of the word "natural" as a violation of "commercial speech." You can actually thank the Supreme Court for this hyperbole, because the rules of commercial speech allow companies to say things that are meaningless. That leaves the FDA no choice but to issue industry-wide definitions for each of these and then sit on their thumbs as they're ignored.

FDA and the Nutrition Facts Label

There's recently been a significant amount of pressure on the FDA to deal with the obesity and diabetes epidemics, and appropriately so. Unfortunately, their response has been far from appropriate. In 2015, the FDA announced there would be a new Nutrition Facts label, which would help consumers decipher what was in each package. The Trump administration killed it. There are a couple of good changes, though—for instance, the FDA proposed a separate line for "added sugar," and have de-emphasized saturated fat by withdrawing its listing on the label. However, juice—which has even more sugar per ounce than soda—doesn't technically "add" sugar, so it's still deceptive. Some companies have voluntarily elected to include the added sugar line, but the majority of industry actors haven't yet taken the plunge, although they would have to if fructose were deleted from the GRAS list.

There are plenty of bad changes, too. The FDA still hasn't woken up to the calorie conundrum and continues to highlight calories above all else; but at least now the label will tell you how many calories are in the entire package, acknowledging that the recommended serving size isn't the recognized eating size (we all know a pint of Ben and Jerry's is one serving). Furthermore, the amount of added sugar will still be listed in grams, not teaspoons, thus obfuscating its meaning for the US population.

Most important, as this whole book is about, it's not what's *in the food* that matters; it's *what's been done to the food* that counts. None of that is on the Nutrition Facts label (see Chapter 17). Oh, and by the way, alcohol is excepted—there's no Nutrition Facts label for beer, wine, or spirits, although the FDA is considering it.

FDA and Nutraceuticals

Currently, 77 percent of Americans take a dietary supplement. Among older adults that rises to 80 percent. Even one-third of children take some form of supplement—perhaps because these micronutrients are missing from food stripped during processing of the fiber fraction.

In 1994, Congress passed the Dietary Supplement Health and Education Act (DSHEA), which turned the $4 billion supplement industry with four thousand products into our current $210 billion nutraceutical industry with eighty thousand products. Are eighty thousand products actually necessary? Either you can look at this as the fountain of youth, or you can look at it as the dumbest fix to a problem that should never have even begun. The key to the passage of DSHEA was employing the threshold of structure-function claim (like food), rather than the threshold of health claim (like drugs). Drugs need testing for safety and efficacy. But, because nutraceuticals are food, there's no need for testing to prove that they're safe.

Why did this happen? The growth of the low-fat movement in the 1980s led to some ambiguous and scurrilous claims on foods and advertising. The Institute of Medicine weighed in to say that claims on foods were "at best confusing and at worst deceptive economically and potentially harmful." In 1990, against food industry lobbying, Congress passed the Nutrition Labeling and Education Act (NLEA), which as we know gave us the first Nutrition Facts label—but this did nothing to stop disingenuous advertising of food and supplements. A tandem bill, called the Nutrition Advertising Coordination Act (NACA), was supposed to do that. But this law threatened the nascent health food industry, because they couldn't back up any of their claims with facts. The supplement industry went into overdrive to win in the court of public opinion and to get Congress to retract the law.

There was only one way to stop the NACA—pass a bill to supersede it. So in 1994, DSHEA was born. Who carried the water for this on the Hill? Orrin Hatch, senator from Utah—and why? Because the dietary supplement market was for the most part based in Utah, and

Hatch's campaign was the recipient of all that lobbying cash. From 2005 through 2010, XanGo was his second biggest contributor, and Herbalife was fourth—plus Hatch's son was a lobbyist for the industry. In 1992, the Utah dietary supplement industry grossed $924 million; by 2012, it was up to $7 billion. After DSHEA, the FDA couldn't block a supplement from reaching the market; they could only take action if there were health or safety problems later.

And the problems started rolling in. For example, one supplement called OxyElite Pro caused forty-seven hospitalizations, three liver transplants, and one death—supporting my contention that the FDA doesn't actively kill people, rather they just let them die. DSHEA is also the source of what's known as the "quack Miranda warning," which absolves nutraceutical companies for any untoward effects from its products. For example, StemGenex is a clinic offering "stem-cell therapies" for conditions such as multiple sclerosis and Parkinson's disease, except they hide behind a website that states that its treatment "is not a part of FDA approved stem cell therapies and is not considered a cure for any medical condition." Do you want anything in your body that neither the USDA nor the FDA has passed judgment on?

USDA, FDA, and the Third *Immoral Hazard*

Since when has government led the public astray (before Trump)? And why? There's a long history of screwups, but usually when the screwup becomes evident, someone fixes it. The cost of inaction is greater than that of action. Nonetheless, there are a few instances where the problem went unabated, and it's instructive to understand why. Let's start with lead poisoning.

The toxicity of lead was first examined in 1892, yet it wasn't until the Lead Contamination Control Act (LCAA) of 1988 that it was removed from gasoline and paint. Why the ninety-six-year hiatus before action? Because the victims of lead poisoning were overwhelmingly people of color and poor. Let's take an even more recent example—the Flint water crisis. This wasn't government complicity, it was government duplicity—people of color and the poor again. The fact of the matter is that social disparities are a primary risk for disease. While some disparities are difficult to address and out of the government's hands, to find that the government has been willingly behind the disparity for a profit motive is truly unconscionable. Well, the USDA and FDA have fomented our current dietary crisis, which *still* disproportionately affects people of color, and they could (with an assist from Congress) help to get us out.

This is a social justice issue, and the death count is way higher than police brutality. But the government is co-opted by the profits they accrue on selling the industrial global diet to the rest of the world and by the international sale of the medicines of Big Pharma to try to assuage the guilt and the gore. There's also the money that funnels in from think tanks like the American Legislative Exchange Council, a political front group for the food and drug (and oil) industries—which pays off more than half of Congress. Taking money to keep people down—**this is the third *immoral hazard*.**

I'm Going to Kansas City, Kansas City Here I Come (or Not)

The icing on the cake of this third *immoral hazard* is that the USDA is doing everything it can to disavow its role by reducing its regulatory footprint, in order to give the food industry carte blanche. Trump Agriculture secretary Sonny Perdue moved the entire USDA brain trust from Bethesda to Kansas City to get scientists to leave the agency by attrition—specifically to lessen its regulatory authority, essentially declaring open season for the food industry to prey on the public at large. It's as simple as shooting farmed fish in a barrel.

CHAPTER 25

Real Food Is Good for the Planet

There's no getting around it. The Earth is doomed unless we change many things to save the environment. Banning plastic straws may feel good, but spitballs were never a match for a thermonuclear weapon. Climate change (e.g., wildfires and cataclysmic storms) generate the most press and angst, but our environmental nightmare also includes soil erosion, water contamination, superweeds, superbugs, and microplastics. The problems with all five can, at least in part, be traced back to our processed food supply.

To feed the country by the year 2040, we're going to need four Central Valleys of California, but we won't even have one, because of the change in temperature and the soil erosion. Some dark humor—the obesity epidemic is going to take care of itself, because the environmental result of our processed food addiction will ultimately be famine. Well, maybe that's a little too macabre—after all, this isn't a Stephen King novel, but it just might be a Jared Diamond prophecy. So, how could Real Food actually fix our planet?

110 in the Shade

Let me say at the outset that I completely agree climate is *the* issue of
the twenty-first century. Let me also say that there's no doubt that agriculture is part of the problem. However, some equate agriculture with
cows, and cows with methane, and methane with, well, farting (although
it's actually the cows burping that releases more methane). However,
pinning our problems on cow farts and burps is a bit of hyperbole because this is a symptom and not a cause of the problem. According to
the Food and Agriculture Organization (FAO), livestock—including
cows, pigs, sheep, and other animals—are responsible for about one-
seventh (14.5 percent) of global greenhouse gas (GHG) emissions. Ten
percent of that is methane production due to natural sources (e.g., de-
caying vegetation and bacteria in swamps). But human activity makes
up a whopping 75 percent.

In another study, GHGs were responsible for 9 percent of all emissions, as compared to transportation (29 percent), electricity (28 percent), industry (22 percent), and commercial/residential (12 percent).
To be sure, GHGs from agriculture could be improved. And animals
(both livestock and fish) are about half of that 9 percent.

Vegan activists want to rid the food supply of all animal-based
products. Would it work? Could it work? A recent report asked that
question. Animal-derived foods currently provide 24 percent of total calories, 48 percent of total protein, 34 to 67 percent of essential
amino acids, and 23 to 100 percent of essential fatty acids for Americans. Also, the bioavailability of iron and zinc is better from animal-
derived products. However, these are just the direct effects of animals
on our health. The USDA estimates that a plant-only dietary paradigm could produce 23 percent more food (as it could repurpose
grazing land for crop growth); but it would meet fewer of the US population's requirements for essential nutrients, making our nutritional
quality worse, particularly for the poor. Thus, removing animal
products from the human diet is a bit dicey in terms of physiology and
health.

Gaslight

But would it make a difference in terms of climate change? This is definitely a give-take proposition. There are three different greenhouse gases—methane, carbon dioxide, and nitrous oxide. All three matter, but to different degrees, as they also have different sources and causes and solutions.

Methane (CH_4) always gets the worst rap, because its heat-trapping effects are twenty-five times that of carbon dioxide, and because it's in part derived from animals. Some want the ruminants (e.g., cows, sheep, and goats) off our plates, in part because they turn the carbohydrate in grass into methane through the process of *enteric fermentation*. They burp up about 95 percent of the methane that they produce, while about 5 percent ends up in the manure. Of these ruminants, 80 percent of the methane is generated by the meat industry, while 20 percent comes from the dairy industry. In a Nebraska beef production study, methane accounted for 50 percent of ruminants' emissions (carbon dioxide and nitrous oxide being the rest), but the amount of methane created by ruminants is only 10 percent of the total GHGs that come from the entire agriculture sector. In 2014, 89 million head of cattle generated 169 billion tons of methane—equivalent to the weight of 74 Golden Gate Bridges—for an average of 1,900 kg/head. Yet in 1968, 109 million cows generated only 40 billion tons of methane, for an average of 366 kg/head. Why do they make more now? This is the crux of the issue that relates climate to processed food, because the problem isn't really the cows. It's what the humans have done to the cows.

When it comes right down to it, most methane emissions derive, either directly or indirectly, from humans. And no one is talking about getting rid of humans—we're doing that on our own. Human burping and farting itself also contributes methane to the atmosphere; not as much as cows, but ultimately for the same reason.

How many of you went to summer camp and lit farts after curfew (the adolescent in me still giggles at this)? What did you think that combustible gas was? Each human generates about a quart of gas per day.

About 10 percent is carbon dioxide, and 5 to 10 percent is methane. A sizeable proportion of the methane is manufactured by the gut bacterium *Archaea*, which, due to current food production practices, especially giving antibiotics to cows, is becoming a more frequent denizen of both the human and ruminant microbiome. Currently, human farts globally contribute about 1 teragram per year of methane. But not every human generates methane, because not everyone is populated with *Archaea*. So what determines if you are a methane producer?

While gastrointestinal diseases render you susceptible, the big determinant is whether you've been exposed to oral antibiotics. If you have ever gone on oral antibiotics, you'll have noticed that your bowel movements change. After your course is complete, you usually go back to normal. However, if you keep eating antibiotics at each meal, don't expect your gastrointestinal tract to bounce back. *Archaea* in the intestine are very hearty; they can survive virtually any antibiotic onslaught that a gastroenterologist throws at them. The rest of the microbiome dies, leaving the *Archaea* to grow, making methane, and causing metabolic problems. If you eat processed food (especially meat whose feed was laced with antibiotics), then your chances of being populated with methanogenic *Archaea* go way up. So, is it your fault if you are an *Archaea* host and a methane producer? And should we get rid of you if you are? Well, it's the same for the cows. If we stopped the antibiotics in the animal feed, their methane production would decline.

And, of course, human's industrial activity is a much bigger source of methane than our farts. Since 1750, the amount of methane in the atmosphere has doubled because of human activity. The oil and gas industry is the top contributor, creating one-third of methane emissions, leaking 60 percent more than government estimates predicted. Another source is the plastic bags formerly found in supermarkets. Polyethylene plastic bags emit methane when exposed to light, and even more when submerged in saltwater. These human sources dwarf that which the cows make. In fact, the UN International Panel on Climate Change (IPCC) argues that 5 percent of methane emissions are directly from the ruminants while 14 percent comes from the transportation of the food. Rather, the EPA adds up all the emissions involved in the life cycle of our food, and argues that the levels are 50 percent higher, due to the addition of the growing of the feed, the petroleum products involved in fertilizer development, packaging, shipping, and food distribution. In other words, it's not the animals, it's the whole processed food system. Most of these non-animal methane sources could be eliminated if we stopped feedlots, went back to locally sourced farming, and improved transport.

Carbon dioxide (CO_2) isn't nearly as bad as methane in terms of heat trapping, but there's five times as much of it. Most of agriculturally derived carbon dioxide is created during animal feed production. Yet the risks of carbon dioxide are immediately offset by the fact that it's an essential nutrient for plants; they need it for photosynthesis. We could live perfectly fine without methane, but we'd be dead without carbon dioxide. The problem isn't the carbon dioxide itself, but that there aren't enough plants to metabolize it, due to deforestation.

This is where the deforestation of the Amazon—the "lungs" of the Earth—comes into play. About 15 percent of the Amazon rain forest has already been cleared for cattle farming. But the biggest danger in Brazil is the "next big thing"—sugar farming. Because of the world's sweet tooth, the Bolsonaro government has approved 19 million hectares of Amazon rain forest to be plowed over to make way for sugar farms. People worldwide were horrified by the Amazon "burning" in 2019, which they attributed to climate change. This is untrue—the real reason was to feed our hunger for processed food.

But back on the farm is where the most egregious GHG of all is manufactured—**nitrous oxide (N_2O)**, which has three hundred times the heat-trapping capacity of carbon dioxide and twelve times the heat trapping capacity of methane. Most US livestock are fattened on fish-meal, corn, soybean meal, or other grains. So is farmed fish. To make animal/fish feed for the US, it takes 149 million acres of cropland, 167 million pounds of pesticides, and 17 billion pounds of synthetic nitrogen fertilizer (usually ammonium nitrate) to grow the feed. When you apply synthetic fertilizer to the soil, it generates big-time nitrous oxide, trapping heat, and seeping into and contaminating groundwater. And the pesticides and herbicides (like glyphosate and atrazine; see Chapter 20) that are necessary to keep the feed from succumbing to the weeds and the locusts will run off into the groundwater as well.

Once upon a time on the family farm, the feed was made on site (dried grass called hay), and cow manure was a combination fertilizer/pesticide—essentially a GHG break-even process. But now, with monoculture farming, the feed is on the factory farm in Iowa, and the manure is left on the concentrated animal feeding operation (CAFO) in Kansas (there's triple the animal manure versus human feces produced each day in the US). Furthermore, on the CAFO, the manure isn't repurposed as fertilizer. Instead it decomposes into methane and other pollutants— including nitrogen, phosphorus, antibiotics, and metals—which leech into groundwater when manure storage facilities inevitably leak.

Cowspiracy

According to the Environmental Working Group, 90 percent of beef's emissions, 69 percent of pork's, 72 percent of farmed salmon's, and 68 percent of farmed tuna's emissions are generated in the production phase, meaning before the animal leaves the farm. In the case of beef and dairy, this is due to the high methane (CH_4) emissions from the ruminants' digestion and manure, as well as the nitrous oxide generated from growing feed. For farmed salmon and for chickens, the emissions in the production phase come from manufacturing the feed.

But wait, it gets even more complicated. It's not just animal feed; it's what kind of feed. Here are two different scenarios to consider:

1. Cattle on the CAFOs are stationary, eat corn, and belch a little less methane (because corn means less roughage than grass)—but the farm in Iowa that grew the corn needed pesticides and synthetic fertilizer, spreading a lot more nitrous oxide. On top of that, the cows get excess omega-6s and branched-chain amino acids to make a fatty, marbled American steak. It's cheap and tasty, but will also contribute to human metabolic

syndrome. The advantage is that grazing land isn't a requirement—that's why CAFOs were invented in the first place.

2. Cattle on the rural farm graze, eat grass, and belch methane—but their manure is the fertilizer. The cows get the right amount of omega-3s, omega-6s, and branched-chain amino acids to make a pink, homogeneous low-fat Argentinean steak (see **Fig. 18–1**), which is more expensive to raise and purchase, but won't contribute to human metabolic syndrome. It's even better if they're munching on legumes like alfalfa and clover. But again, making grazing land available would be the key issue. Cows that graze on pastures with legumes belch 21 percent less methane—and their manure will fix nitrogen in the ground. There will be some nitrous oxide, but way less than with synthetic fertilizer. The problem here is the space needed for grazing.

All agriculture and food policy experts decry the current CAFO-monoculture model, because it switches out animal manure (which fixes nitrogen in the ground) for synthetic nitrogen fertilizer (which ends up in water runoff and generates nitrous oxide).

Our current mode of divided monoculture farming creates climate change. And yes, it's all in the service of feeding livestock in CAFOs, especially ruminants, to make meat cheap. It's not the animal as much as it is the type of feed, the need for fertilizer, the antibiotics, plus the availability of grazing land, and the by-products of transportation. That being said, it's not like plants are GHG-free. They're just like animal feed—without manure, they need synthetic fertilizer. Therefore, even though they don't make carbon dioxide or methane, producing synthetic fertilizer generates a whole lot of nitrous oxide.

Furthermore, plants themselves aren't emission-free; they're just generated after the crops leave the farm (processing, transport, cooking, and waste disposal). Post-farm emissions account for 65 percent of dry beans' and 59 percent of lentils' total emissions, primarily because of the heat energy needed to cook them. Ninety percent of potato emissions occur after the crop leaves the farm, leaving 10 percent due to the synthetic fertilizer. Bottom line, Real Food means less GHGs from both animals and plants, because it means less fertilizer, better manure management, shorter transport, and perhaps less waste.

The Shape of Water

All that pesticide and fertilizer ends up in the groundwater, which the EPA tracks—you can see by satellite the toxic plume from Iowa to the Missouri River, to the Mississippi River, and all the way to the Gulf of Mexico, where there is a dead zone due to the nitrogen runoff. In many countries, agriculture is the leading cause of *eutrophication* (nutrient pollution of waterways), and it's expected to worsen as the global population increases and the demand for food grows.

Nitrogen in solid form (e.g., manure) grows crops, while nitrogen in liquid form kills freshwater and coastal ecosystems. Fertilizers and manure from agricultural fields, as well as sewage and runoff from our urban centers, are increasingly polluting our waterways. Too many nutrients in the water can fuel large algae blooms, including toxic algae. The algae can smother the coral reefs and sea grasses, kill fish, and shift aquatic ecosystems. Then, when these toxic algae blooms die, they suck oxygen out of the water. Under the right conditions, these die-offs create hypoxic areas or dead zones, areas where fish and other aquatic creatures can't survive.

Globally, eutrophication of coastal systems has risen from fewer than seventy-five systems in 1960 to more than eight hundred today. Eutrophication can also render freshwater sources unfit to drink. The Environmental Working Group estimates that the US already spends $4.8 billion per year to treat drinking water contaminated by nitrogen fertilizer, while additional treatment for drinking water affected by toxic algae blooms costs between $12 million and $66 million for a town of one hundred thousand people. Synthetic fertilizer can't be completely banned, but restoring local regenerative farming practices to produce Real Food could go a long way to reduce our dependence on it.

Phosphorus is another fertilizer component, but is particularly notable around sugar plantations, as it increases yield of sugar cane. The phosphorus runoff from the Fanjul brothers' U.S. Sugar and Florida Crystals plantations at Lake Okeechobee, as well as other ranches and dairy farms, is responsible for both toxic algae blooms and the loss of large amounts of wetlands in the Everglades. During 2018's severe flooding in Florida, state planners had to release the locks on Lake Okeechobee; the runoff spilled along the Gulf Coast, where it destroyed the coastal ecosystem.

Shadowlands

There's a big difference between soil and dirt. Soil has carbon, nitrogen, and bacteria. Dirt, on the other hand, is just dirt. It's dead. There's only so much carbon, nitrogen, and bacteria in the ground, and we have to replenish it or we get dirt. More people means more extrication of those elements.

As intensive agriculture came into being in the twentieth century, it allowed the world's population to increase from 1.9 billion to 7.7 billion. Thus, a premium is placed not only on housing all those people but also feeding them—in the cheapest and most profitable way possible. As stated earlier, nineteen million hectares of Amazon jungle are to be cleared to make way for sugarcane planting. This will have disastrous consequences for the Amazon ecosystem to be sure, but also for carbon dioxide recoupment—driving even more global warming.

Monoculture crop planting, like what has occurred in both Iowa and the Amazon, has taken its toll on land use, with increased soil erosion and reduced amounts of organic material in the ground. An estimated five to six million hectares of cropland is lost annually due to severe soil erosion and degradation. Unlike dirt, soil is a living, dynamic resource, made up of different sized mineral particles (sand, silt, and clay), organic matter, and a diverse community of living organisms. Different soil types display different properties, including vulnerability to erosion, salinity, acidity, and alkalinity. Sugar crops uniquely contribute to soil degradation (by increased rates of erosion and soil removal at harvest) and reduced soil quality. Erosion is a significant issue in areas planted with sugarcane or beets, particularly in tropical areas (where most cane is grown), since the tropics erode faster than soil is formed. Soil erosion is also influenced by a range of factors including rainfall and irrigation, wind, temperature, soil type, and topography. Couple this with the loss of coastline from rising oceans, and you'll come to see that sugar and corn may not be the only culprits, but they are definitely the top two.

Amazingly, there is an easy fix to all this. There are eleven million unplanted acres in the state of Michigan alone that could be made arable, and food could be produced there with a simple technology: a big white fabric tent to allow sun rays to penetrate and warm the soil. You can grow green vegetables almost anywhere—and it's Real Food. And you can turn dirt back into soil. It's called regenerative farming. You just need a cow.

Weeds—Dude, Have You Got Any?

Similar to the indiscriminate use of antibiotics, the excessive and widespread use of glyphosate and atrazine in fields planted in monoculture (and therefore without the natural pesticide of manure) over the past four decades has led to the development of resistance to these herbicides, and the rise of "superweeds." Superweeds can't be exterminated through standard chemical methods, and almost 50 percent of farms surveyed have exhibited infestation, which is only likely to worsen each successive year. Soon it won't matter that the crops are Roundup Ready—because we'll either need to find the next best herbicide, or the superweeds will have crowded out the crops. We'll be selling the weeds for food instead!

Garbage Warrior

Plastic was an environmental problem even before processed food, but soda was the reason for the two-liter plastic bottle. Processed food notoriously uses a lot of plastic. Containers and packaging alone contribute over 23 percent of the material reaching landfills in the US, and some of these discarded materials are food-related containers and packaging. Tons of that plastic ends up in the ocean, and some of it even ends up in the snow of the Arctic.

Food comprised 22 percent of all waste in 2019, and over forty million tons reached landfills in the US—equivalent to half a pound per person per day. That's enough food waste to fill the Rose Bowl every day. Worse yet, the EPA argues that 23 percent of the methane emissions come from solid waste—and that's not just the meat. The bacteria chomping on rotting food waste will make methane just as easily as a cow's stomach.

Have you ever noticed that gummy bears don't go rancid? Why do you think that is? Food waste is primarily Real Food. And that's the point. It becomes food waste because it *can* go rancid. That means the bacteria can metabolize it. Well, our mitochondria are refurbished bacteria, and that means that we can metabolize it, too. That's a whole lot better than eating it and not being able to metabolize it—like what happens with *trans*-fats (see Chapter 20)—as mitochondrial dysfunction is a primary cause of NCDs.

Sustainable Nation

Between soil erosion, waste, water contamination, pollution, and GHGs, the industrial processed food system is wreaking havoc on ecosystems all over the globe. Monoculture means fossil fuels, nitrogen contamination, and dead zones. Antibiotics and pesticides mean superweeds and superbugs. Plastics mean pollution and more GHGs. And there's no EPA-sponsored superfund cleanup for any of these, because after all, it's food, right?

In the fifty years since President Richard Nixon told his agriculture secretary Earl Butz to "make food cheap," through political and economic and technological efforts, American agriculture has produced lower market prices for commodity crops like corn, wheat, and soybeans, all driving NCDs. Yes, we got cheap food, but we also got expensive and ineffective Modern Medicine that's breaking the bank on healthcare.

In the Introduction, I argued that you can't fix healthcare until you fix health, you can't fix health until you fix diet, and you can't fix diet until you know what the hell is wrong. These same cheap food policies have now brought us environmental changes that are breaking the planet. Health and sustainability don't exist in a vacuum. They are inextricably related through the food. And, as it turns out, so is the economics.

===

CHAPTER 26

Real Food Is Good for the Wallet

Countries are in the throes of economic crisis for many reasons, not least of which is rising healthcare costs. Governments are trying to figure out how to stem the tide in the cheapest way possible. But no one wants to revamp the food supply because they'd then have to retool the system and the model. They want a quick fix to a systemic problem.

Show Me the Money

In August 2015, I traveled with a team of academics from UCSF and UC Berkeley to Mexico City, where we engaged in a discussion with the Enrique Peña Nieto government to study the health and economic aftermath of their recently enacted 1-peso-per-liter soda tax. We were ushered into a conference room at the President's Palace, where we met behind closed doors with twenty ministers representing Social Security, Labor, Health, Education, the Instituto Nacional de Salud Pública (Public Health Institute), and last but not least, Hacienda—their Treasury minister. The first thing the deputy minister of the Treasury said to us was, "We don't care about how many lives the soda tax saves. It's about the money. Show us how much money we save."

Indeed, governments often don't care about lives—until Election Day, of course. Then they'll say anything to get your vote. The quantitation of lives saved and diseases saved is already clear and unassailable. But lives are not factored into those costs, even though they should be, because productive, healthy individuals pay taxes, while sick, infirm individuals extract money from government health programs like Medicaid and Social Security. Such savings are only evinced long-term, after the administration in question is out of office and will get no credit. It's all about the short-term balance sheet and immediate political capital.

I heard the deputy minister loud and clear—it's only about the money. So let's look at the US numbers. The entire food industry (grocery and restaurant) grosses $1.46 trillion per year with a profit of $657 billion, to yield a gross profit margin of 45 percent. Yet US medical costs total $3.5 trillion per year, of which 75 percent are food-related chronic disease. Of that $2.67 trillion, 75 percent or $1.9 trillion is conceivably preventable if we could roll back rates of disease to 1970 levels, before metabolic syndrome took hold.

Conversely, the pharma industry generates $771 billion in gross revenue annually, of which 21 percent is gross profit. One company made $19 billion in annual profit from diabetes drugs alone. Big Food is even bigger and badder—and with an even larger clientele.

You do the math: between food and pharma, you've got $2.1 trillion per year going down a rathole—into shareholder pockets—while the public gets sicker and healthcare is collapsing. We lose triple what the food industry makes cleaning up their mess. This is unsustainable. We could slash disease rates and medical costs and even budget deficits just by reducing the consumption of processed food. And don't even think of listening to pharma's promises—there's no drug for this, because those eight subcellular pathologies are not druggable.

How about the nutraceutical market? That's a $210 billion business. Some people have to take dietary supplements—they've got a bona fide eating disorder, a gastrointestinal malabsorption problem, or they're taking medications that either inactivate or waste those micronutrients. I'm not going to diss the entire nutraceutical market, as it serves a valid purpose, because many of us need micronutrients that aren't in abundance in the Western diet to help prevent those eight subcellular pathologies. But if you don't have one of these preexisting conditions or an eating disorder, then the only reason you need a dietary supplement is that you're not getting the micronutrients you need from your food. This only happens if you're eating processed food, in which the vitamins, minerals, micronutrients, and especially the fiber have been stripped out. Yes, some processed food is fortified to try to make up the difference (for instance, adding folic acid to bread to prevent neural tube defects), but even these foods are a far cry from having an adequate diet to support metabolic health. Therefore, the cost of adding an inadequate antidote to the poison adds $210 billion to our debt sheet; so now we're at $2.3 trillion.

What about the energy sector? Aside from the money spent cleaning up the climate change problems that it creates, does food processing produce or suck energy? Nitrogen fertilizer production uses large amounts of natural gas and some coal, and can account for more than 50 percent of total energy use in commercial agriculture. Oil accounts for between 30 percent and 75 percent of energy inputs, depending on the cropping system. It appears that nonorganic farming uses at least 10 percent more energy than organic, and as the cost of crude oil goes up, more money is wasted. Turning corn into ethanol doesn't result in any energy yield, and may end up costing more money than it saves; the real reason ethanol exists is to create more demand for corn and support price hikes.

OK, so does food processing produce or suck water? There's no question that water use is way higher for processed food; just ask developing countries about how their water systems are diverted to manufacture Coca-Cola. And, of course, the nitrogen runoff contaminates water tables worldwide and makes the water unfit to drink. All of these increase inherent costs.

And, finally, let's have a look at the real estate market. There's $26 billion in reduced property values from water contamination, and a loss of $4.1 billion in soil and groundwater contamination from animal manure leakage. That $30 billion is chicken feed compared to the costs of healthcare. But still, no one wants to live near a factory farm or a concentrated animal feeding operation (CAFO), because it stinks to high hell. The chance for contamination of the water supply due to a flood is imminent, as was seen in North Carolina after Hurricane Florence.

Food and Farm—Two Four-Letter Words Beginning with "F"

Bottom line: there's no sector that escapes unscathed from the scourge of processed food—except for the food and drug industries. Big Food escapes, not because of its own practices, but because of the food subsidies embedded within the annual $173.4 billion Farm Bill. Rural representatives vote for the SNAP program, only if urban representatives vote for crop insurance (8 percent of the Farm Bill) and commodity subsidy programs (5 percent of the Farm Bill). The last is soil conservation (6 percent), which isn't very controversial.

Farming (at least in a market economy) approaches perfect competition. Therefore, winners in the farm sector are those enterprises that are the least-cost producers, regardless of the commodity—and that means industrial agriculture. There's no incentive for quality, just quantity. The cost of a basket of commodities will most likely be cheaper in the future (after inflation) than it is today. Furthermore, low-cost production will benefit any enterprise that's downstream of the resultant commodity (i.e., the processed food industry). There's no easy way to stop food processors from having access to cheap inputs, unless you differentially subsidize by stopping the commodification of crops. Some people think this is impossible, and any such cure (think Soviet Union, Venezuela) would likely be worse than the disease. But we really have no other choice.

Fig. 26-1 explains the political problem in simple terms. The state of Iowa accounts for 0.95 percent of the US population, and two-thirds

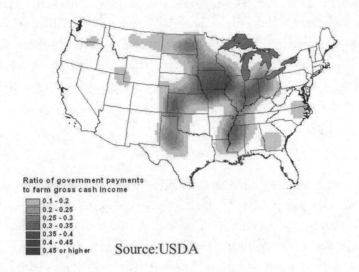

Ratio of government payments
to farm gross cash income

	0.1 - 0.2
	0.2 - 0.25
	0.25 - 0.3
	0.3 - 0.35
	0.35 - 0.4
	0.4 - 0.45
	0.45 or higher

Source: USDA

Figure 26–1: Ratio of US government payments to farm gross income, 2007. Iowa receives the lion's share of government subsidies, produces corn but receives little revenue for it, and Iowans have more than double the representation in the U.S. Senate based on state population.

of Iowans farm, have farmed, or have relatives who farm. However, they send 2 percent of the senators to Washington and those senators make sure that Iowans are taken care of. The figure depicts the ratio of government payments to farm gross income. Clearly, it's not about the money; it's about the votes. When there are more votes than dollars, that's when things will change.

Pharma—Doesn't Start with an "F," but Might as Well

Big Pharma, well, they've got more and sicker patients who are prescribed their medicines by doctors, so they're making out like bandits. Even Obamacare couldn't stop the party—all it did was cap insurance company profits at 15 percent, not pharmaceutical company profits, which can be any amount, whatever the market will bear. For diabetes drugs, a 1,000 percent increase in price over twenty years generates a

pretty hefty profit. Indeed, the two sectors who win this game are two
of the three that are guilty of the *immoral hazards* outlined in this book.

And government? Well, it's fronting the costs of both of these
debacles—but doesn't realize they're inexorably linked, so it continues
to apportion the benefits to the industry and the costs to the public
into two different buckets.

Rock the Boat, Baby

In May 2011, I shared the dais at a Culinary Institute of America meeting with Sam Kass, Michelle Obama's personal chef and her point person for her Childhood Obesity Task Force. I got twenty minutes in the
Green Room alone with him, and he admitted to me that everyone in
the White House, including the president, had read the April 2011 *New
York Times* Magazine article "Is Sugar Toxic?", in which our UCSF
research was featured. They wished me well—but they would do absolutely nothing to help. No endorsement, mention, not even a wink or
a nod. They didn't want the fight with the food industry; the Obama
administration had enough enemies. Don't rock the boat.

Well, sometimes you have to rock the boat to turn it around. This
fight is long overdue. Blaming the victim hasn't worked. Magical thinking hasn't worked. It's time for something that does. In the next chapter, I offer you a veritable smorgasbord of policy principles designed
to foment food system change, all of which are tried and tested in the
field. I'll explain what works and what doesn't, based on the science.
Then you get to choose.

———

CHAPTER 27

Un-processing Our Food Supply

How do you change behavior? For UK Prime Minister Boris Johnson, self-avowed libertarian who in 2018 called the UK soda tax "a continuing creep of the Nanny State," it took landing in an ICU due to COVID-19 compounded by his obesity. Now he's spent $13 million on an educational campaign to reduce obesity nationwide. Will it work? Don't bet on it, because none of the measures actually change the food.

So how do you truly change a whole country's behavior? Or a whole world's? In the US we reduced smoking and drunk driving. Could we reduce processed food and sugar consumption in favor of Real Food consumption? Well, we don't have to smoke, and we don't have to drink alcohol. But we do have to eat. Still, there are lessons to be learned from tobacco and alcohol control. There are two general strategies: *personal intervention* (i.e., rehab), and *societal intervention* (i.e., laws). They're both important, but neither works without the other.

What Doesn't Work—Education Alone

One the most important things we've learned from tobacco and alcohol policy research is that public education, despite being the most popular and necessary component of prevention, doesn't work alone. Evidence from the US suggests that government labels warning consumers about the health effects of excessive drinking have no effect on alcohol consumption, but might have limited effect on risky drinking patterns, such as drunk driving.

How about those unsettling pictures of people with tracheotomies on packs of cigarettes? Barely touched the problem. The most popular approaches—school-based health education, public information campaigns, product labeling, and government guidelines—have very little evidence supporting their efficacy in isolation. Finally, as has been shown in the field of alcohol, the record of long-term successes in obesity prevention also leaves little cause for optimism.

Education *alone* hasn't solved any substance abuse. It didn't solve alcohol and it didn't solve tobacco. It didn't solve heroin or crystal meth or cocaine. And it's not going to solve sugar. A "Just Say No" campaign targeting the other kind of Coke would be just as ineffective by itself. Indeed, that's the definition of *abused*—you can know that a substance is hurting your life, health, family, your pocket, but you're powerless to do anything about it. The biochemical drive of wanting, needing, and proclivity to abuse is just too great.

Nonetheless, education is the cornerstone of successful intervention—it just doesn't work alone. Rather, it softens the playing field, so that societal policy interventions can become acceptable and take hold.

What Does Work—the *Iron Law*

Remember, we're dealing with an inherently addictive compound in sugar, and it's been infused into the majority of processed foods (see

Chapter 21). Caffeine is also addictive and added to individual food-stuffs such as SSBs, while other hedonic substances have it naturally (e.g., chocolate, coffee). Those foods with sugar and/or caffeine are also price-inelastic, because people will still buy them even when the cost goes up, precisely because they're addicted.

We must take a look at what works to reduce the consumption of addictive substances. Research on alcohol policy demonstrates that regulatory controls on pricing, marketing, and distribution are highly effective worldwide in reducing the negative impacts of consumption. This strategy has also been effective with tobacco—not perfect, but clearly better. Fewer cases of lung cancer and emphysema. All of these policies build upon the premise of the *Iron Law of Public Health*, which clearly states: *reducing availability reduces consumption, which reduces health harms*. If you make bad stuff (like processed food) harder to get, people won't get sick in the first place.

There are three ways to reduce availability: pricing strategies (e.g., taxation), restriction of access (e.g., blue laws), and interdiction (e.g., banning). No one thinks interdiction is a good idea—can you imagine ice cream speakeasies? We tried prohibition with the Eighteenth Amendment; the Twenty-first Amendment is a testament to how well that strategy worked. But the other two—pricing and restriction of access—are very real, very deployable, and have proven very effective.

One assumption of the *Iron Law* is that decline in consumption is a good thing. And for morally or metabolically hazardous products and behaviors, decline in consumption is generally good for society, and ultimately good for the individual—only the individual likely won't see it that way. And the investor certainly won't. In 2017, the FDA announced it would require cigarette makers to reduce nicotine levels in cigarettes sold in the US. Upon release of this news, the stock price of all major tobacco companies tanked. Why? Doesn't reduced nicotine in cigarettes mean that they are less dangerous? Maybe more people would want to try them?

The Original Sin Tax

As we explored above, hedonic substances are uniformly price-inelastic (see Chapter 21). Caffeine may be addictive, but it's not under threat of regulation because it's not toxic. In fact, it increases the positive side of the ledger (e.g., productivity, GDP), and doesn't affect the negative side (e.g., disability, medical costs). Indeed, when hedonic substances don't exact a cost to society, we let the market do its job. The public health criteria for regulation of a substance are:

1. **Ubiquity.** Sugar has been added to virtually every processed food, limiting consumer choice. Evolutionarily, sugar as fruit was available to our ancestors for only one month a year (harvest time) or as honey, which was guarded by bees. Nature made sugar hard to get, while man made it easy (see Chapter 20). Now it's in everything that we eat.

2. **Toxicity.** Every country consuming the Western diet has increased its prevalence of NCDs, and sugar is the driver. Fructose increases liver fat, drives the glycation reaction, and inhibits mitochondrial function, all of which underlie NCDs (see Chapters 7 and 8).

3. **Abuse.** Sugar is clearly abused, because it's addictive in a percentage of the population. Like tobacco and alcohol, it acts on the reward center to encourage subsequent intake. It also meets the criteria for tolerance and dependence (see Chapter 21).

4. **Externalities.** Your consumption affects me, therefore I get to say something about it (see Chapter 23).

If a substance meets these four criteria, the *Iron Law* should kick in. That means the local, state, and federal government have to participate (hence the Bureau of Alcohol, Tobacco, Firearms and Explosives). So far, there's been no such movement on processed food, because there's too much money involved—except more money is wasted than generated. Which is why we're in this ridiculous mess.

The prevalence of cigarette smoking in the US reduced from 24 percent in the Clinton era to 15 percent in the Obama era, and cigarette consumption reduced by 37 percent in those same twenty years. Yet tobacco company revenues increased by 32 percent, and stock prices increased commensurately, because there will always be addicted hardcore customers, and investors know that hedonic substances sell. Addictive substances follow their own economic precepts.

Sin Taxes Aren't about Sins, They're about Dopamine

Which addictive substance is the cheapest to produce and procure, yet the most expensive burden to society? Nicotine used to be the cheapest. At its worst, lung cancer claimed 443,000 people a year and cost healthcare $14 billion annually. But it also made the US government lots of money, because the median smoker died at age sixty-four, before they started collecting Social Security and Medicare.

Even after the removal of ads from television, Big Tobacco still scored big; cigarette taxes netted $12.5 billion for the government. Even after we learned nicotine was addictive, tobacco consumption didn't appreciably change. It was only after the Master Settlement Agreement in 1996 that regulation of tobacco was taken seriously, and consumption started to decline; yet, despite all the data and warnings, the US government continues to subsidize tobacco farming.

How about alcohol? Each year, alcohol causes ten thousand deaths from drunk driving and twenty-five thousand deaths from cirrhosis and other diseases, and underlies many other disorders—costing the medical system $100 billion annually. But it generates $5.6 billion per year for state and local governments in taxes. No one wants to turn off that spigot (except when you realize the Feds cough up 62 percent of the costs of healthcare).

Sin taxes have been around for about as long as there's been sin. And they work. Society accepts them because they affect only people who use those products. In fact, when individual states run a deficit, a sin tax is often the first tax to which lawmakers turn to help them fill the budget gap.

The question is, what's the real goal? Making money for the state? Or reduction in consumption? Because if you reduce consumption, you limit revenue generation. And it's been shown that for a sin tax to work, it has to hurt.

By far and away, the most expensive burden to society is sugar. Soft drinks are the consumable with the second lowest price elasticity, just up from fast food. Raise the price 10 percent (e.g., with taxes), and consumption drops 7.6 percent, mostly among the poor, as we saw in Mexico. But an Oxford group modeled that a soda tax would have to be at least 20 percent to significantly reduce general consumption. Chronic metabolic disease (type 2 diabetes, cardiovascular disease, fatty liver disease, chronic renal failure) currently accounts for 75 percent of all healthcare costs ($3.5 trillion); and 75 percent of that is preventable, caused by our sugar overconsumption (yes, you read that right). Sugar and processed food wastes $1.9 trillion in healthcare spending, drives diabetes, dialysis, and disability, and knocks people off over a forty-year period, thus reducing economic productivity and driving our Social Security trust fund to depletion.

Defizzing the Soda Stream

Despite concerted efforts by the beverage industry to the contrary, soda taxes are now a fact of life in many countries. In fact, twenty-eight countries around the world have passed some form of sugar taxation—the most notable in the UK. Even the tax-cutting prime minister David Cameron proposed it, and the Tory Party bought into it because it raised money for the NHS. However, Boris Johnson is now eschewing that same soda tax—not because of Brexit (for which the soda tax would help offset governmental losses), but because Tate & Lyle (a UK sugar company) sponsored the UK Conservative Party Conference. Once again—money, power, politics.

In the US, the sugar tariff is the second oldest piece of legislation, dating back to 1790, yet the US government continues to quota its production and props up the industry in return. Why? Population-wide sugar reduction would prevent premature death, save economies billions, and improve quality of life for millions across the globe. I worked with UCSF health economist Jim Kahn, who used advanced Markov modeling (a method for projecting into the future) to quantitate this, using nonalcoholic fatty liver disease because it's the "new" phenomenon attributable to processed food. If we removed 20 percent of sugar from the average American Diet, data showed we could reduce obesity, type 2 diabetes, heart disease, death rates, and medical expenditures within three years, saving $10 billion annually in healthcare costs. A 50 percent reduction could save $31.8 billion.

On the productivity side, Morgan Stanley modeled US economic growth rates from 2015 through 2035 in low-sugar and high-sugar simulations. If the US reduced its sugar consumption, economic growth would be maintained at 2.9 percent, while if we maintained our Krispy Kreme high-sugar craze, economic growth would slowly decline to 0.0 percent. However, to reduce consumption, the tax would have to be high enough to hurt.

The problem with the soda tax is that it's really three taxes in one:

1. There are federally mandated market controls on sugar production, which involve tariff-rate quotas limiting the amount of sugar that can be imported. There are also domestic product quotas, and a federal price support program extending loans to sugar processors who pay growers a minimum price. The net result of this prop-up is that US taxpayers pay billions more for sugar than they should. A tax accomplishes the same thing; it's just that the revenue goes to the government and not the sugar growers. Even Senator Ted Cruz in the 2016 presidential primary thought we needed to end this practice.

2. The cost of chronic disease is built into healthcare. We don't call that a tax; instead we call it a premium. If your employer pays for a blue-chip

health plan, then you get a lower salary—and if your employer doesn't, then you pay it instead.

3.   Soda is a tax in itself. It seems pretty ridiculous for states to tax something that's already being propped up with federal dollars. Robbing Peter to pay Paul? Why not remove all the food quotas (both production and import quotas) and all the associated taxes? Which really means, why not remove all the food market controls and subsidies on other foods? Let the market work as intended.

A Corny Issue

The same is true for corn, which is highly subsidized. Forty percent of the corn crop is converted to ethanol to extend gasoline, yet this doesn't result in any energy yield, and may end up costing more money than it saves. The real reason ethanol in gasoline exists is to create more demand for corn and support price hikes. Of the rest of the corn crop, 36 percent goes to feeding domestic cows, chicken, and pigs (increasing their branched-chain amino acid consumption and therefore their metabolic syndrome that then requires antibiotics). The last 10 percent is exported.

Bottom line is that right now, only 17 percent of the corn grown in this country is for human consumption, and most of that goes into HFCS. So why are we subsidizing it? So you can afford a corn dog at the state fair? So you can have corn on the cob on July 4? Unfortunately, the use of corn for ethanol and HFCS is so ingrained in the economic fabric that if the subsidy were abruptly eliminated, the price of corn would increase markedly, which could precipitate another Tractor March on Washington like that of the early 1980s. Corn and ethanol subsidies do need to be phased out, but slowly to avoid agricultural collapse.

Subtract the Subsidies

The bigger question is, why do we have food subsidies in the first place? Agricultural subsidies are payments and other kinds of support extended by the US federal government to certain farmers and agri-businesses. While some people consider subsidies vital to farmers and the economy, others consider them a form of corporate welfare. They're essentially a holdover from the original Farm Bill of 1933, when it was necessary to provide cheap food to a destitute population across the country—and the way to make it cheap and transportable was to process it. As a result, we bolstered the commodities market of the US, which up to that time was heavily dependent on cotton.

Storable food is also a commodity. Back in 1930, nearly 25 percent of the population, or thirty million people, lived on 6.5 million farms, and they had considerable clout in Washington. Today three million people live on 2.1 million farms. Seven states are awarded 45 percent of the subsidies: Texas 9.6 percent, Iowa 8.4 percent, Illinois 6.9 percent, Minnesota 5.8 percent, Nebraska 5.7 percent, Kansas 5.5 percent, North Dakota 5.3 percent. These are also the states that are the largest producers of corn, soybeans, wheat, and rice, which are the basics for processed food production. While humans don't eat the vast majority of the corn and soybeans directly, we do ingest branched-chain amino acids, high-fructose corn syrup, and omega-6 fatty acids laden in processed food, and get sick doing it.

While the Farm Bill was supposed to preserve the family farm, it was no match for the inevitable wave of technology, which killed it off anyway. Today, the largest 15 percent of farm businesses (also the most technologically advanced) receive 85 percent of the subsidies. Small commodity farmers qualify for a pittance, while producers of meat, fruits, and vegetables are left holding the bag. A 2017 USDA report states that only 14.6 percent of the money spent on food goes to the farmers, the sixth straight year farmers have earned a smaller share of domestic food spending. Conversely, 85 percent is for everything else (e.g., labor, packaging, transportation, advertising). For example, a loaf of bread that sells for $2.55 required $0.16 of commodities to produce it, or 6.3 percent of the loaf's retail value, while the farmer made $0.004 of profit, 0.15 percent of the loaf's retail value. That's because the subsidies aren't for the farmers, they're for the processed food producers. Subsidies are the anchor that weighs food progress down.

Subsidies took hold because they inflated land prices in rural America; but this is now hurting, as land prices are too expensive, and is one reason to rethink them. Despite more money in the Farm Bill than ever before, the net farm income between 2009 and 2018 dropped by $4.3 billion or 6.7 percent. Now the commodities farmers are even more adamant about maintaining these subsidies. Once you give out government goodies, taking them away is like taking a toy from a baby, even when it's not placating them.

Bottom line is that there's no economist on the planet who believes in food subsidies, because they distort the market. They make the wrong stuff available while making the right stuff harder to afford. As long as commodities are cheap, Real Food will stay out of reach for much of the population.

Furthermore, the American commodities market is rife with hedonic substances. In fact, numbers one (crude oil), two (coffee), four (sugar), five (cocoa), and eight (corn, which is turned into alcohol) are all hedonic. It drives our economy. Today, we tax cigarettes and alcohol, but the US government still subsidizes tobacco production. We toy with a carbon tax. And now six cities have soda taxes, on an item for which the government exerts price controls. How about just ending the food subsidies, quotas, and price controls? People say that the price of food would go up, but the Giannini group at UC Berkeley modeled what food would actually cost, and the only two items that would increase in price are sugar and corn. Not surprisingly, these are two of the major industries fighting to maintain the status quo.

Still, people will argue, the overall price of food will go up. Well maybe it should, at least a little. Out of all the countries, the US spends the least percent of GDP on food at 7 percent—that's because all the food is commodity crop-based and processed. The next two smallest spenders are the UK at 9 percent and Australia at 11 percent. All three of us are the sickest nations.

Real Food costs more than processed food—usually double—so

they're selling cheap food that's subsidized and making an enormous profit on it. The annual profit margin of the food industry prior to 1970 was 1 percent. Well, the population increased annually by 1 percent. In other words, they made money by selling the same per capita amount of food to more people.

Since 1980, the annual profit margin of the food industry has been 5 percent. Yet the rate increase in annual population has reduced to 0.7 percent. Their rate of revenue increase has gone up despite the rate of population decrease. These are the economic benefits you can achieve when you add addictive substances to food.

Once upon a time at least one soft drink manufacturer added cocaine to its product. Now they just put in sugar and caffeine—still, people are hooked.

Workplace Bans

The workplace presents an educational moment and venue. This is especially true when the education matches up with its mission. For instance, where were cigarettes first banned? Medical centers. Hospitals and hospital employees are supposed to model good health practices for the general public. So, what does it say to the public that 28 percent of all children's hospitals have a fast food venue in their lobby?

At UCSF, we asked the same question, and decided to put up or shut up. From 2013 to 2015, the UCSF Wellness Committee slowly twisted arms around campus to push for a workplace ban on sugared beverages. As a result, all sugared beverages—soda and flavored coffee drinks alike—were banned from sale in the cafeterias, vanished from patients' meal trays, and disappeared from the menus of any outside vendors. According to policy, if an employee wants to drink a soda, they can bring it from home (though diet soda and juice are still available; baby steps . . .).

Obviously, we were interested in the aftermath, so we studied a subgroup of 214 employees who regularly drank sugar sweetened beverages (SSBs) before and one year after the ban was put in place. They reported a daily intake of 35 ounces of SSBs at baseline and 18 ounces at follow-up—a 17-ounce decrease, a cut by almost half. Furthermore, reduction in sugared beverage intake correlated with improvements in waist circumference, insulin sensitivity, and a pattern of reduction in blood lipids. Oh—and no one complained. Seriously. But what about revenues? The UCSF cafeteria just sold more water—there was no decline.

At the societal level, private sector–driven change through workplace bans solves a lot of political obstacles that governmental reform can't. Of course, there are issues of contractual arrangements and so-called pouring rights contracts that require decisions regarding on-campus marketing, promotion, and sales. Some employers may face challenges in implementing a workplace culture where SSB sales bans are perceived as paternalistic. Nevertheless, this proves the *Iron Law of Public Health* is indeed a *law*. Reducing availability reduces consumption, which reduces health harms. Period. We can fix this if we want to.

A Uniquely UK Proposal

In the US, at least one presidential candidate campaigned on a platform of a universal basic income. The catch is that this is where socialism meets libertarianism. After all, you can use that basic income to buy whatever you want: weed, sex workers, Fortnite, and of course donuts—lots of donuts.

In the UK, they've got a better idea. Invest in a local and sustainable agriculture system, which will cut down on obesity and disease. Give people a monthly stipend in the form of "beetroot bonds," which can only be exchanged for Real Food. It would also allow each person to use their beetroot shares (and the shares of their dependents) to vote on local food policy, and in so doing, promote local farmers and organic practices.

The Best Nudge of All

If that's too socialist for you, another tactic that could offset the increased cost of food, as well as serve the interests of farmers, the food industry, and public health alike, is called *differential subsidization*. Yoke the carrot with the stick—the inducement with the punishment. Differential subsidization was employed in 1977 in Nordic countries, including Sweden, Denmark, and Norway, to curb the increasing number of alcoholics in their respective countries. The three countries collectively adopted two pieces of legislation: first, they nationalized the liquor stores, resulting in the same products sold at the same price everywhere; second, they taxed high-alcohol spirits, and then used the money from the tax to subsidize low-alcohol beer. In doing so, they were able to nudge the public away from hard spirits and toward the low-alcohol beer, thus reducing alcohol consumption. In the process, hospitalizations decreased, car accidents were reduced, cirrhosis of the liver declined, and economic productivity improved. All of these policies are still in place today.

Here are two ways to put this concept to use. First, tax soda (twenty-eight countries around the world are already doing that), and use the revenue generated from the tax to subsidize water. The beverage makers won't care, because they're also selling the water. It's just a straight-up exchange, nudging people to a healthier option with a zero-sum scheme. Second, instead of subsidizing corn and soy, tax the corn and soy, and use the revenue to subsidize fresh fruits and vegetables. This would force commodity farmers to rethink their land use, which is urgent considering the imminent disaster of climate change. Promotion of high-fiber foods in US low-income food programs, such as WIC, SNAP, and the NSLP, would be the most expedient place to begin. In so doing, you can nudge people in a healthier direction, and they won't complain. Most of the time, they won't even notice.

CHAPTER 28

The Case for Real Food

Processed food kills people (eventually). Processed food kills pocketbooks (eventually). Processed food kills budgets (eventually). Processed food kills the planet (eventually). It's a slow process, even glacial, but we know it's happening—or at least some of us do. Others of us keep doing it anyway because it's mindless, seemingly cheap, convenient, tasty, and most of all, addictive.

One could make the argument that food processing has saved countless people around the world from dying of starvation (in the same way it saved the population in the Southwest from the ravages of the Dust Bowl, from 1930 to 1936). Or that it has contributed to the vitality of the global economy by strengthening the commodities market, and by creating corporate behemoths like Nestlé, PepsiCo, Coca-Cola, Mars, Danone, Kellogg's, and Unilever. All true. But if processed food is so good, why are so many countries interested in its antithesis—sustainable agriculture and regenerative farming? Why are European banks and financiers starting sustainable food equity funds? Maybe because they know processed food isn't so good after all?

Does Real Food Work?

Processed food is short-term gain for long-term pain. This is true for any toxic and addictive substance at personal and societal levels. Does Real Food mitigate that long-term pain? Also, does Real Food interfere with the experience of the short-term gain?

I can personally attest to the fact that Real Food improves health— because it's how I took care of obese children for two decades. We published our results so that people could replicate our success. The UCSF Weight Assessment for Teen and Child Health (WATCH) clinic sees twelve to sixteen new patients every month. At each patient's intake visit, the parent fills out a bunch of forms and meets with the doctor, a fasting blood specimen is drawn for assessment of comorbidities, and then, most important, the patient and parent attend our communal Real Food "teaching breakfast," a one-hour sit-down and narration where we feed six patients and six parents together, staffed by one of our clinic dietitians. They explain why each food is on the menu, and why others aren't. We show them what breakfast should look like. This was the most important and effective thing we did, provided the parent sees their kid will eat the food, sees that the other parents will eat the food, sees that other kids will also eat the food, and finally understands that they can afford, access, and cook the food. If we checked all four boxes, that patient lost weight and kept it off, and their metabolic health improved. If not, then we had to start finagling with other modalities, including medicine in certain cases.

The goal of our imperative was to educate the parent with enough science to tie the environment to the biochemistry, the biochemistry to the behavior, and then the behavior to the disease state, so that they could see that altering the environment would alter the behavior, which would then alter the health harms. This is the *Iron Law of Public Health* applied to clinical medicine. We estimate that 50 percent of the patients we saw needed nothing more than this nutritional education along with real-world strategies for implementation. If we could enact these precepts across the country, a significant portion of childhood chronic disease would be ameliorated—and rapidly.

Switching kids to Real Food doesn't sound like a big deal—but it is a *huge* deal, especially in lower-income families. Processed food is cheap, it's what SNAP covers, and it's what's given out in food banks. It's the path of least resistance—even if parents can see that it's hurting their kids. I saw this time and again in the WATCH clinic at UCSF. You need to make the changes easy and sustainable. That's the only way it will work.

Incentivizing Real Food

In 2018, there were 127.6 million households in the US, which spent $779 billion buying food that was consumed at home, of which approximately $617 billion was purchased from traditional US grocery stores. The average income before tax of those grocery stores in 2018 was a meager 1.3 percent. Therefore, the net income food retailers accrued was a paltry $63 per household. Processed food might be good for the processed food producer, but not for the retailer. Yet, the consumption of processed food is causing chronic metabolic disease that costs American healthcare payers $1.9 trillion annually, or just over $14,000 per household. Who's funding the discrepancy? More important, who's going to pick this up going forward?

When a company pollutes or causes sickness or death, people can file class action suits to hold the company accountable. Similarly, governments can sue, using a legal instrument called *parens patriae* (the state as the parent). Think Big Tobacco, *Exxon Valdez*, and Purdue Pharma. But who's holding Big Food accountable? Should Coca-Cola be paying your insurance bill? Should companies who make commercial salad dressing also be liable? That might make technical sense, but can you imagine the cry of the politicians and their lobbyists over it. Nonetheless, there is a case to be made for individual states to sue beverage companies to recoup Medicaid costs for diabetes.

In the meantime, the only viable approach is for healthcare payers/insurers to provide food retailers with financial incentives to encourage consumers to choose Real Food. Given the huge disparity between the income earned by the food retailer and the cost to society of selling highly processed food products, it's in both their best interests. If the insurer underwrites the cost of Real Food, the improved health and lower healthcare costs to the healthcare purchaser could be several times the $63 the food retailer earns per household. By increasing the net income of the food retailers to incentivize Real Food sales, we could nudge people in the right direction. The prospect of doubling or tripling a grocery store's income should get its attention.

Foogal-Perfact

The only way to relegate chronic disease to the dustbin is to make Real Food the standard within all households in America and around the world. This is obviously a heavy lift, because of cost, accessibility, and Big Food practices of questionable or misleading advertising and availability.

The industry blames the consumer for choosing processed food over Real Food. Based on the percentage of food consumed in the US (62 percent processed), they have a point. But why do people choose processed food? Because it tastes better? Reduced spoilage and depreciation? Cost? Cooking and cleanup time? Marketing? Or maybe it's just addictive? Big Food simultaneously exploits the two laws of marketing—*give the public what it wants*, and *if you build it they will come*.

My colleagues at a startup food delivery system called Foogal focus-grouped the question "Why do people eat junk?" It turns out, most people think that deciding what to make for dinner and then buying the ingredients is an enormous hassle. They want what is good for their household, but trying to pick out food based on health and ingredients is impossible, and the inadequacy of our current food label becomes overwhelming. They don't know how to read packaging (wonder why—because there's nothing on the label that's worth reading? See Chapter 17), and they certainly don't know how to make food choices based on it. When they enter the supermarket, it's like walking into the opium den with a cacophony of voices on the endcaps of the aisles, shrieking "buy me." They fall prey to the siren songs of the tortilla chips, soft drinks, and cookies.

To combat this, my colleagues at Foogal have developed a digital platform that ties together four stakeholders: the patient-consumer, the doctor-provider, the supermarket, and the insurance company. Here's how it works: First, your doctor-approved biochemical profile is inputted into the Foogal platform (e.g., do you have high lipids, do you have hypertension, do you have diabetes, do you have celiac disease, what medications are you on). This information is combined with preventative nutrition (i.e., avoidance of processed food) and then used to determine which foods would optimize your health. For example, let's say you want to select something for dinner—Foogal will present you with tens of thousands of recipes that can be made from groceries that conform to your biochemical profile to promote metabolic health. Foogal is able to do this by using a comprehensive food database developed by Perfact, another startup. Perfact checks each Nutrition Facts label on each food item and then uses this information to create filters (e.g., no sugar, low salt, low glycemic load, gluten-free) that correspond to various biochemical profiles. So, if you decide you want chicken cacciatore and type it into the search engine, the Foogal app accesses a database of hundreds of thousands of recipes to find the one chicken cacciatore recipe that best fits your biochemical profile. Foogal then orders the groceries to be delivered to your home with the recipe. Instead of the grocery store sending you the bill, they charge the insurance company. And the insurance company should be happy to pay it, because the cost of the food— even Real Food—is one-tenth the cost of the medications for which they won't have to pay. You get better, the doctor can spend less time with you (thus increasing the number of patients the doctor can see— more profit for them), and the supermarket sells more outer-store, high-margin perishables (reducing waste and increasing profit). Everyone wins.

There are only two potential losers in this game: Big Food and Big Pharma. The reason they currently make out like bandits is because of our current food model, which subsidizes the commodity crops that are the backbone of processed food, as well as our pharmaceutical model, which rewards pharma companies for abandoning acute care medicines like antibiotics in favor of chronic care medicines. It punishes pharma companies for innovation via the U.S. Patent Office giving them twenty years of patent protection and seven years of drug exclusivity, with an extra six months for pediatric studies. Big Pharma makes its money doing the wrong thing; it must make its money doing the right thing.

We all need to eat. The food industry can adapt. They could instead supply fresh food meal kits; locally sourced produce to cut down on transport time, costs, and waste; and quick freeze liquid nitrogen to prevent food fiber disruption. Currently, the upper economic stratum of society has access to deliverable meals in a box; we just need to make this available at all tiers of society. If food companies are going to take the risk of inventing Real Food products, they should be rewarded (maybe with subsidies), while those companies who stick to their processed habits should pay a tax, raising prices, which could dissuade people from purchasing. Similarly, if pharma companies are going to take the risk of inventing new therapies, they should be rewarded, while those who develop similar drugs shouldn't be able to jack up the price indiscriminately.

Eat REAL

There's only one place in America that's completely devoid of Real Food—our nation's schools. And we made it that way. Once upon a time, the National School Lunch Program (enacted in 1946) required that all public schools serve meals to the poorest students. Thus, the advent of the "lunch ladies"—women wearing blue hairnets who prepared and served food in school cafeterias nationwide. Some of the food was tasteless, some of it was nasty, but it was real. Then, in the early 1970s, financial pressures on boards of education nationwide took their toll, and forced schools to rethink their concept of food service. The fast-food industry rode to the rescue, offering precooked "heat and eat" options for children (like pizza), all of which were processed in some fashion. The contracts were cheaper, requiring less labor (bye-bye lunch ladies), and also allowed repurposing of kitchen space for other school uses. Of course, this was the industry's plan all along—to get schools to remove their kitchens. Once the kitchens were gone, schools were dependent on processed food. The kids got sicker, and their school test scores declined (see Chapter 15).

In 2009, the Obama administration, and especially Michelle, roared out of the gate—reform kids' lunches! The Healthy, Hunger-Free Kids Act (HHFKA) of 2010 was supposed to get real food into schools and kids' stomachs, but didn't succeed for two reasons. First, the increase in price for each lunch went from $2.80 to $2.86—enough for two grapes. Second, the schools don't have kitchens anymore—the space has been repurposed into classrooms—so where and how were they supposed to cook? So the Obama administration settled. The big reveal—they put a salad bar in every school. But as I've told you throughout the book, the processed food is still poison, and a salad bar isn't the antidote to bad food, especially when kids will always opt for pizza or fries (but, hey, they're both vegetables, right?).

Schools need a new model. We're working on developing one. Two nonprofits, Eat REAL, in partnership with like-minded LifeLabs, have developed a nutrition curriculum, using the school cafeteria as an education center. Working with the head of food service, Dominic Machi, at the Mount Diablo Unified School District (MDUSD) in Contra Costa County east of San Francisco, we've developed an off-site kitchen for the entire district, so every school gets hot meals produced that very day. We're also teaching fourth graders nutrition and culinary skills at lunchtime—so we're serving up both education *and* implementation at the same time. Jamie Oliver dumped 57 tons (114,000 pounds) of white sand (substituting as sugar) on top of a school bus. Thus far, we've removed 10 pounds of sugar from 27,000 students' diets over a nine-month school session, for a total of 270,000 pounds of actual sugar removed. Jamie, eat your bus out.

Eat REAL at Home

The trick is to do this at home as well. Real Food doesn't take much longer to prepare than processed food. Yes, there will be a little more cutting up of ingredients, so you'll need a sharp knife. As a demonstration project, my colleague and cookbook coauthor Cindy Gershen and I made a Real Food six-course meal for twenty people in under thirty minutes. The difference is you have to plan for it. Get a recipe. As a service during the COVID-19 pandemic, Eat REAL posted the entire contents of our *Fat Chance Cookbook* (2013) online at www.eatreal.org. Real Food is a primary prevention.

But you can't eat Real Food at home if you didn't buy it in the first place. It all starts with the point of contact—the grocery store. In the midst of COVID-19, Americans put their addiction to processed food on display—the supermarket aisles were devoid of pasta, breakfast cereal, chips, and candy. The store itself is the problem: it's a minefield, and it's really easy to blow yourself up. Here are the seven shopping rules to abide by, even before you walk into the store (or order online), that will keep you from stepping on any of the landmines the store has placed in your way.

1. Don't go shopping hungry.

2. Shop the edges of the supermarket. If you've gone into the aisles, you've gone off the rails.

3. If a product is on the endcap of the aisle, the company paid to have it placed there. Don't be a stooge.

4. Any food that has a logo you've heard of or any food with a Nutrition Facts label has been processed.

5. If a product lists a structure-function claim on the package, don't buy it. Example: any food that says *low-fat* or *no trans-fats* is poison, because something else is in there instead.

6. If it doesn't say *whole grain*, it isn't. And even if it does say *whole grain*, it probably isn't. If the carbohydrate to fiber ratio is greater than 10 to 1, don't buy it.

7. If any form of sugar is one of the first three ingredients, it's a dessert.

When Sugar Goes Away, So Will Processed Food

Sugar is both the marker and the hook for processed food. Therefore, we need real efforts at food revision, not just lip service. Here are seven proposals that could be implemented immediately, if we had the political will to do it:

1. Nutrition education for the public should emphasize that there's no biological requirement for, or nutritional value of, added sugar.

2. The industry should be forced to label "added sugars" (because that's what they added!) on food products in teaspoons rather than grams, which will make it easier to understand.

3. There should be a complete ban of companies associated with sugary products from sponsoring sporting events. Further, as Golden State Warriors star Stephen Curry and Indian cricket team captain Virat Kohli have done, we should encourage other sporting role models and those within the entertainment industry to publicly dissociate themselves from endorsing sugary products, including product placement.

4.   Like alcohol and tobacco, there should be a ban on loss leading (discounting products) in supermarkets of processed foods and drinks.

5.   Soda taxes should be everywhere, and should extend to sugary foods as well. The tax should be on the amount of the sugar, not the volume of the soft drink.

6.   There should be a complete ban of all sugary drink advertising (including fruit juice) on TV and internet demand services.

7.   There should be a discontinuation of all governmental food subsidies, especially commodity crops such as sugar, which have been shown to contribute to health detriments. As stated in Chapter 26, subsidies distort the market and increase the costs of nonsubsidized crops, making them unaffordable for many. Either let the markets do their work or use differential subsidization to tax soda and subsidize water.

The Power of Public Ideas

I hope I've convinced you that processed food is the culprit, and that Real Food is the only answer at the molecular, biochemical, medical, psychological, economic, environmental, and societal levels.

Even more important, I hope I've shown you that Real Food is achievable. Right now, the only things standing between us and success are: sugar addicts in the population, hubris addicts in the medical and ancillary professions, money addicts in the food and pharma industries, and power addicts in Washington and beyond. But things can change, when the culture changes.

How do you change an entire culture? In the last forty years, we've witnessed four separate cultural tectonic shifts in America: 1) smoking in public places; 2) drunk driving; 3) bicycle helmets and seat belts; and 4) condoms in bathrooms. In 1980, if any elected official stood up in a State House or in Congress or in Parliament and proposed legislation to combat any of these, he or she would have been laughed right out of office. Today, they're all facts of life.

We also taught the children who grew up and started voting. And the naysayers, well, they're all dead. That's why culture shifts are generational shifts. You're seeing it now with climate change. We need a global reckoning around food. It's already started, but it has to pick up more steam.

What can you do today? You have the vote—instead of a ballot box, you have your fork. Your vote is tallied immediately. And you get to vote twenty-one times a week—every meal, three times a day, every day.

Vote early, vote often. Change your grocery buying habits. If you have a local butcher or produce store, shop there—your choices are limited to the healthy stuff. Unfortunately, so many convenience stores around the country don't sell fresh produce, so go to the proprietor and tell them what you want. Get all the parents in your kids' school to do the same.

You'll also have to change your mindset about food and money. One way or another, you're going to pay. You can either pay the farmer or the doctor—which would you prefer? Make a conscious choice.

What you can do tomorrow? Nelson Mandela noted that politicians lead from behind—you can't wait for them. The petroleum industry/climate change is an *immoral hazard*. The Stanford Research Institute warned the American Petroleum Institute that fossil fuel emissions represented an existential environmental threat as early as 1968. Yet the industry hid behind fifty years of propaganda. It took Superstorm Sandy, the California wildfires, and Greta Thunberg to wake us from our torpor, and now we're making it a voting issue.

Food started the same way. First, there was a guy named César Chávez, and he exposed the farming industry for what it was. Yet the *immoral hazard* of the processed food industry and chronic disease has remained hidden behind fifty years of propaganda. The public needs the same level of discourse. The next wave of the food revolution is long overdue. We have to make food a voting issue, just like the populace has made climate change a voting issue.

Once upon a time, you would walk down the street, see someone smoking, and think they were cool and hip. Today you see someone smoking and feel pity for them. I believe that ten years from now, you'll walk down the street, see someone drinking a Coca-Cola, and feel pity for them as well.

That cultural tectonic shift—you can feel it under your feet—that's how you change the world.

Epilogue

Recently, *Annals of Internal Medicine* reported a case of a thirteen-year-old boy who went blind eating only junk food. Even after the cause of the blindness was determined and shown to be due to micronutrient deficiencies resulting in retinal and neural dysfunction, replacement of these micronutrients didn't restore the boy's eyesight. Now, this is an isolated event, but it explains the power of food—and foreshadows what will happen if we don't address the problem.

In some ways, devising and planning this book was easy. I've been preparing for it for forty-five years, and I've either learned or lived everything in it. In other ways, the actual writing of this book was the hardest thing I've ever had to do, because no matter what I say, I'm going to piss somebody off. Food is *everyone's* business, and so everyone has an opinion, informed or not. There's a lot of "heresy" in these pages, and in today's intuitive, antagonistic, and viral environments, I anticipate more heat than light from the blogosphere. The science had to be right in order to stand up to the onslaught of scrutiny and attempts to discredit that this book will no doubt engender, from the medical establishment, scientific community, policy wonks, food industry, and, of course, the general public.

I'm a name dropper, but not for self-aggrandizement. Rather it's to impress upon people that we're not alone in these views or warnings for society. I'm going to drop the names of four colleagues, compatriots, and acquaintances who've got their own takes on our current global food disaster.

In 2014, at the LA premiere of *Fed Up*, I had the great fortune to meet Jane Seymour. From *Solitaire* to *Dr. Quinn, Medicine Woman* to *Wedding Crashers*, she's always been at the top of her game. At the time she was sixty-three, but looked thirty-six, and with virtually no makeup. She confided in me that her father was a country obstetrician/gynecologist in the UK, and he was very wary of the processed food industry. She said she owed her good looks to the fact that she had *never* consumed processed food in her entire life. Knowing what I know about sugar, glycation, and wrinkles, she was a living testament to the work that I was doing.

I've mentioned some personal heroes in this book, including Weston Price, John Yudkin, and Fred Kummerow. Another is Raj Patel, author, journalist, activist, and former Eat REAL board member. He's put his life on the line to expose the inequity of the world's food systems and to stump for Real Food. In his book *Stuffed and Starved* (2007), he describes the obesity and food insecurity pandemic as a social inequality, and as one of moral hazard—those who are stuffed versus those who are starved. Right he was: it is about being stuffed and starved—and for a different, more innately biologic reason. Our livers are stuffed and our intestines are starved—because of processed food.

World-famous journalist Michael Pollan, author of *The Omnivore's Dilemma* (2006) and *In Defense of Food* (2008), has warned against the concept of *nutritionism*, that is, the scientific reductionism of food to its individual nutrients and components, as that often leads industry actors to use sleight-of-hand maneuvers to relabel a food so it doesn't look as bad, or to supplement a food so it looks like it's healthy. Well, I'm a scientist, and a reductionist. It's because of that reductionist mindset that I can "reverse engineer" these individual dietary components, and turn them back into Real Food. In fact, the reductionism described in this book has led us right back to constructionism—and the simple thesis that only Real Food will work. My hope is that now both the scientists who have held sway with the clinicians and the food activists who have held sway with the public can embrace whichever philosophy they wish, and still come to the same conclusion.

Last, I want to tell you about my friendship with Professor Jeffrey Sachs, Columbia University economist and president of the UN Sustainable Development Solutions Network. Jeffrey pointed out our problem in stark economic terms, which I think resonates well. John Maynard Keynes documented the behavior of the "rational actor"—the person who can rationally assess value (utility divided by cost)—while Daniel Kahneman and Amos Tversky documented the behavior of the "irrational actor," or the person who's driven by risk aversion and thinks the cost is too high, and therefore consistently underestimates value. Jeffrey effectively argues that we have plenty of evidence for a third actor—the "hedonic actor"—or the person who knows exactly what things cost, but can't assess value because they need their fix. It's the hedonic actor who's driven the tobacco epidemic, and who now drives the gun, opioid, and processed food epidemics. All you need to do is superimpose the county-by-county maps for each of these, and you'll see how they overlap. The hedonic actor responds to things that are, well, hedonic. And that's what processed food is, plain and simple.

Solving the processed food problem is going to require more than just making Real Food available. We also need to understand and embrace the science, not the propaganda. We need to think critically about where and how "healthy" statements, claims, and ideas are coming from, and who they are sponsored by. We need to adopt the addiction paradigm into our medical treatment plans and laws to "nudge" people toward healthy decisions. Every substance or behavior of abuse has required both personal intervention (i.e., rehab) and societal intervention (i.e., laws). One doesn't work without the other. We have both for tobacco and alcohol. We're finally getting there on opioids, now that Purdue Pharma is bankrupt and Johnson & Johnson has given up the ghost. But we have nothing for processed food. The phalanx of consumer anger hasn't materialized yet—but it must, and it will.

Acknowledgments

I have many people in my personal and professional lives that lived through this book with me. Some of them read early drafts of chapters and provided feedback. Each was singularly helpful, and they all deserve credit for their contribution in bringing this work to fruition.

First and foremost, I must thank my fellow UCSF/Touro University research team members. We truly are a team, and everyone contributes equally. Drs. Alejandro Gugliucci, Jean-Marc Schwarz, Kathy Mulligan, Sue Noworolski, Grace Jones, Ayca Erkin-Cakmak, and members of the GOD (Glycation, Oxidation, and Disease) Lab are my colleagues and good friends. When we get together to talk science, it is always the highlight of my day. The concepts espoused in this book are the product of our collective brains working as one.

Next, I must thank my American colleagues in diet and chronic disease, especially Dariush Mozaffarian, Tim Harlan, Ron Krauss, Ethan Weiss, Marcelle Cedars, Paolo Rinaudo, Suneil Koliwad, Michele Mietus-Snyder, Kimber Stanhope, Gary Taubes, Peter Attia, Monica Dus, and Bill Grant; my British colleagues Aseem Malhotra, Zoe Harcombe, Michael Yudkin, David Unwin, Ivor Cummins, and Alan Ebringer; and my Australia/New Zealand colleagues Gary Fettke, Grant Schofield, Maryanne Demasi, Simon Thornley, Gerhard Sundborn, and Kieron Rooney. All of them have helped move the field of metabolic disease along in various ways and venues, all of them have been extremely forthcoming, and I am indebted to each of them. Drs. Mark Hyman, Rachel Abrams, Joe Mercola, David Perlmutter, Andreas

Eenfeldt, and Jason Fung are also on the same metabolic page, and help to disseminate and amplify the message.

I also have a group of comrades active in diet and mental health, including my American colleagues Bill Wilson, Joan Ifland, Nicole Avena, Mark Gold, Daniel Amen, Georgia Ede, and Dale Bredesen, and my British compatriots Alex Richardson, Michael Crawford, Patrick Holford, Kirkland Newman, Rachel Gow, and Fiona Fay. I thank them for their open-mindedness and counsel.

Writing about dietetics proved to be the hardest chapter, as I am not trying to take down a field, but rather help to build one up. Patrika Tsai, Kathryn Smith, Emily Perito, Luis Rodriguez, Nancy Guardino, Andrea Garber, and my teammates at the UCSF Weight Assessment for Teen and Child Health (WATCH) clinic helped me more than anyone in formulating the message. I also owe a debt of gratitude to Pat Crawford, Ken Hecht, Laurel Mellin, Tara Kelly, Leslie Lee, Belinda Fettke, and Patty James for making sure I hit the right tone.

My colleagues in dentistry and myofunctional sciences have been indispensable in understanding the relationship between oral, airway, and systemic health. Thank you to Kevin Boyd, Susan Maples, John Featherstone, Yasmi Crystal, Kim Kutsch, George Taylor, Brian Hockel, Jacob Park, Marc Moeller and Samantha Weaver, Paul Ehrlich, Sandra Kahn, Georgia Rodgers, Karen Sokal-Gutierrez, Michael Glick, David Williams, and Huda Yusuf.

As you might imagine, the science of food processing can be quite arcane, and matching that science with the diseases of metabolic syndrome can also be daunting. Therefore, I must thank Carlos Monteiro, Jean-Claude Moubarac, Serge Hercberg, Kelly Brownell, and Yogi Hendlin for their insights. I must acknowledge Brenda Eskenazi, Kim Harley, and my colleagues at the UC Berkeley Center for Environmental Research and Children's Health for their pioneering work in endocrine-disrupting chemicals and metabolic syndrome. And I want to specifically acknowledge Mitchell Weinberg, a pioneering New York attorney who is leading the charge against food fraud worldwide, and who co-drafted that chapter.

You can't complain about a problem if you don't have a solution. My friends at the UCSF Institute for Health Policy Studies have been instrumental in helping to formulate and test various policy initiatives. Our UCSF advocacy subgroup has an unofficial moniker, "The Sugar Hill Gang," of which Elissa Epel, Laura Schmidt, Claire Brindis, Cristin Kearns, Ashley Mason, Janet Wojcicki, Dean Schillinger, and Stan Glantz are all proud members. My British colleagues at Action on Sugar, Graham MacGregor, Jack Winkler, and Katharine Jenner, as well as my Dutch friends at Voeding Leeft (Food Lives), Martijn Van Beek, Barbara Karstens, Peter Voshol, Hanno Pijl, and Albert Van de Velde (deceased), carry the torch across the pond, and Simon Barquera, Arantxa Colchero, and Juan Rivera-Dommarco south of the border.

My legal colleagues, David Faigman and Marsha Cohen at UC Hastings College of the Law, and Michael Roberts and Diana Winters at the UCLA Resnick Center for Food Law and Policy have been instrumental in helping to analyze policy. And I owe Jim Kahn, Rick Vreman, Travis Porco, Todd Knobel, Alainn Bailey, and Rory Robertson a huge debt in helping to explain and vet the economic and environmental arguments in this book.

Many people in the food/health system are trying to make a difference, and they have shared their expertise, including Eric Smith, Jessie Inchauspe, Wolfram Alderson, Andreas Kornstadt, Ken Nochimson, Alan Farago, Ricardo Salvador, Nadja Pinnavaia, Paolo Costa, Sarah Wilson, Chantal Bonneau, and Daniel Menard. My nonprofit Eat REAL colleagues Jordan Shlain, Nora LaTorre, Beth Seligman, Kristin Zellhart, and Sarah Friedkin, and board members Laura Modi, Jim Warren, Tesha Poe, Riva Robinson, Lawrence Williams, and Alan Greene do the heavy lifting for kids in the Bay Area. And to cookbook coauthor Cindy Gershen, who's stuck by me through some very difficult times.

My academic friends from around the globe always bring their A-game to bat around scientific ideas. This is by no means an exhaustive list, but I want to acknowledge Ram Weiss, Sonia Caprio, Ania Jastreboff, Christopher Gardner, David Ludwig, James Johnson, Richard

Johnson, Jack Yanovski, Michael Goran, Martin Wabitsch, Uma Pisharody, Bruce Alpert, and Pedro Velasquez-Mieyer for their camaraderie. And to my French colleagues Francois Taddei, Ariel Lindner, and Xavier Desplas at the Center for Research and Interdisciplinarity (CRI) in Paris, and Philippe Gaussier, Francois Germinet, Arnaud Le-Franc, and others at the Université de Cergy-Pontoise.

Three people stand out in terms of my never-ending gratitude. To my "goombah" Stefano Natella, a brilliant and self-effacing polymath who helped to crystallize the need for, and the scope of, this book. And I must personally thank my two academic mentors, Walter Miller and Howard Federoff, each friends for over thirty years, who taught me that good science and good ethics are indistinguishable, and for always believing in me, no matter what.

My final thank-yous go to the people who directly made this book possible—my long-time editor Amy Dietz, my graphic designers Glenn Randle and Jeannie Choi, my agent Janis Donnaud, and my Harper Wave publishers Karen Rinaldi and Rebecca Raskin, for believing in me and the message. And, of course, to my wife and kids for putting up with my foibles and faults, especially under the close quarters of the pandemic. I love you all.

Glossary

ACE2: angiotensin-converting enzyme-2, a receptor on cells that regulates water balance and which the coronavirus uses to inject its RNA into a cell to infect it.

ACLM: American College of Lifestyle Medicine, a physician-based vegan advocacy group.

ADA: American Dental Association or American Diabetes Association (also, formerly the American Dietetic Association, now called the Academy of Nutrition and Dietetics, or AND).

Addiction: a strong and harmful need to regularly have something (such as a drug) or engage in a specific behavior (such as gambling), due to an overwhelming biochemical drive, and which cannot be controlled by behavioral restraint.

AGE: advanced glycation end product, the result of the Maillard reaction either in the food or in the body.

ALEC: American Legislative Exchange Council, a nonprofit that crafts legislation and lobbies governmental entities on behalf of industry clients.

ALT: alanine aminotransferase, a blood test that tells about liver function and is sensitive but not specific for the amount of fat in the liver.

AMP-kinase: adenosine monophosphate-kinase, an enzyme that routes energy to mitochondria for burning.

Amygdala: part of the stress-fear-memory pathway. This walnut-sized area of the brain generates the feelings of fear and stress, which tells the hypothalamus to tell the adrenal glands to make extra cortisol.

Anandamide: a naturally occurring neurotransmitter that binds to the CB_1 endocannabinoid receptor and reduces levels of anxiety.

AND: Academy of Nutrition and Dietetics (formerly the American Dietetic Association).

Apoptosis: Programmed cell death, in which proteins in the cell are activated to cause self-destruction.

ARDS: acute respiratory disease syndrome, a lung disease due to an overwhelming inflammatory cytokine response.

ATP: adenosine triphosphate, the chemical in which energy is stored inside the cell.

Autonomic nervous system: the part of the nervous system that controls unconscious functions of the body. It consists of two parts: the sympathetic system controls heart rate, blood pressure, and temperature; while the parasympathetic system (the vagus nerve) controls eating, digestion, and absorption, slows the heart rate, and lowers blood pressure. The two together control energy balance.

Autophagy: the process of clearing away and resorbing old and dysfunctional cellular debris to keep cells functioning optimally—in the brain, this occurs during sleep.

BCAA: branched-chain amino acid, either leucine, isoleucine, or valine, necessary for muscle growth, but can be metabolized in the liver into energy.

BMI: body mass index, an index of excess adiposity, computed from the weight and height.

BP: Blood pressure.

BPA: bisphenol A, a chemical found in food and household goods that acts like an estrogen.

CAFO: concentrated animal feeding operation (animals confined specifically for food production).

CDR: Commission on Dietetic Registration, the entity that certifies and protects clinical dietitians.

CGM: continuous glucose monitor.

Cortisol: the stress hormone released from the adrenal glands, which acutely mobilizes sugar for use, but which chronically lays down visceral fat.

COVID-19: coronavirus disease 2019, the disease caused by the virus SARS-CoV-2.

CVD: cardiovascular disease.

Cytokine: a protein made by one cell that travels elsewhere and leads to inflammation.

Depression: a mental condition characterized by feelings of severe despondency and dejection, inadequacy, and guilt, often accompanied by lack of energy and disturbance of appetite and sleep often needing medical treatment.

Developmental programming: alterations in brain or body functioning due to alterations in the environment that occur in the fetus prior to birth.

DGAC: Dietary Guidelines Advisory Committee, convened every five years to advise the USDA on population dietary recommendations.

DNA: deoxyribonucleic acid, the molecule inside the cell that carries genetic information.

DNL: *de novo* lipogenesis, or the process of turning carbohydrate into fatty acids, occurring in the liver.

DO: doctor of osteopathy, a medical degree conferred by schools of osteopathy.

Dopamine: a neurotransmitter that when released acutely can cause feelings of reward, but when released chronically reduces the number of its receptors, leading to tolerance.

Dopamine receptor: the protein that binds dopamine to generate the reward signal, and when reduced in number leads to tolerance.

EC: endocannabinoid, a kind of neurotransmitter (e.g., anandamide) that binds to brain receptors and acts like marijuana, driving reward and reducing anxiety.

EDC: endocrine-disrupting chemical, a chemical that binds and either activates or inhibits a cellular hormone receptor.

EFSA: European Food Safety Authority.

Endogenous opioid peptide (EOP): a neurotransmitter made in the brain that binds to its receptor to signal the consummation of reward or euphoria.

Endogenous opioid peptide (EOP) receptor: part of the reward pathway. A protein that binds either opiates (e.g., heroin) or endogenous opioid peptides (e.g., beta-endorphin) to signal the consummation of reward or euphoria.

Epigenetics: modifications in DNA without changes in the DNA genetic sequence, usually occurring prior to birth.

ER stress: endoplasmic reticulum stress, a cell metabolic defect leading to abnormal production and misfolding of proteins.

Estrogen: female sex hormone, made either in the ovary or in fat tissue.

EWG: Environmental Working Group.

FDA: US Food and Drug Administration.

Fructose: a monosaccharide, half of dietary sugar or high-fructose corn syrup, the molecule that makes sugar taste sweet, causes the reward system to activate, and is the addictive component.

FTC: US Federal Trade Commission.

Galactose: a monosaccharide, half of lactose or milk sugar, a molecule that contributes to brain structural components.

GGT: gamma-glutamyl transpeptidase, a liver function test that signifies liver damage.

GHGs: greenhouse gases, specifically methane, nitrous oxide, and carbon dioxide.

Ghrelin: a hormone made by the stomach that conveys a signal of hunger to the hypothalamus.

Glucose: a monosaccharide, half of dietary sugar or high-fructose corn syrup; also the molecule found in starch, the molecule that every cell on the planet burns to liberate energy.

Glycogen: starch stored in cells; a string of glucose molecules that are easily cleaved to liberate glucose.

HbA$_{1c}$: hemoglobin A$_{1c}$, a blood test of glucose control in diabetes management.

Hcy: homocysteine, a metabolic by-product of the Krebs cycle, whose excess is associated with heart disease.

HFCS: high-fructose corn syrup, isolated from corn, which has undergone enzymatic reaction with glucose oxidase, converting some of the glucose into fructose, so that the product contains varying amounts of fructose and glucose.

Hippocampus: part of the stress-fear-memory pathway. The part of the brain where memories are housed, and which exerts influences on the amygdala and prefrontal cortex.

HOMA-IR: homeostatic model of insulin resistance, an index computed based on the fasting glucose and insulin level.

Hypothalamus: the area at the base of the brain that controls hormones of the body, particularly cortisol.

IEA: UK Institute of Economic Affairs, a political action group.

ILSI: International Life Sciences Institute, a nonprofit representing the food and drug industries.

Insulin: a hormone made in the pancreas that tells fat cells to store energy, and interferes with the leptin signal to increase food intake.

Insulin resistance: the state in which insulin signaling is reduced, requiring the beta-cells of the pancreas to make more insulin, which drives both obesity and chronic disease.

Insulin secretion: the process of insulin release in response to both rising blood glucose and the firing of the vagus nerve.

IRKO: insulin receptor knockout, an animal model of insulin resistance in different tissues.

Ketogenic diet: a diet in which little to no carbohydrate is consumed, so the body will generate ketones as an energy source instead of using glucose.

LCHF: low-carbohydrate, high-fat diet, also known as the low-carb diet.

LDL-C: low-density lipoprotein cholesterol concentration.

LDL-P: low-density lipoprotein particle number.

LDL: low-density lipoprotein, a blood lipid that contributes to heart disease.

Leptin: a hormone released from fat cells that travels in the bloodstream to the hypothalamus to report on peripheral energy stores.

Leptin resistance: the state where the leptin signal is dampened, leading to the hypothalamus interpreting starvation.

Maillard reaction: the naturally occurring binding of a simple sugar (glucose or fructose) to a protein, making the protein less flexible and generating oxygen radicals in the process.

Metabolic syndrome: a cluster of chronic metabolic diseases characterized by energy overload of the mitochondria.

Micronutrient: vitamin or mineral found in Real Food, usually isolated with the fiber fraction.

Mitochondria: subcellular organelles specialized to burn either fat or carbohydrate for energy.

mTOR: mammalian target of rapamycin, an enzyme that controls cell survival vs. cell death.

NAFLD: nonalcoholic fatty liver disease.

NCD: noncommunicable disease.

Necrosis: cell death due to exposure to a toxin or lack of blood or oxygen.

Neurotransmitter: a chemical in the brain made in one nerve cell, which when released causes other nerve cells to fire or stop firing.

NNT: number needed to treat, a measure of the population efficacy of a given treatment.

NSLP: National School Lunch Program, an entitlement program sponsored by the USDA.

Nucleus accumbens (NAc): the area of the brain that receives the dopamine signal and interprets the feeling as reward.

Obesity: excess body fat deposition.

Obesogen: a chemical that increases the amount of fat stored, to a greater extent than the calories released when it is burned.

OECD: Organisation for Economic Co-operation and Development, the thirty-seven richest countries.

OGTT: oral glucose tolerance test, a test to screen for diabetes and hyperinsulinemia.

Omega-3 fatty acids: a fatty acid found in wild fish and flax that is an important component of neuronal membranes, and which reduces inflammation.

OSA: obstructive sleep apnea, a lack of oxygenation during sleep due to obstruction of the airway either due to obesity or tongue placement within the pharynx, often leading to metabolic dysfunction.

PAH: polycyclic aromatic hydrocarbon, a cancer-causing chemical that is a product of burning coal, petroleum, tobacco, wood, or meat.

PBDE: polybrominated diphenyl ether, a chemical added to mattresses and pajamas as a flame retardant, and which causes insulin resistance.

PCRM: Physicians Committee for Responsible Medicine, an anti-meat advocacy group.

Peptide YY$_{(3-36)}$: a hormone made by the small intestine in response to food that signals satiety to the hypothalamus.

Peroxisome: an area of the cell that contains antioxidants to detoxify reactive oxygen species.

Phenylalanine: a dietary amino acid that can be converted into dopamine.

PI3-kinase: phosphatidylinositol-3-kinase, an enzyme that increases glucose transport into the cell.

Prefrontal cortex (PFC): part of the stress-fear-memory pathway. The part of the brain, located in the front (above the eyes), that inhibits impulsive and socially unacceptable and potentially dangerous behaviors and actions.

Pyruvate: a metabolic breakdown product of glucose, which can be further broken down by mitochondria to carbon dioxide and water, generating ATP.

Reactive oxygen species: chemicals generated from cellular metabolism that can cause protein or lipid damage and can lead to cell dysfunction or death if not detoxified by antioxidants.

RNA: ribonucleic acid, the molecule that codes for specific protein synthesis inside the cell.

ROS: reactive oxygen species or oxygen radical, a metabolic by-product of cell metabolism or inflammation, which can inflict damage if it is not quenched by an antioxidant.

SARS: severe acute respiratory syndrome, caused by a coronavirus, first noted in 2002.

Satiety: the feeling of fullness that stops further eating.

SDA: Seventh-day Adventists, a Christian sect advocating vegetarianism or veganism.

Serotonin: part of the contentment pathway. A neurotransmitter made from the amino acid tryptophan, which, when it binds to its 1a receptor on neurons, transmits feelings of contentment; and when it binds to its 2a receptor, evokes the mystical or psychedelic experience.

Stress: an uncomfortable state of mental or emotional strain or tension resulting from adverse or demanding circumstances. Accompanied by neural output from the amygdala, which tells the hypothalamus to signal the adrenal glands to make the hormone cortisol.

Subcutaneous fat: the fat outside of the abdomen, which is a storehouse of extra energy, but which does not signify an increased risk for metabolic syndrome.

Sympathetic nervous system: the part of the autonomic nervous system that raises heart rate, increases blood pressure, and burns energy.

TEF: thermic effect of food, the energy released from the process of digestion and metabolism.

Telomere: the ends of chromosomes, which confer stability and shorten as the cell ages.

TG: triglyceride, a blood lipid that contributes to heart disease.

THI: True Health Initiative, an anti-meat advocacy group.

TOFI: thin on the outside, fat on the inside, referring to increased visceral fat.

Tolerance: the state where the signal for reward is dampened and can only be generated by consuming more substrate (in the case of obesity, palatable food) or engaging in more behaviors (e.g., gambling).

Transcription factor: a protein in cells that turns on genes to make the cell change its function.

Tryptophan: the rarest dietary amino acid in the diet, which is converted into serotonin.

Type 1 diabetes: a disease of high blood sugar due to inadequate insulin production by the beta-cells of the pancreas.

Type 2 diabetes: a disease of high blood sugar due to defective insulin action on tissues.

Tyrosine: a dietary amino acid that is converted into dopamine.

Uric acid: a breakdown product of nucleic acids, which causes gout and is a contributor to high blood pressure, and is sensitive to sugar and meat consumption.

USDA: US Department of Agriculture.

Vagus nerve: the part of the autonomic nervous system that promotes food digestion, absorption, and energy storage, and slows heart rate.

Ventral tegmental area (VTA): part of the reward pathway; the area of the brain that sends the dopamine reward signal of signifying reward to the nucleus accumbens.

Ventromedial hypothalamus (VMH): the area of the hypothalamus that receives hormonal information from the body to regulate energy balance.

Visceral fat: the fat around the organs in the abdomen, which is a risk factor for diabetes, heart disease, and stroke, and a marker for metabolic syndrome.

Index

About the Author

ROBERT H. LUSTIG, MD, MSL is the editor of the academic volume *Obesity Before Birth*, and is the internationally acclaimed author of the popular works *Fat Chance*, *Sugar Has 56 Names*, the *Fat Chance Cookbook*, and *The Hacking of the American Mind*. He is Emeritus Professor of Pediatrics in the Division of Endocrinology and member of the Institute for Health Policy Studies at UCSF. He lectures globally, and consults with numerous medical societies and policy organizations to improve population health. He lives with his family in San Francisco.